Pediatric Orthopedics
of the
Lower Extremity

Pediatric Orthopedics
of the
Lower Extremity

An Instructional Handbook

John D. McCrea, D.P.M.

Diplomate, American Board of Podiatric Surgery
Diplomate, American Board of Podiatric Orthopedics
Associate Clinical Professor, Department of Pediatric
  Orthopedics, Dr. William M. Scholl College of
  Podiatric Medicine
Fellow, American College of Foot Orthopedists

FUTURA PUBLISHING COMPANY, INC.
MOUNT KISCO, NEW YORK
1985

Library of Congress Cataloging in Publication Data

McCrea, John D.
    Pediatric orthopedics of the lower extremity.

    Includes bibliographies and index.
        1. Foot—Abnormalities. 2. Extremities, Lower—
Abnormalities. 3. Pediatric orthopedia. I. Title.
[DNLM: 1. Leg—abnormalities. 2. Orthopedics—in
infancy & childhood. WE 850 M478p]
RD781.M33 1985   617'.398   84-81645
ISBN 0-87993-230-9

Copyright © 1985
Futura Publishing Company, Inc.

Published by
Futura Publishing Company, Inc.
P. O. Box 330, 295 Main Street
Mount Kisco, New York 10549

L.C. No.: 84-81645
ISBN No.: 0-87993-230-9

*T*his book is dedicated to my deserving wife Jane, and to my three children, Megan, Mac, and David, who provided me the enthusiasm to produce this manuscript

FOREWORD

T he design of this book is to collect, organize, and present a vast array of information on pedal problems of the growing child. The author adroitly blends information gleaned from diverse sources and then incorporates his particular insights and methodology, thereby making the text didactically informative and clinically practical.

The chapter covering history and examination readily identifies the necessity for "getting to know" the patient in order to evaluate and understand the cause of the problem. The anatomy and biomechanics of the developing child are stressed in relation to identifiable generalized pathomechanical aberrations and isolated foot problems.

Dr. McCrea's treatment plans are founded on historically proven regimens; however, his modifications and individualized alterations of therapy make for interesting and contemplative reading.

The book is a much needed composite on podopediatrics that can readily serve as an instructional text for the student, resident, and neophytic practitioner. For the seasoned practitioner, it can serve as an excellent resource, with concise and clinically appropriate information for contemporary practice.

Charles L. Jones, D.P.M.
Chairman of the Residency Program
Thorek Hospital and Medical Center
Chicago, Illinois

PREFACE

*I*t's about time! Not since Herman Tax and Philip Brachman has a text on Podopediatric been published.

I've had the privilege of knowing John McCrea for about ten years—as a student, resident, and a respected colleague. I am, therefore, not surprised that he undertook this challenge.

In the late sixties and early seventies, biomechanics, as applied to the foot, became a clinical science. For this, our profession will always be indebted to Dr. Root and his two disciples, Weed and Sgarlato. They deserve the full credit for developing and propagating this new applied science. It has revolutionized our approach to pedal problems. This applied science has: refined our examination techniques, based on a systematic approach; led to the development of a sophisticated classification system for foot deformities; produced a universal terminology that we all understand; and ultimately, treatment regimes have become more predictable and sophisticated.

Dr. McCrea represents that first generation of podiatrists, who have graduated from our colleges where biomechanics have been incorporated as an integral part of the curriculum.

Armed with the proper background and training, coupled with long-term experience, Dr. McCrea has filled a void in our podiatric literature. He has condensed into one text the state-of-the-art knowledge of what we know, from a podiatrist's viewpoint, about pediatric foot and related problems.

Thank you, from all of us.

Stephen D. Smith, D.P.M.
Des Plaines, Illinois

Acknowledgments

*F*or being able to produce a book encompassing the topics herein provided, I must thank many people from both the present and the past for their research and knowledge, which I was able to draw upon. The synthesis of this information into one text required the help of several individuals to whom I must deeply and appreciatively express my gratitude and thanks.

To Dr. Charles Jones for his help, encouragement, and direction during my residency training I am deeply indebted, and I must extend my thanks to the administration and staff at Thorek Hospital and Medical Center for providing an environment in which my interest in pediatric orthopedic problems was nurtured. I wish also to express my appreciation to the Dr. William M. Scholl College of Podiatric Medicine for their excellent Podopediatric's Department and for their help in providing some of the photography work encorporated in this book. A special thanks goes to my secretary Kathy Carter who persevered and completed all of the typing and retyping of this manuscript. She extended herself above and beyond my highest expectations.

To Jay Harris, who labored tirelessly creating the numerous drawings to my exact requests goes a deep feeling of indebtedness. And my sincere appreciation goes to the Futura Publishing Company for their patience and generous help in guiding me to the completion of this book.

Finally, and most important to me, a profound and warm thank you to my loving wife Jane, and our three children, Megan, Mac and David, for the patience, understanding and encouragement they have shown for many years through to the completion of this book.

INTRODUCTION

*T*his textbook has been written with knowledge and appreciation for the rapid development of the medical specialty of podiatric medicine and its subspecialty of podopediatric orthopedics.

As a podiatric medical student I became very much interested in the subject of podopediatrics. I became aware of the fact that many deformities are more easily correctible or at least controllable in the early years of life. I also appreciated the problems and complications that arise later in life with the fixation of these deformities resulting in a poorer response to treatment. I began seeking a text that would offer the needed didactic information along with a pictorial description and clinical application useful to a student and a practitioner who is seeing and treating children. Unfortunately, a concise and comprehensive text offering this needed information regarding everyday problems of the lower extremities could not be found. During my ensuing years of private practice, as well as instructing students in the care, prevention, and treatment of various pediatric lower extremity deformities, a text of this nature still did not appear. With the opportunity to lecture on this subject extensively to both students and practitioners, a question persistently arose, "Where can this information you are talking about be found?" The only answer available was that the information was extrapolated from numerous articles, textbooks, monographs, manuals, handbooks, outlines, synopses, and the like. The desire by many to have this information compiled and accessible in a text prompted this undertaking. I have felt an obligation to these students, practitioners, my profession, and myself to compile this information into one book.

The primary purpose of this book is to provide the reader with the necessary information to examine an infant or child and to make an intelligent diagnosis of the cause or causes for the more common lower extremity orthopedic disorders encountered. I think most would agree that one textbook cannot offer every conceivable aspect of podopediatric orthopedics without exceeding several volumes. It is therefore my intention to provide the reader a handy text that will offer the basic knowledge providing a solid foundation from which to build. If you review the organization of the chapters first, you will realize they are organized in a logical progression to help the reader develop a system in the examination of a youngster.

It becomes imperative that the examiner acquire a good working knowledge of the normals encountered for each level of development. Without this background, an examination can easily become disorganized and an erroneous conclusion may be drawn.

This author feels that the reader who completes this book will be comfortable and able to provide a basic, but comprehensive, pediatric orthopedic examination of the lower extremities. To achieve this, it is paramount that a detailed history and physical examination including a comprehensive neurological and musculoskeletal investigation of a child be performed. The text is organized in such a way that will allow the examiner to develop an outline to follow for a proper evaluation. Because it is understood that every practitioner develops his own methods and patterns of examination, the information available within these chapters provides for the needed help to a proper diagnosis of an orthopedic condition. The author feels and hopes that the materials offered will fulfill the needs and demands to maintain good lower extremity health in children.

One final area to be discussed is the scope of our profession of podiatric medicine and its constant changes. The realm of practice is significantly variable from one state to another and from region to region. The training and abilities of our present students and young practitioners are exceeding the furthest concepts of our forefathers in podiatry. To provide these practitioners with a full spectrum of knowledge in the examination, management, and treatment of basic orthopedic disorders of the lower extremities, this text has encompassed the hip, knee, leg, and foot. This information is presented with the realization that a diagnosis is 90 percent of dealing with a problem and treatment only 10 percent. I am not professing that podiatrists should treat deformities of the lower extremities that are not included in the licensure of a podiatric physician; however, the ability to determine and recognize the level and degree of the abnormality is significantly important. Additionally, a knowledge of the types of treatments available is helpful. The practitioner must proceed in his treatment in accordance with his training, licensure, and personal capabilities.

CONTENTS

Chapter 1

PEDIATRIC HISTORY

*I*n attempting to arrive at a proper diagnosis, it is imperative that a proper clinical history be obtained skillfully. Most certainly, there are numerous incidences where a misdiagnosis is the result of an inaccurate or incomplete clinical history. Therefore, the history should initially include the basic statistical information usually obtained from the data sheet completed by the parents. Included should be the name, date of birth, place of birth, address, etc. In addition, the parents' ages, especially that of the mother, are of importance in that a higher incidence of birth trauma exists in mothers under 16 years of age. Also, mothers over the age of 35 have a higher risk of having babies with Down's syndrome.[1]

Knowing the parents' height is important in attempting to evaluate the potential development of the child. **Figures 1 and 2** relate the average weights and heights for a given age relative to their physical development.[2] Also included should be the development of any progeny within the family.

The socioeconomic background of the parents is especially important to note in cases of premature births. It has been found that mothers from below-average socioeconomic backgrounds have a higher rate of premature deliveries than mothers from average or above-average environments. The mother's general background is certainly of importance regarding her education, marital status, social habits (alcohol, cigarettes), and economic situation.

Doctor–Child Relationship

Your first encounter with a child is likely to make a strong impression and should be pleasant. When you enter the examination room, you should be noting and observing the reactions of the parents to the child, the child to the parents, the child to his siblings, and so on. This is certainly important in developing a proper understanding and relationship between you, the doctor, and the parents and child. Many musculoskeletal problems in children are factitious, brought on by a need for attention or due to a child's mimicking a sibling with a similar condition.

1

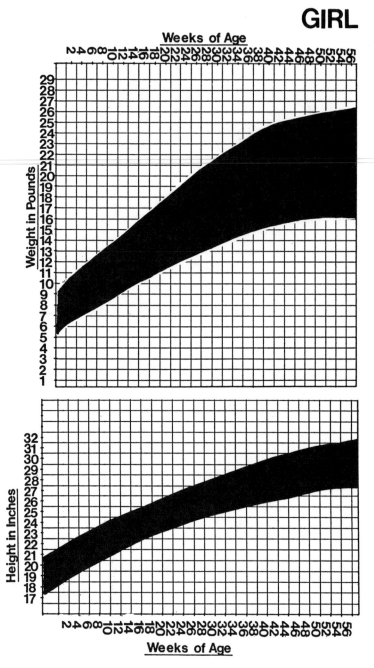

Figure 1

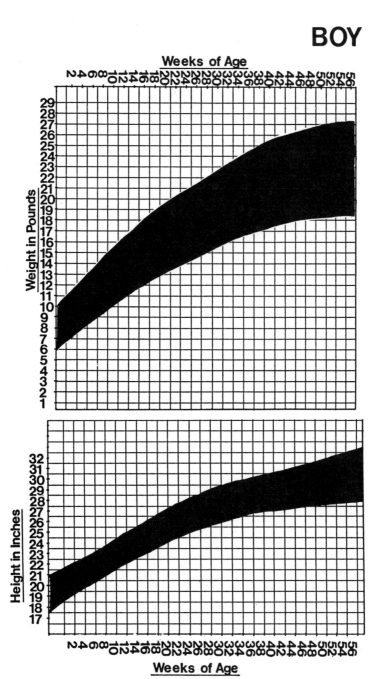

Figure 2

The doctor initially should attempt to establish a good rapport with the child to allow any fears to be overcome. To accomplish this, one may employ a variety of methods. This author finds that by not wearing a lab coat when examining certain children, he is not stereotyped. This has been extremely effective. Keeping the examination room free of instruments or unusual equipment has also been helpful.

Spending five minutes with the child prior to an examination discussing topics other than his presenting problem tends to reduce any fears of your presence. Smiling, being courteous and pleasant are very effective in establishing a good relationship. By trying not to talk loudly or to move too quickly or forcefully, you will put your patient more at ease. In many cases the child is more comfortable and secure in the parents' lap than on the examination table. If this is so, then attempts on your part to complete the examination in this manner are encouraged. Certainly this situation is age-dependent and should be dealt with discreetly.

Patience is also essential when dealing with infants, especially if they have been frightened by an experience elsewhere. In these cases it may take numerous visits before complete confidence in you, the doctor, is accomplished. It cannot be emphasized strongly enough that the initial impression the child develops about the doctor is long lasting and in many cases irreversible.

Chief or Presenting Complaint

The information derived here concerns the specific musculoskeletal problem the patient is presenting. The symptoms should be determined by the doctor as carefully and in as much detail as possible. The chronology of events leading to the problem with the approximate dates, the type of onset, any history of trauma, and the duration of the problem should be determined. Included should be questions concerning the amount of disability, the severity of the problem, factors that aggravate or reduce the symptoms, and any previous occurrences. Also, any types of previous treatment that may have been instituted, the results of this treatment, and any problems or complications should be investigated.

Family History

This part of the history should include such common illnesses as mumps, measles, and chickenpox, as well as any congenital or genetic anomalies. Also to be included in this history are:

- allergies to medications, foods, or pollen, etc.;
- familial birth defects;
- blood dyscrasias such as hemophilia, anemia, or leukemia;
- bone and joint disorders;
- cancer;

- chronic asthma or bronchitis;
- glandular diseases such as diabetes or thyroid;
- kidney disorders;
- heart problems;
- mental retardation;
- muscle diseases which are usually congenital in origin such as the dystrophies;
- nervous disorders such as brain tumors, cerebral palsy, or epilepsy;
- psychiatric disorders which may be familial due to environmental conditions;
- tuberculosis, venereal diseases, rheumatic fever, etc.

The Prenatal History

The prenatal period is that time prior to delivery. It is imperative that the mother's history before delivery be recorded to help determine any potential factors that may have affected the infant. Information elicited should include how often the mother was seen by her obstetrician; frequent or infrequent visits may help you to determine whether there was proper care, or possibly a problem, during the pregnancy.

The doctor should also determine if the pregnancy had been planned by the parents or if the mother had considered terminating it. This may affect the parents' attitude toward the child.

Any history of toxemia should be noted if present during the pregnancy. The triad of proteinuria, high blood pressure, and a large weight gain are indicative of pre-eclampsia. If these three symptoms also have associated convulsions, then this is termed eclampsia.[3]

Any bleeding noted during any of the trimesters is of importance. You should note the amount of bleeding and any type of treatment that may have been rendered. If bleeding occurred during the first trimester this could have been a signaled abortion.[4]

Infections during the pregnancy, especially in the first trimester, should be documented. Viral infections, such as rubella, can cause congenital heart problems, microcephaly, mental retardation, and potential ophthalmologic problems. Any history of diseases, such as diabetes or tuberculosis, should be recorded if present during the pregnancy.[3]

The mother should be questioned thoroughly regarding the matter of drugs. There are numerous drugs that can cause significant alterations or problems in the fetus and should be known to the doctor. A few of the more common drugs and their potential side effects are:

- *Antihistamines*—Can cause some congenital problems.
- *Analgesics* (aspirin)—These may have the propensity to produce neonatal bleeding.
- *Thyroid drugs*—They can result in a hypothyroid child due to their ability to cross the placenta.

TABLE 1
Teratogenic Drugs

Maternal Medication	Fetal or Neonatal Effect
Established human teratogenic drugs	
Thalidomide	Fetal death or phocomelia, deafness, cerebrovascular, gastrointestinal, or genitourinary anomalies
Sex hormones	
androgens, progestogens, estrogens	Masculinization, advanced bone age
Antineoplastic agents	Multiple anomalies, abortion
antimetabolites: amethopterin, 5-fluoro-uracil (5-FU), DON, 6-azauridine, etc.	
alkylating agents: cyclophosphamide, etc.	
antibiotics: amphotericin B, mitomycin, etc.	
Possible human teratogenic drugs	
Vitamin D	Cardiopathies
Antihistamines	Anomalies (?)
Hallucinogens	"Fractured chromosomes,"
lysergic acid (LSD), mescaline, etc.	Anomalies (?)
Antidiabetes drugs	Anomalies (?)
sulfonylurea derivatives	
Corticosteroids	Cleft palate, harelip (?)
Insulin (shock or hypoglycemia)	Anomalies (?)
Antithyroid drugs	Goiter, mental retardation
thiouracils, inorganic iodides (potassium iodide, etc.)	
Human fetotoxic agents	
Analgesics, narcotic drugs	
heroin, morphine	Neonatal death or convulsions, tremors
salicylates (excessive)	Neonatal bleeding
Anticoagulant drugs	Fetal death or hemorrhage
the coumarins	
Anti-infective drugs	
chloramphenicol	Neonatal death ("gray syndrome")
chloroquine	Death or deafness or retinal hemorrhage
erythromycin	Hepatic injury
nitrofurantoin	Hemolytic reactions
novobiocin	hyperbilirubinemia
quinine, quinidine	Nerve deafness, thrombocytopenia
streptomycin	Nerve deafness
sulfonamides (Kynex, Medicil)	Kernicterus
tetracyclines	Hemolysis, hepatotoxicity, inhibition of bone growth, discolored teeth

TABLE 1 *Continued*

Maternal Medication	Fetal or Neonatal Effect
Cardiovascular drugs	
ammonium chloride	Acidosis
hexamethonium	Neonatal ileus
reserpine	Nasal congestion, drowsiness
thiazides	Thrombocytopenia
Polio vaccine (Sabin)	Death or neurologic damage
Sedatives, hypnotics, tranquilizers	
meprobamate	Retarded development
phenobarbital (excessive)	Neonatal bleeding
phenothiazines	Hyperbilirubinemia
Smallpox (cowpox) vaccine	Death or fetal vaccinia
Tobacco smoking	Undersized babies
Vitamin K (excessive)	Hyperbilirubinemia

- *Heroin, morphine*—These drugs are associated with death, convulsions, depression, and withdrawal symptoms by the infant.
- *Tetracycline*—Has the ability to cause teeth staining in the child if given to the mother during her pregnancy. This drug will also affect children if given up until the ages of 8–10 years.
- *Alcohol*—Has the potential of causing various congenital anomalies.
- *Tobacco*—Can affect the baby's size and development.

Refer to Table 1 for other fetotoxic medications.[3]

To conclude, it should be realized that any drug given during pregnancy, especially during the first trimester, could have teratogenic effects on the developing fetus.

The Natal History

The natal period is the time when delivery occurs. Some important information to be noted about this period is the duration of labor, any cephalopelvic disproportion, whether the child was born via a caesarean section, and whether it was a breech or cephalic delivery. If labor was excessively long, then the stress on the baby could have deleterious effects. If the "water bag" was ruptured for more than 24 hours, it could have caused an in-utero infection.[6]

Cephalopelvic disproportion pertains to the size of the fetal head in relation to the mother's pelvis. If the birth canal was narrow or the child's head enlarged, then trauma to the skull could have ensued.

If the child was born by caesarean section, one should question why this procedure was necessary and at what point the decision to operate was made. In most cases, mothers who have had a C-section may not be able to have subsequent children by natural means.

TABLE 2
Developmental Milestones

1 month—Spontaneous motor activity generalized
Lifts head when prone; poor supine head control
Beginning to regard surroundings
Follows objects to midline

2 months—Motor activity generalized
Smiles and coos socially
Follows objects past midline

3 months—Follows well with eyes
May wave at toy: beginning to regard hands
Good control of head when prone and looking around
Head control improved when in sitting position
Moro's reflex disappearing
Smiles: coos in more sustained fashion

4 months—Beginning to reach for toys symmetrically
Regards toys and may pull them to mouth
Removes cloth from face
Control of head good when sitting
Plays with hands
Laughs

6 months—Reaches with either hand and begins to transfer objects
Rolls over
May sit briefly when placed in sitting position
Laughs and plays with examiner

8 months—Prehensile function palmar
Sits alone
Beginning to creep reciprocally
Vocalizes with infantile rhythms and polysyllabic vowel sounds
Regards self in mirror

10 months—Crawls reciprocally
Pulls up on rail
May begin to cruise
Uses thumb and index finger in opposition
May say "mama" or "dada"
Feeds self crackers and holds own bottle

12 months—Walks with support
Stands alone
Places cube in cup; tries to build tower of two cubes
May have two words in addition to "mama" or "dada"
Begins to feed self with fingers

15 months—Walks alone (toddles)
Creeps upstairs
4- to 5- word vocabulary
Pats pictures
Drinks from cup
Beginning to feed self with spoon
Makes wants known by pointing or vocalizing

TABLE 2 *Continued*

18 months—Walks well
        Sits in chair
        Throws a ball
        Climbs on furniture
        Stacks 3 to 4 cubes
        10-word vocabulary
        Begins to identify pictures
        Pulls toy on string
        May be toilet-trained during day

2 years—Runs well
        Negotiates steps one at a time
        Uses pronouns and 3-word sentences
        Feeds self with spoon
        Refers to self by name
        Toilet-trained during day

2½ years—Undresses self partially
        Attempts to put on socks
        Draws horizontal or vertical lines but does not cross them
        Refers to self as "I"
        Knows full name
        Helps to put things away

3 years—Alternates feet going upstairs
        Pedals tricycle
        Builds tower of cubes
        Names drawings
        Uses plurals and obeys propositional commands
        Feeds self well
        Buttons and unbuttons clothes and puts on shoes

4 years—Runs and climbs well
        Walks downstairs alternating feet
        Hops on one foot
        Throws a ball overhead
        Attempts to catch ball or kick it in the air
        Pedals tricycle rapidly
        Draws man with head, trunk, and arms or legs
        Counts 3 objects
        Names one or more colors

5 years—Skips, alternating feet
        Draws a man
        Copies a square, cross, and a circle
        Dresses and undresses without assistance
        Knows the names of 4 or more colors
        Counts to 10 or higher

6 years—Draws a man with hands and clothes
        Repeats 4 digits
        Knows morning and afternoon
        Knows right from left side

Establishing whether the birth was breech or cephalic is of importance. If a breech presentation occurred, then you must consider the possibility of an umbilical strangulation. This cannot be determined at the time of birth because the baby may have appeared normal. Later in life the child may exhibit mental retardation or cerebral palsy, which could have been due to cerebral hypoxia during the delivery.[5] Also to be considered is the potential for a congenitally dislocated hip in this type of presentation. The child should be examined for this at the time of birth.[5]

Postnatal History

This portion of the history is concerned with events after delivery. The three most important parameters in determining the child's growth are weight, height, and head circumference. At birth, the average values are 7.5 lbs. (3.4 kg), 20 inches in length, and an average head circumference of 14 inches.[1] Refer to Figures 1 and 2 for weight and height development.[2]

Developmental milestones also help in evaluating the child's mental and physical maturation. Although these milestones are variable, they do help to establish an index from which to judge. It must be noted that none of these milestones should be rigidly adhered to, but rather should be interpreted in view of the whole picture. Refer to Table 2 for the developmental milestones.[6]

Systems Review

Respiratory System

A frequent disorder of this system is the upper respiratory tract infection, which can be either viral, bacterial, or allergic in origin. Viral infections will produce an increase in lymphocytes and may present with an associated elevated temperature. Conversely, a bacterial infection will show fever with an increase in polymorphonuclear leukocytes and a positive throat culture. Allergic infections do not always demonstrate a fever and are usually seasonal or related to house dust, mold, or animals. You may see an increase in eosinophils with this condition.

Cystic fibrosis can also cause recurrent upper respiratory infections and, if suspected, should be tested.

A third cause of upper respiratory tract infections is immune deficiencies. These are due to a decrease in the immunoglobins in the system which in turn cause a decrease in resistance.[3]

Cardiovascular System

You should determine any family history of congenital heart problems and note any familial cyanosis. Also to be asked is any history of rheumatic fever, etc.[1]

Gastrointestinal System

Diarrhea should be noted and its cause determined. Some causes are baby formula, allergies, and infections. The infections can include bacterial, associated with a fever; parasitic, which is determined by stool culturing; and viral, which is the leading cause of diarrhea.[1]

Genitourinary System

Urinary tract infections are more common in females, because of their shorter urethra. Any history of hematuria, dysuria, pain, or edema could indicate cystitis or nephritis. Additionally, marked edema is indicative of a nephrotic syndrome. Also to be noted is any polydipsia or polyuria, which may suggest a possible diabetes mellitus or insipidus.[1]

Musculoskeletal and Neurological Systems

These areas will be the topic of discussion in the ensuing chapters of this book.

References

1. Barness, L.A.: *Manual of Pediatric Physical Diagnosis.* Chicago, Year Book Medical Publishers, 1969.
2. Frankenburg, W., Dodds, J.: *Denver Developmental Screening Text Manual.* Denver, University of Colorado Medical Center and Mead Johnson, 1968.
3. Graham, B.D.: *Pediatric Examination in Physical Diagnosis.* St. Louis, C.V. Mosby Co., 1969.
4. Kempe, C.H., Silver, H.K., O'Brian, D.: *Current Pediatric Diagnosis and Treatment.* Los Altos, California, Lange Medical Publication, 1972.
5. Tachdjian, M.O.: *Pediatric Orthopedics.* Philadelphia, W.B. Saunders Co., 1972.
6. Spivek, M.L.: *Examination of the Child In Practice of Pediatrics,* Edited by J. Brennemann and I. McQuarrie. Hagerstown, Md., W.F. Prior, 1970.

Chapter 2

NEUROLOGICAL EXAMINATION

*T*he neurological examination is a very important part of a pediatric evaluation. It is imperative that the examiner realize that findings on the neurological examination of infants, especially in the newborn period, differ markedly from those present in children and adults.[1] In infancy the subcortical level is the mediator of behavior patterns due to its more rapid maturation. In the older child the cerebral cortex is the controlling level. The cerebral cortex, as it develops, will suppress some of the functions of the subcortical nuclei, although certain subcortical responses remain throughout life. Taking into consideration the fact that cortical function develops slowly after birth, it is therefore impossible to test its capacity adequately until early childhood.[5] In addition, the development in infancy occurs from cephalocaudal resulting in advancement of the motor control, coordination, and reflexes of the upper extremities in relation to the lower appendages.[7]

To be appreciated is the fact that a normal brain stem and spinal function do not ensure an intact cortical system in an infant. Conversely, abnormalities of the brain stem and spinal cord may exist without cortical defects.[3]

The neurological evaluation in infancy will allow the examiner to detect any extensive disease of the central nervous system but it will not enable one to pinpoint a minute lesion or specific functional deficits.[5]

In the examination of an infant one should include an evaluation of mental status, motor system, sensory system, reflexes, and coordination. The mental status of the child can be evaluated by observing alertness, the type of cry, feeding habits, amount of irritability, tremors, and seizures. The motor system should be tested for muscle tone, power, and coordination. The motor function is tested to determine whether muscle tone is normal, spastic, or flaccid in nature. This is best accomplished by putting each major joint through its respective range of motion. In doing this the examiner should note symmetry of mobility, spasticity, tone, and any fasciculations present. Being that infants have a considerable amount of fat over their muscles, and that fasciculations are therefore difficult to exhibit, one should use the tongue for this evaluation.[12]

Sensory examination should include testing pain, touch, temperature, vibration, and position sense. Pain, touch, and temperature thresholds are con-

13

siderably higher in the infant than in the older child; one must realize this when examining an infant and not assume that the infant is insensitive to testing. Stronger stimuli and greater temperature gradients are necessary to elicit a proper response. It should also be noted that infants have a much slower reaction time to stimuli. This is easily exhibited when a pinprick is used and the interval of time between the actual stimulus and the withdrawal is measured. There will be a delay of a second or two before the response is produced.[3]

When testing an infant for sensations the examiner should be cognizant of the movements produced and the facial expressions of the child. Absence of withdrawal when a noxious stimuli is applied to an extremity may indicate anesthesia of the limb possibly with a paralysis. If, however, a change in facial expression or a cry is elicited in the absence of withdrawal, paralysis, rather than an anesthetic limb, is indicated. With spinal cord lesions, the extremities will withdraw in response to pain but there will be no concomitant change in the baby's facial expressions or cry.[15]

Coordination can best be evaluated by using the developmental milestones presented in Chapter 1 (Table 2) as a guide. Discrepancies in motor and communication areas may suggest a deficit in the motor as well as the sensory or intellectual levels of the child.

The reflexes to be examined are the deep tendon reflexes and the subcortical reflexes, including the infantile automatisms and mass reflexes. These reflexes will be described and discussed individually. The examiner needs to be cognizant of the specific age levels at which these reflexes exist and when they disappear, if applicable. It is essential to elicit the reflexes properly in order to make a valid determination. Many parents have been misled or children misdiagnosed because of the examiner's inability to produce the proper responses during an examination.

Subcortical Reflexes

Deep Tendon Reflexes

Because the corticospinal pathways are not fully developed in infants, the spinal reflex mechanism, i.e., deep tendon reflexes and plantar response, are variable. The degree of their presence and exaggeration, as well as their absence, has little diagnostic significance unless there is asymmetry of the response or change in response from a previous testing. These reflexes can be elicited by using your bent index finger as a neurological hammer with the tip of the bend as the striking point. Also, your finger or thumbnail is an adequate stimulus for eliciting the plantar response.

Deep tendon reflexes are elicited in the same manner as in an adult. Of importance is to note symmetry of response in the knee jerk (patellar reflex) and ankle jerk (Achilles' reflex). (**Figure 3**). If there exists an absence or diminished response in one or both limbs, one should suspect a possible paralysis or spinal cord injury. Asymmetry is most easily noticed in an exami-

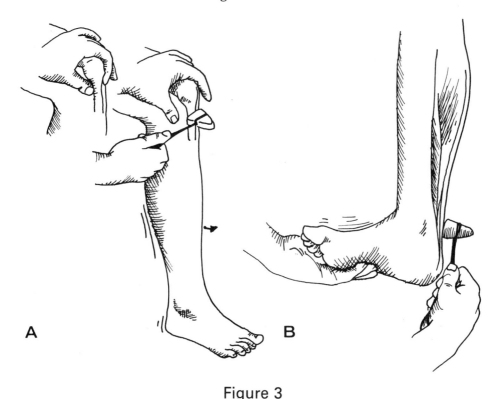

Figure 3

(A) Patellar Reflex. (B) Achilles reflex.

nation, but one must be more astute in the bilaterally symmetrical diminished response. Most infants will have a reasonable amount of hyperreflexia, although the response will vary from one moment to the next. Absence of a response by one attempt is certainly not conclusive. If this does occur, the examiner should attempt many times throughout the examination to elicit the reflex. If the reflex still does not exist then a more supportive conclusion can be made.[16]

Plantar Response   L4 5 S1 2

This is oftentimes referred to as the Babinski sign or reflex. It is a normal reflex in infants from birth to the age of six months to one year of age. It can, though, exist up to the age of two in some children and still be considered normal. The response is elicited by stroking the plantar surface of the outer border of the foot with a blunt point or fingernail. The response is a slow dorsiflexion of the great toe accompanied by fanning of the lateral toes. After approximately one year of age this reflex should no longer be existent and a response of plantarflexion of the toes should be present. If this sign is persistent, then a strong indication of a disorder of the pyramidal system exists[6] (**Figure 4**).

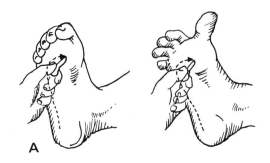

A

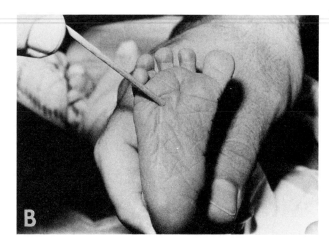

B

Figure 4

Babinski sign.

Test pyrimidal system

Infantile Automatisms

There are certain reflex phenomena that exist at birth or shortly thereafter which are referred to as infantile automatisms. Some exist for only a couple of weeks and others will continue until two to three years of age. The value of these responses has been debated as to their prognostic value for central nervous system integrity. Although the question is still unanswered, the responses do help in initially recognizing the presence of a disorder. A list of the more common reflexes will be presented.

PLANTAR GRASP REFLEX

The plantar grasp reflex is a response which produces flexion and adduction of the toes when light digital pressure on the plantar surface of the foot is performed. This is a subcortical reflex and exists from birth to approximately one year of age. Its presence past this age may suggest a birth injury or possibly a delay in development[10] (**Figure 5**).

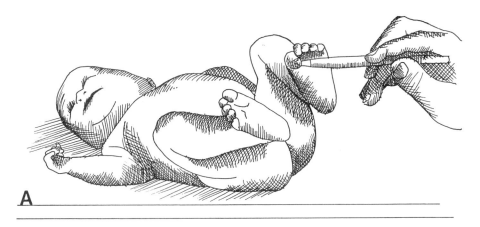

A

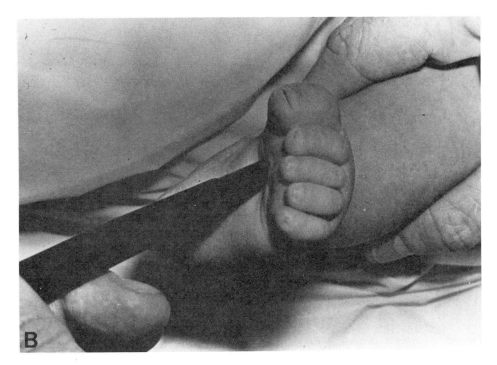

B

Figure 5

Plantar grasp reflex.

HAND GRASP REFLEX

The hand grasp reflex responds similarly to the plantar grasp reflex in that stimulation of the hand muscles produces flexion. This is achieved by stimulating the ulnar side of the baby's hand with finger pressure to the palm. The infant will automatically grasp either your finger or the object being used for stimulation, i.e., a pen or pencil (**Figure 6**). It should be noted that the

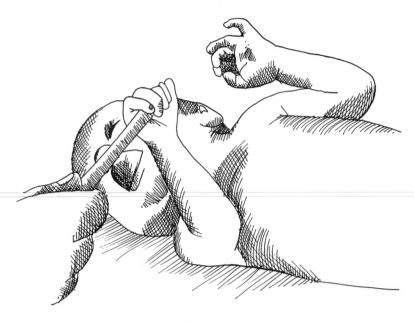

Figure 6

Hand grasp reflex.

head should be in the midline as the reflex will be more pronounced on the side the child's head is facing.[2] There also exists an *extensor reflex* that can be produced by stroking the ulnar surface of the hand and the fifth or little finger. The fingers will respond with extension.[15]

The hand grasp reflex usually exists from birth to two to four months. If its existence is noted beyond this age, one may suspect a spastic cerebral palsy, or if on one side you may consider a spastic hemiplegia. In cases where the response is absent at birth, then an indication of a flaccid paralysis may be present.

ACOUSTIC BLINK REFLEX

This reflex is present from birth to approximately one to one and one-half years of age. The response is elicited by producing a very loud sharp noise, i.e., clapping hands, slapping the side of the table. The reflex will be one of blinking of both eyes. This response tests the infant's ability to hear. If the reflex is absent one should seriously consider some degree of deafness or loss of hearing to be present.[12]

ROOTING REFLEX

The rooting reflex is one in which the infant is placed on his back with his head in the midline and his hands against the chest. To produce a response,

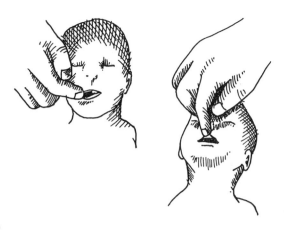

Figure 7

Rooting reflex.

stimulate the corners of the mouth by stroking away from the corner. The infant will open its mouth and turn to the side that was stimulated. In addition, by stroking the upper or lower lip the child will bend its head backward or forward, respectively. The upper lip stimulation will result in extension while the lower lip will produce flexion of the head. This reflex is present from birth to three to four months. If the response is absent during this period then a severe central nervous system disorder is indicated[10] (**Figure 7**).

TRUNK INCURVATION (GALANT'S) REFLEX

This reflex exists from birth to approximately two months of age. It is elicited by stroking either one side of the back or the other approximately 1–2 inches from the midline of the spine. The reaction will be one of curving of the back and torso toward the stimulated side. Both sides should be tested to ensure symmetry of response. In cases where this reflex is nonexistent, a suspicion of a spinal cord lesion should be investigated[15] (**Figure 8**).

VERTICAL SUSPENSION REFLEX

This reflex will exist until about four months of age. To produce this response, hold the infant around the chest under the axilla and keep his head maintained in the midline of the body. A normal response is one of flexion at the knees and hips. If the child exhibits a fixed extension with adduction of the legs, i.e., scissoring effect, then an indication of a spastic paraplegia or diplegia may exist[15] (**Figure 9**).

PLACING REFLEX

To elicit this reflex, the examiner should hold the baby around the chest and support the head with his thumbs. The dorsum of the baby's foot should then be brought to touch the underside of a tabletop edge. Care should be taken to avoid plantarflexing the foot. The baby will respond by flexing the

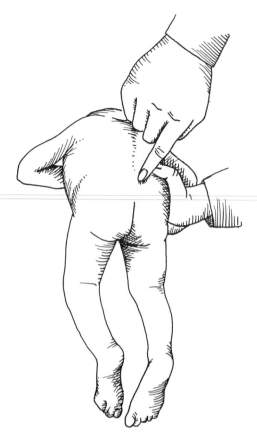

Figure 8

Trunk incurvation reflex (Galant's).

hip and knee and placing the stimulated foot on the top of the table. This should be tried 2–3 times and performed on each side. Its presence will exist from approximately the second to the fourth day after birth to age six to eight weeks of age. Absence of this reflex may indicate brain damage[9] (**Figure 10**).

STEPPING REFLEX

This response is present from birth to one to three months of age. To accomplish this reflex, the examiner should hold the child around the chest. With light pressure on the feet the child is moved in a forward progression. The response is flexion of the knee and hip on one side and extension on the other. This is simulating walking. It must be remembered that this is merely a subcortical reflex producing a reciprocal action of the extensor and flexor muscles and does not constitute actual weight-bearing walking. If this reflex is not present, then paralysis should be considered, or possibly some type of brain dysfunction[14] (**Figure 11**).

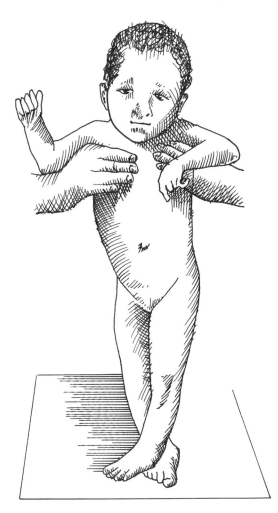

Figure 9

Vertical suspension reflex (scissoring effect).

ASYMMETRIC TONIC NECK REFLEX

To perform this reflex, place the baby supine and maintain the head in the midline. As you rotate the head to either one side or the other, a reflex of extension of the arm and leg will occur on the side on which the head is facing. Flexion will concomitantly occur on the opposite side. This response is existent from age two months to approximately six months. Occasionally a newborn will exhibit this response but most often it is found past one and one-half to two months. If present past the page of 6–8 months one could expect a possible major cerebral disorder or damage[14] (**Figure 12**).

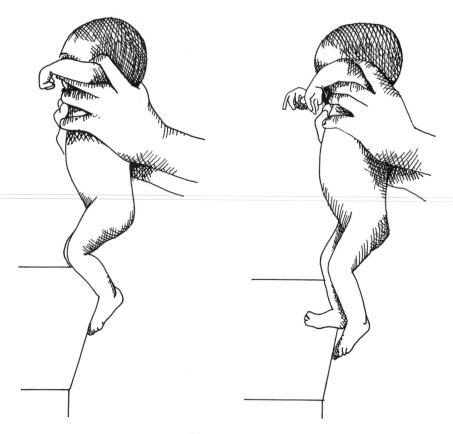

Figure 10

Placing reflex.

WITHDRAWAL REFLEX

This reflex should exist from birth to adult life. If a noxious stimulus is applied to the plantar surface of the foot, i.e., a pinprick, then a withdrawal response of dorsiflexion at the ankle and flexion at the knee and hip will occur. If this reaction is absent or weak, a meningiomyelocele or paralysis due to an intraspinal lesion may be present[4] (**Figure 13**).

LANDAU REFLEX

To produce this reflex, hold the child under its stomach with one hand and keep the body as close to parallel with the ground. With the other hand flex the head. A response of flexion of the head and extension of the limbs should be noted. This reflex is normal for children from the age of six months to two and one half years of age. The presence of delayed maturation will exist if present past the age of two and one half to three years[3] (**Figure 14**).

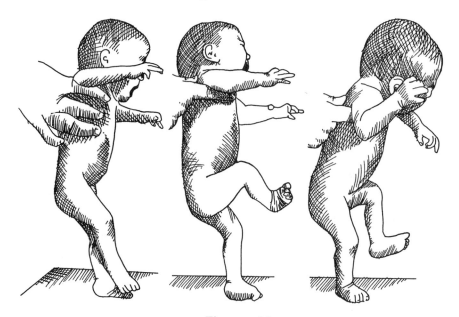

Figure 11

Stepping reflex.

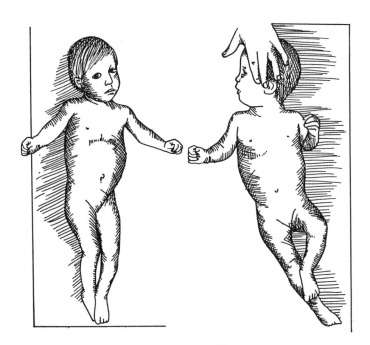

Figure 12

Asymmetric tonic neck reflex.

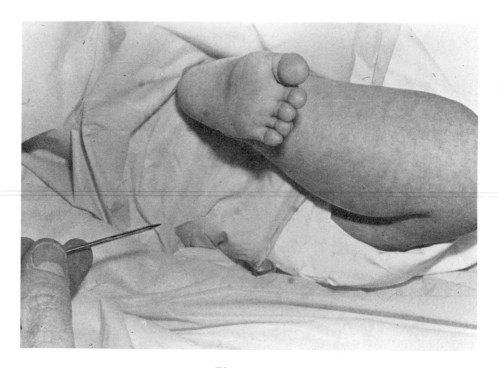

Figure 13

Withdrawal reflex.

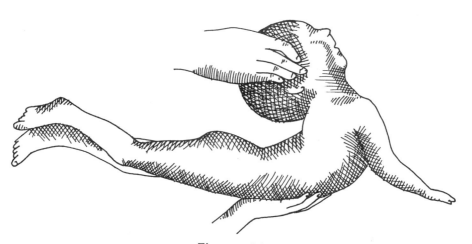

Figure 14

Landau reflex.

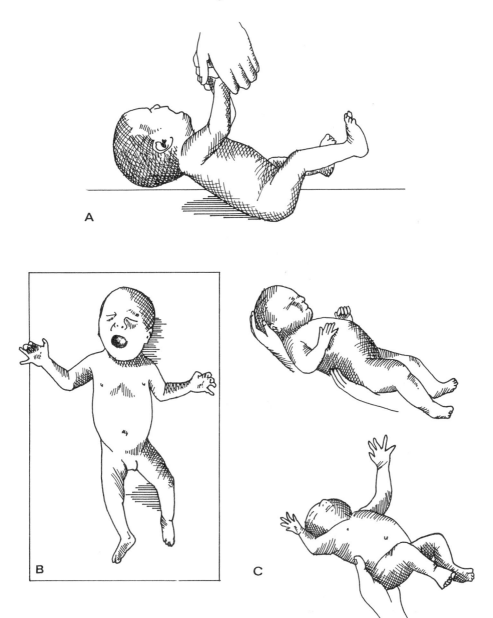

Figure 15
Moro reflex.

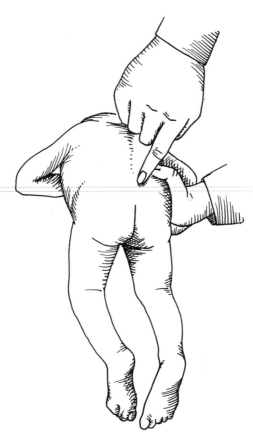

Figure 16

Perez reflex.

Massive Reflexes

There exist two massive reflexes in infants that are normal to approximately the age of 3–5 months. These reflexes are the *Moro* and *Perez* reflexes.

Moro Reflex

This reflex can be elicited by a variety of methods including the holding of the infant by the hands, raising him approximately 6–8 inches and dropping him (**Figure 15A and B**). Another is to hold the baby supine while supporting the back and pelvis with one hand and dropping him several inches with a sudden rapid movement (**Figure 15C**). The response in both of these maneuvers is an abduction and extension of the arms and hands. The legs will extend with abduction of the hip. This is then followed by flexion and adduction of the extremities with usually an accompanying cry. Asymmetry of this response will suggest hemiparesis, possible spinal cord injury, or even a congenital hip dislocation. The presence after six months may indicate delayed maturation of the central nervous system or possibly cerebral palsy.[9]

PEREZ REFLEX

To produce this response hold the infant prone in one hand. With the other hand stroke firmly the length of the spine from the sacrum to the head with your thumb. Observation of extension of the head and spine with flexion of the knees against the chest and a cry with emptying of the bladder will exist. Absence of this response indicates cerebral damage or spinal cord injury and persistence of the reflex indicates a delayed maturation of the central nervous system[3] (**Figure 16**).

The neurological evaluation in early and late childhood should be performed in a different manner. Motor development and sensory development, as outlined by the *Developmental Milestones* in Chapter 1, are a good basic measuring stick to determine the progress of a child. Such signs as *Gower's sign for muscular dystrophy* should be kept in mind when muscular development is not consistent with the age of the child.

Gait Analysis

In evaluating a child's neurological development there must not be forgotten the observation of his walking patterns. Abnormal gait patterns can be suggestive of many types of muscular and neuromuscular disorders. With the assumption that the reader has a basic knowledge of the determinants of gait and the biomechanics of walking, I will describe the abnormal gait patterns and the types of disorders correlated to them. If you do not feel you have a basic background in the biomechanics and determinants of gait, then refer to the article by Saunders, Inman, and Eberhart on the determinants of gait and to the *Compendium of Podiatric Biomechanics* for the mechanics in walking.[11,13]

Tip-Toe Gait

This gait presents with the child persistently ambulating on the ball of the foot while the heel rarely comes in contact with the weight-bearing surface. The youngster needs to be observed at various times to determine its constancy. It is of value to view the child's walking when no attention is being placed on the problem such as when entering or leaving the office. Observation on two or three separate occasions is beneficial. The continuance of this gait abnormality for any period of time is suggestive of a contracted tendoachilles, which may be secondary to a possible neuromuscular disorder. Spasticity may be the causative factor. If suspected, further evaluation is warranted.[9]

Circumducting Gait

In patients presenting with a spastic hemiparesis, a circumducting gait pattern can be observed. This presents with a rotating and swing pattern of each leg when ambulating. This gait is also observed in stroke patients.[2]

Waddling (Trendelenberg) Gait

In this type of gait the patient will present with a dropping of one or both hips when walking. This will take on a "duck waddling" characteristic in ambulation. It is suggestive of a possible congenital hip dislocation or possibly a paralysis of the musculature on the affected side. Further evaluation is required.[4]

Wide Base of Gait and Ataxic Gait

A suspicion of a central nervous system disorder such as an anterior horn cell disorder or a peripheral nerve disorder, i.e., peripheral neuritis, may produce this type of gait. The patient will walk with a wide-based, unsteady and irregular pattern. Often the person will stagger and be unable to walk in a straight line. It will be noticed that a slapping of the foot during heel-to-toe contact is present.[8]

Foot-Drop Gait

This abnormal gait is frequently due to a peripheral neuropathy causing paralysis of the muscles needed for dorsiflexion of the foot. What will be observed is an external rotation of the lower limb and a flexion of the hip and knee to a higher level than normal. This occurs to allow the foot to come through the swing phase of gait without contacting the ground. Testing is necessary to determine the degree of functional impairment.[8]

References

1. Andre, N.: L'Orthopedie àu l'art de prevenir et de Corriger Clans les Enfants les Deformites du Corps. Paris 1741, London 1743, Philadelphia, reproduced by J.B. Lippencott Co., 1961.
2. Chusid, J.G.: Correlative Neuroanatomy and Functional Neurology, 15th Edition. Los Altos, California, Lange Medical Publications, 1973.
3. DeJong, R.N.: The Neurological Examination, 3rd Edition. New York, Hober Medical Division, Harper & Row, 1967.
4. Denny–Brown, D.: Handbook of Neurological Examination and Case Recordings, Revised Edition. Cambridge, Mass., Harvard University Press, 1967.
5. Farmer, T.W.: Pediatric Neurology. New York, Hoeber Medical Div., Harper & Row, 1964.
6. Gatz, A.J.: Manter's Essentials of Clinical Neuroanatomy and Neurophysiology, 4th Edition. Philadelphia, F.A. Davis Co., 1970.
7. House, E.L., Pansky, B.: A Functional Approach to Neuroanatomy, 2nd Edition. New York, McGraw-Hill Book Co., Inc., 1970.
8. Haymaker, W., Woodhall, B.: Peripheral Nerve Injuries. Principles of Diagnosis, 2nd Edition. Philadelphia, W.B. Saunders Co., 1953.

9. Paine, R.S.: Neurological examination of infants and children. *Pediatr. Clin. N. Am.,* 7:471–510, 1960.
10. Prechtl, H., Beitema, D.: *The Neurological Examination of the Full Term Newborn Infant.* London, National Spastics Society Medical Education and Information Unit, 1964.
11. Saunders, J.B., deC, M., Inman, V.T., Eberhart, H.D.: The major determinants in normal and pathological gait. *J.B.J.S.,* 35-A:543–558, July 1953.
12. Steegman, A.T.: *Examination of the Nervous System. A Student's Guide.* Chicago, The Year Book Publishers, Inc., 1969.
13. Sgarlato, T.E.: *A Compendium of Podiatric Biomechanics.* San Francisco, California College of Podiatric Medicine, March, 1971.
14. Thomas, A., Chesni, Y., Dargassies, S.S.: *The Neurological Examination of the Infant.* London National Spastics Society Medical Education and Information Unit, 1960.
15. Tachdjian, M.O.: *Pediatric Orthopedic.* Philadelphia, W.B. Saunders Co., 1972.
16. Van Allen, M.W.: *Pictorial Manual of Neurological Tests.* Chicago, Year Book Medical Publishers, 1969.

Chapter 3

SCOLIOSIS AND LIMB-LENGTH DISCREPANCY

A proper pediatric history and a neurological examination have been discussed in the preceding two chapters to prepare the examiner for the third area of analysis—musculoskeletal system of the lower extremities. An examination should start with the spine and continue down through the segments of the lower extremity to include the hips, thighs, knees, legs, ankles, and feet.

This chapter will discuss the most common spinal disorder, scoliosis, and will relate the effect(s) of a limb length discrepancy on this condition as well as its effects on other segments of the body. The ensuing chapters will progressively examine the other components of the lower extremity in a logical order necessary for a comprehensive evaluation.

Scoliosis

Abnormal curvatures in the spine have been present since man first assumed an erect posture. Unfortunately, the etiology of idiopathic scoliosis still evades us. The condition can only be treated at present by correcting the curvatures that developed without any known method of prevention.[5]

Since podiatrists examine a reasonable number of children and infants for lower extremity disorders, they should be aware of and examine for the presence of this abnormality. If any suspicion of scoliosis exists, then consultation with an appropriate specialist is paramount.

Anatomic Considerations

The spine maintains its stability by the: vertebrae, disc, anterior-posterior-interspinous ligaments, articular facets and their capsules, musculature; and the stability of the rib cage and abdominal muscles. The articular facets of the lumbar vertebrae have a more vertical inclination allowing for extension, forward flexion, and lateral bending. The facets of the thoracic and cervical articulations are more horizontal allowing for more rotational movements to occur. The condition of scoliosis is complicated by the existence of not only lateral bending, but also rotation of the vertebral column around its longitudinal axis.[5] The presence of lordosis and kyphosis will also complicate the total condition (**Figure 17**).

With rotation of the column, the ribs attached will rotate in an anterior-posterior direction causing a "rib hump."[7] The posterior rotation causes the hump while the anterior rotation may cause an anterior prominence of the chest wall. This is most often noted in thoracic scoliosis particularly when the patient is asked to bend over and the spine is viewed as in **Figure 18**.

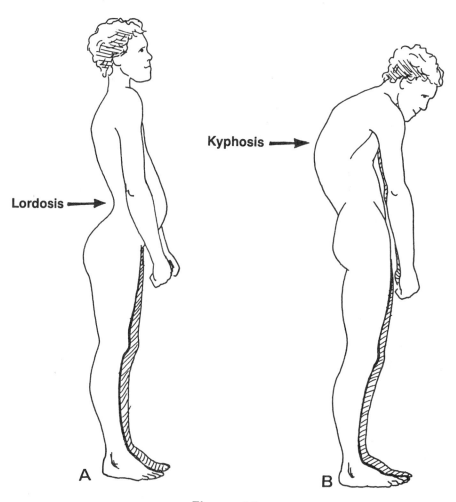

Figure 17

(A) Lordosis. (B) Kyphosis.

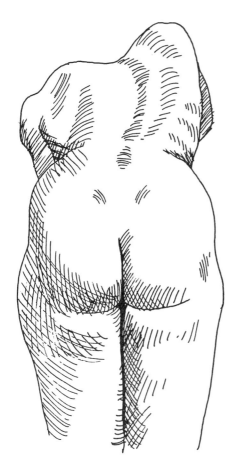

Figure 18

"Rib Hump" from the posterior rotation of the rib cage noted with bending over. Adapted from an original painting by Frank H. Netter, M.D., from Clinical Symposia, © *CIBA Pharmaceutical Company, Division of CIBA-GEIGY Corporation. With permission.*

These characteristic findings are most common in idiopathic scoliosis. The paralytic or congenital curvatures will present with the ribs assuming a vertical position on the convex side.[6]

Classification

STRUCTURAL

Idiopathic Scoliosis:

This form is primarily considered the result of an unknown cause, although recent evidence indicates that genetic transmission may be a valid consideration. Approximately 70% of all scoliosis is classified as idiopathic with the prevalence being 8:1 females to males in the adolescent group.[2]

The curvature(s) can occur at the: lumbar area; thoracic and lumbar area; thoracic area; and cervico-thoracic area (**Figure 19**). The onset of these curves can be divided according to the age in which the curve is first seen.[5]

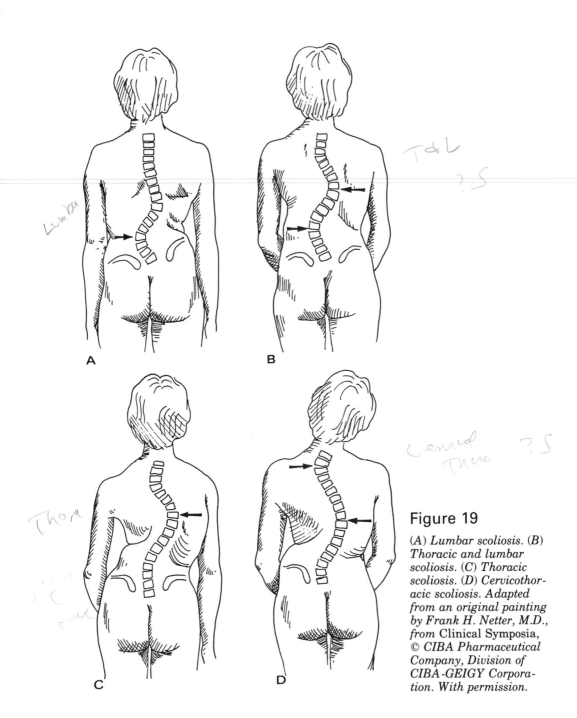

Figure 19

(A) *Lumbar scoliosis.* (B) *Thoracic and lumbar scoliosis.* (C) *Thoracic scoliosis.* (D) *Cervicothoracic scoliosis. Adapted from an original painting by Frank H. Netter, M.D., from* Clinical Symposia, © *CIBA Pharmaceutical Company, Division of CIBA-GEIGY Corporation. With permission.*

Infantile form—occurs from birth to approximately 3 years of age. It is most often noticed in the first year of life with males being more prevalent than females. A high incidence has been found in children from the northern European areas. Etiologically it is felt to be the result of uterine position. Its prognosis is usually good with resolution occurring spontaneously. On occasion, these may progress to a more severely rigid curve and the result is a very poor prognosis. This form is not considered to be genetically transmitted.

Juvenile form—is noted between 4 and 9 years of age with the male to female ratio being equal. The progression of this type usually does not allow its recognition until after the age of 6–7 years. This is felt to more likely be an inheritable condition.

Adolescent form—commonly occurs after the age of ten or from the onset of puberty to full skeletal maturity. Frequently these curves have existed prior to this age of recognition. The adolescent growth spurt, however, brings the abnormality to the attention of the patient or parents. As mentioned earlier, the prevalence is 8:1 females to males during the adolescent period. *Note:* the younger the child in whom an idiopathic structural curve is found, the more serious is the prognosis. The exception is the infantile type.

CONGENITAL

This form of scoliosis is not the result of genetics but is, rather, due to developmental failure of the vertebral or extravertebral structures. These can be subdivided into the *open type* of failure in development, such as a myelomeningocele, or a spina bifida, or the *closed type* of failure, as in: failure of proper vertebral formation; failure of segmentation; fusion of the vertebrae or ribs; failure in development of the transverse process (hemivertebrae) (**Figure 20**). One or more of the closed-type failures may occur together to form a more serious disorder.

The congenital type of scoliosis usually does not progress significantly as does the idiopathic, although some may become severe and irreversible.

NEUROMUSCULAR

Several known causes for scoliosis have been documented. Disorders causing muscular imbalance of the paravertebral musculature will ultimately result in a scoliotic condition. Examples of these disorders are: poliomyelitis, neurofibromatosis (Von Recklinghausen's disease), intraspinal tumors, Friedreich's ataxia, syringomyelia, spastic paralysis (cerebral palsy), muscular dystrophys, arthropathies (i.e., rheumatoid arthritis), osteoid osteomas of a vertebrae, congenital heart problems (i.e., Marfan's syndrome), traumatic conditions (i.e., fractures, burns).

J. DAVIS

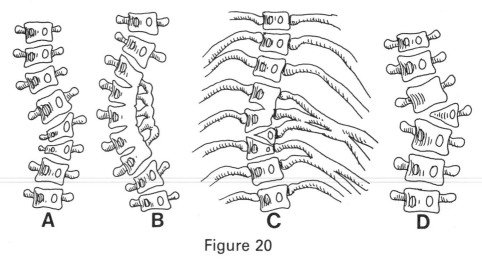

A   B   C   D

Figure 20

(A) Failure of proper vertebral formation. (B) Failure of segmentation. (C) Fusion of vertebrae or ribs. (D) Failure in development of the transverse process (hemivertebral). Adapted from an original painting by Frank H. Netter, M.D., from Clinical Symposia, *© CIBA Pharmaceutical Company, Division of CIBA-GEIGY Corporation. With permission.*

FUNCTIONAL

This form of scoliosis is the result of a postural imbalance. This is most commonly due to a leg length discrepancy forcing the pelvis on the shorter side to drop and producing a curve in the spine. The curves are flexible and reducible and there are usually no compensatory curves, rotational changes, or structural changes. These curves will reduce when the person is asked to lie down or the stretch test is employed by lifting the child off the ground by his chin. (**Figure 21**).

Clinical Examination

When examining a child for scoliosis, a thorough history is mandatory to derive pertinent information relative to the condition. It will also help in determining any medical conditions contributing to the disorder (i.e., Marfan's syndrome, arthropathies, etc). Physical examination may reveal skin changes (café-au-lait spots, pigmented or patches of hair at the lumbar region) which could signal a Von Recklinghausen's disease or a spina bifida, diastematomyelia, or spinal dysraphism. Alterations in the cardiopulmonary status, eyes, genitourinary system, and teeth may also provide evidence of an underlying congenital disorder.

The examination of the spine will not only reveal the degree of flexibility or rigidity but also determine the direction of the curve(s) and any rotation.

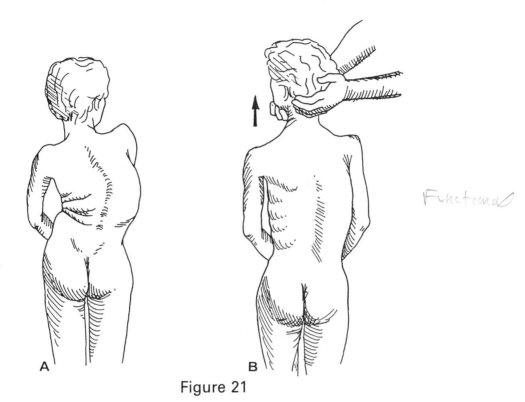

Functional

Figure 21

(A) Flexible curve present before the "stretch test." (B) Raising the child by the chin shows reduction of the curve.

The flexibility (reducibility) is evaluated by having the patient bend towards the convex side of the curve to determine if the curve reduces (**Figure 22**). Another method used is the stretch test. The child is lifted gently by the head and a determination as to the degree of reduction of the curve is assessed (**Figure 21**).

The curve patterns may include a right thoracic curve, thoracolumbar curve, double curve, lumbar curve, and/or a cervicothoracic curve. These primary curves, which are usually structural, may have an accompanying secondary curve that is compensatory to the primary curve (**Figure 19**).

Further examination should include determining: scapular and shoulder symmetry; the presence of a "rib hump" when the child bends over (**Figure 23**); pelvic obliquity as a result of a short leg syndrome, muscular contractures, or habit (**Figure 24**) (further described in the section on *leg length discrepancy*); neurological findings—including reflexes, motor strength and skills, and sensory; hip range of motion for any congenital hip dysplasias.[7]

Radiographic evaluation is equally important in the evaluation of a scoliotic condition.[2,8] This should be performed by a radiologist in conjunction with an orthopedist trained in the treatment of this disorder (**Figure 25**).

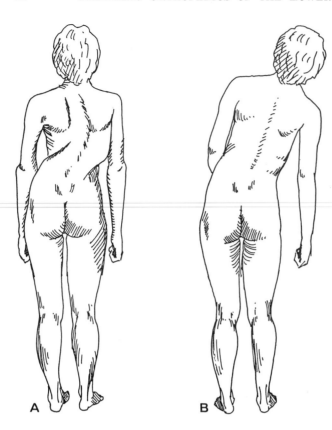

Figure 22

(A) *Flexible curve prior to stretching toward the convex side of the curve.* (B) *Reduction of the curve with bending toward the convex side of the curve.*

Treatment

It has been determined by most authors treating scoliosis of all types that only two methods of treatment are effective: the Milwaukee brace with exercises and surgical realignment.[1,7,8,9] Most agree that exercises alone will never improve a scoliotic curve and should be avoided as a sole method of treatment. Congenital scoliosis proves to be one of the more difficult types to treat although promising advances are forthcoming. Limb length discrepancies should be treated according to the cause when feasible. This will be discussed in further detail under the section *Limb Length Discrepancies*.

Limb Length Discrepancy

Length differences in the legs, either actual or apparent, will greatly affect the structural attitude and function of the entire limb including the foot, ankle, lower leg, knees, femur, hip, and lower spine. Compensatory changes are evident with any form of length difference. These changes may involve collapse in the foot structure, rotation at the knee joint, pelvic obliquity, and sacral tilting and rotation. Degenerative changes may eventually occur at these levels

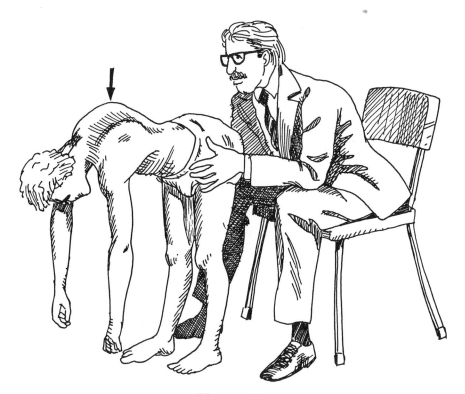

Figure 23

Examination for a "rib hump."

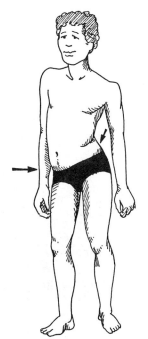

Figure 24

Pelvic obliquity secondary to either a limb length difference, muscular contractures, or habit.

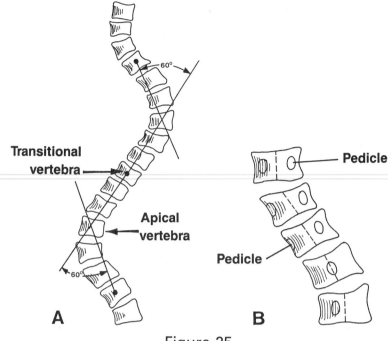

Figure 25

(A) This is the Risser–Ferguson method for measuring curvatures. This method employs using a small dot in the center of the upper and lower end vertebrae of the curves and one dot in the center of the apical vertebrae. Lines are then drawn from dot to dot and the angle formed measured. (B) The pedicles can provide a determination for the amount of rotation present with scoliosis. This is viewed from an AP x-ray. The absence of one pedicle and the position of the viewed pedicle will allow one to qualitatively determine the degree of rotation. Adapted from an original painting by Frank H. Netter, M.D., from Clinical Symposia, © *CIBA Pharmaceutical Company, Division of CIBA-GEIGY Corporation. With permission.*

as a result of the pathomechanics and disalignment. Care must be taken to accurately determine the presence of a length discrepancy and appropriately treat the condition when indicated.

Etiology

Several causes for a limb shortage have been offered and determined. These may include: a congenital hip dislocation; fractures of the femur or tibia; injury to the epiphysis from trauma, infection (osteomyelitis), or from unknown causes as in Legg-Calvé-Perthes disease; slipped capital femoral epiphysis; retardation or overgrowth in epiphyseal development as a result of genetics etc.; neuromuscular disorders causing paralysis and resulting diminished epiphyseal growth; spasm or contractures in the lower back musculature causing an elevation in the pelvis resulting in an apparent shortage; and scoliosis resulting in the elevation of one side of the pelvis.[1-8]

Clinical Evaluation

-functny

A child should be examined for both an apparent or actual (true) limb shortage. It is best to determine first whether any scoliotic condition is present. This was described thoroughly under the previous section on scoliosis. The child should be examined when standing with the feet together. The symmetry of the gluteal creases, popliteal fossae, pelvic heights, and shoulder position is beneficial in determining any discernible changes. Have the child walk and note any dropping down of the pelvis or shoulders on either side. This can possibly be indicative of a limb shortage. View the architecture of both feet while the child is standing. Very often there will be a unilateral collapse in the foot structure of a longer limb. If so, further examination for a limb length discrepancy is in order.

To determine whether an apparent or a true leg length discrepancy is present, one must employ two methods of measurements. To determine an actual (true) limb difference, place the person supine on a table with the legs together and parallel. Measure from the anterior superior iliac spine to the medial malleolus on each side by using a tape measure (**Figure 26**). Be careful not to let clothing or skin slippage affect your measurements. If you use the undersurface of the anterior superior iliac spine for the placement of the one end of the tape measure, and you mark the most medial aspect of the maleolus with an X or a dot, then your measurement should be reasonably accurate. If a discrepancy in the distance measured from left to right occurs, then an actual (true) limb shortage exists.

An apparent limb shortage resulting from muscular contractures and pelvic obliquity must be determined by measuring from the umbilicus to the medial malleoli (**Figure 26B**). If a measurable difference is determined, then one may assume a functional shortage is occurring.

The combination of both actual and apparent measurements must be performed to determine if either or both conditions may be existing. The use of a tape measure does allow for a reasonable amount of inaccuracy, though it is still a valuable tool in an initial evaluation. Radiographic studies by the use of orthoradiography or teloradiography are advantageous in locating the exact area of discrepancy (**Figure 27**). Since 60–65% of growth in a limb occurs at the knee area, with 15–20% at the distal tibia, the most likely area of any true disparity will be the epiphyses at the knee joint. Measurements less than $\frac{1}{2}$ inch should not be evaluated radiographically, due to the exposure, unless the difference has been progressing and treatment would be warranted in the immediate future. Radiologic studies should not be an exercise with no real purpose for a final result or treatment.

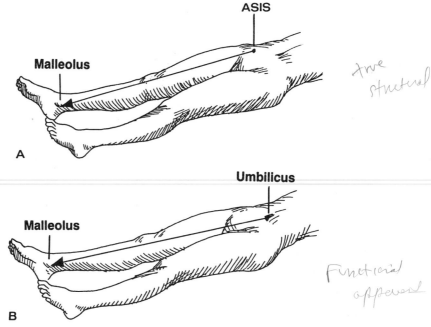

true
structural

Functional
apparent

Figure 26

(A) Measurement is taken from the anterior superior iliac
spine (ASIS) to the medial malleolus. Care must be taken to
avoid the interference of clothing in the actual measurement.
Unilateral deformities such as genu valgum or genu varum
may affect the length measured and should be accounted for
in your evaluation. (B) Measurement is taken from the umbilicus to the medial malleolus for both legs. The pelvic area
should also be observed for obliquity. This will provide information to determine a functional (apparent) shortage.

see
Salter
p. 58

Treatment

Treating a leg length difference requires a proper determination of the
cause and the progressiveness of the deformity. Assuming the length difference
is reasonably constant and a true structural disparity exists less than ½ inch,
then conservative lift therapy is indicated. This can be accomplished by the
use of an orthotic device adding no more than ¼–⅜ inch lift to the heel area. If
a lift greater than ⅜ inch is required, then the additional amount should be
added to the shoe itself. One will find many times a difficulty in seating even
a ¼ inch lift on an orthosis in a shoe. The patient or parents must be encouraged
to buy shoes with an adequate heel-counter height to accommodate for this
rise.

Lift therapy on a shoe without adequate structural control of the foot may,
in most cases, produce secondary changes in the foot and limb. It therefore is
recommended that proper orthotic control of both feet in addition to the lift

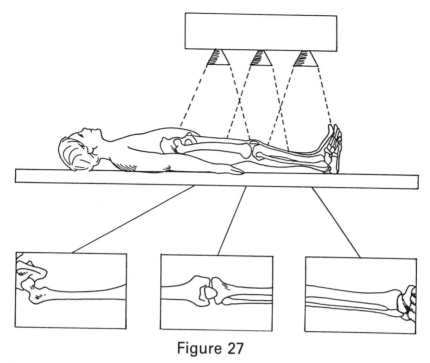

Figure 27

Orthoradiography allows the limb to be sectioned for accurate bony measurement. Using the measured information for each limb and each bony section of the limb, an accurate amount of discrepancy with the exact bony segment(s) involved can be provided.

be used. Care must be taken to add a lift to the shorter limb only in those cases of structural differences in the limb. An apparent (functional) limb difference resulting from a lumbar scoliosis, muscular contractures, or spasm in the spine area may require lifting the longer limb and/or stretching the musculature to reduce the pelvic raising (**Figure 28**). This can be determined by your clinical examination and weight-bearing orthoradiograms. It therefore behooves the examiner to properly evaluate the exact cause before instituting any form of lift therapy. Indiscriminate application of a lift may actually produce pain as well as detrimental effects to the superstructures.

If a limb difference exceeds $\frac{1}{2}$ inch and/or is progressing, then a consideration for a surgical intervention may be suggested. Several methods have been offered to correct a difference including: epiphysidesis or epiphyseal arrest of the longer limb at an appropriate age to balance the length difference; shortening of the longer limb (i.e., femur or tibia) to equalize the shorter limb and usually performed after epiphyseal closure; or lengthening of the shorter limb by slide osteotomies or bone grafting.[2,3,7] This last method has more inherent difficulties and therefore carries a poorer overall prognosis.

Consultation with an experienced surgeon who has performed this procedure is mandatory.

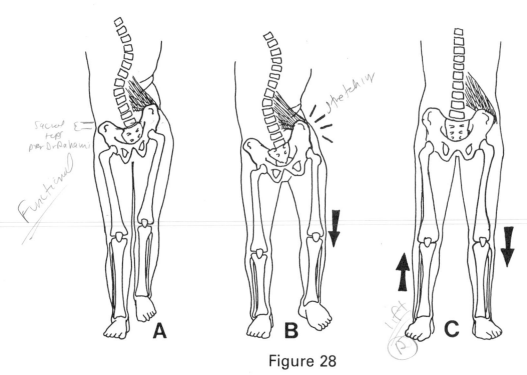

Figure 28

(A) *Short leg syndrome secondary to contractures in the musculature of the lower back attached to the pelvis. (B) If the leg is attempted to be brought to the ground, there will result a stretching of the contracted musculature. Note—If a lift was used on this shorter side, it would not allow the musculature to stretch and achieve a more normal state. (C) A lift should be employed on the longer side to force the pelvis on this side upward therefore causing greater stretching on the opposite side and a straightening of the spine's curvature.*

Because the effects of even a small degree of limb difference may result in knee derangements, hip disorders, and low back syndromes, particularly in the active or athletic person, immediate attention is warranted. It therefore is the duty of the practitioner to recognize this condition and either treat it appropriately or refer the patient to someone who can balance the difference properly.

References

Scoliosis:
1. Blount, W.P., Bolinski, J.: Physical therapy in the nonsurgical treatment of scoliosis. *J. Am. Phys. Therapy Assoc.*, 1967.
2. Hagen, D.P.: A continuing roentgenographic study of rural school children over a 15 year period. *J. Am. Osteopathic Assoc.*, 63: February 1964.

3. Herring, J.A.: Rapidly progressive scoliosis in multiple epiphyseal dysplasia. *J. Bone & Joint Surg.,* 58-A: July, 1976.
4. Jones, C.L.: The damaging effects of a disaligned musculoskeletal system. *J.A.P.A.,* 61: October 1971.
5. Keim, H.A.: Scoliosis. *Clinical Symposia.* Volume 24, Number 1, 1972.
6. Kostuik, J.P., Bentivoglio, J.: The incidence of low back pain in adult scoliosis. *Spine,* 6: 1981.
7. Scott, J.C., Morgan, T.H.: Natural history and prognosis of infantile idiopathic scoliosis. *J. Bone & Joint Surg.,* 37-B:, 1955.
8. Tachdjian, M.O.: *Pediatric Orthopedics.* W.B. Saunders Co., Philadelphia, 1972.
9. Tax, H.R.: *Podopediatrics.* Williams and Wilkins, Baltimore, 1980.

Limb Length Discrepancy:

1. Jones, C.L.: The damaging effects of a disaligned musculoskeletal system. *J.A.P.A.,* 61: October 1971.
2. Langer, S.: Structural leg shortage. *J.A.P.A.,* 66: January 1976.
3. Okun, S., Morgan, J.W., Burns, M.: Limb length discrepancy. *J.A.P.A.,* 72: December 1982.
4. Sanner, W.H., Page, J.C., Tolbot, H.R., Blake, R., Box, C.A.: A study of ankle joint height changes with subtalar joint motion. *J.A.P.A.,* 71: March 1981.
5. Sgarlato, T.E.: *A Compendium of Podiatric Biomechanics.* California College of Podiatric Medicine, San Francisco, 1971.
6. Subotnick, S.I.: The short leg syndrome. *J.A.P.A.,* 66: September 1976.
7. Tachdjian, M.O.: *Pediatric Orthopedics.* W.B. Saunders Co., Philadelphia, 1972.
8. Tax, H.R.: *Podopediatrics.* Williams and Wilkins, Baltimore, 1980.

ADULT   ontogeny   CHILD
                                                     [BIRTH]

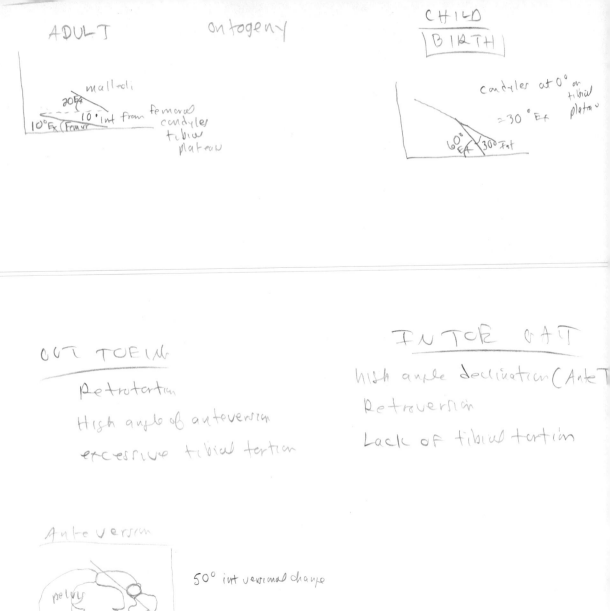

malleoli
20° EF
10° Ex (Femur   10° int from femoral
                 condyles
                 tibial
                 plateau

condyles at 0° or
tibial
            =30° Ex plateau
60°
 EX   30° Fat

OUT TOEING   INTOE GAIT

Retrotortion   high angle declination (Ante T

High angle of anteversion   Retroversion

excessive tibial tortion   Lack of tibial tortion

Anteversion

pelvis

60°
   Exten

50° int versional change

10°
 Ex

Chapter 4

EXAMINATION OF THE HIP

When examining the hips of children, there are many aspects to be considered. Determination of any local deformities in the bony structure and musculature is of importance. The examiner must be reminded that oftentimes metabolic, infectious, or genetic factors may be the true etiology of the presenting complaint. All children with a rotational abnormality should be examined for pathological conditions such as cerebral palsy, myelodysplasia, diastematomyelia, or the subtle beginning of a neurological problem such as Charcot–Marie–Tooth disease. The child who has asymmetric findings or a history of progression is particularly suspect, as these are not characteristic of the usual rotational problems.[21,49] The scope of this chapter is primarily directed toward the basic orthopedic abnormalities frequently encountered in a podiatric or general practice. Therefore, many of the more infrequently encountered disorders will not be discussed. The reader is referred to other more detailed orthopedic textbooks for reviews of the systemic manifestations in the hip in addition to infectious, genetic, and traumatic disorders.

Antetorsion Versus Retrotorsion

In the femur bone there exists a certain degree of torque or rotation. This is determined by the relationship of the head and neck of the femur with the axis of the femoral condyles. As has been described in Dorland's dictionary, *torsion* is an actual twist in whatever it is being related to.[13] Therefore in the femur, torsion means the twisting of the bone itself. Unfortunately, much confusion has been created in the discussion of torsion of the femur. Most orthopedic literature uses the terms *torsion* and *version* synonymously. *Version* has been defined by Dorland as a change in direction.[13] Podiatric literature has differentiated these two terms. The term *torsion* has been accepted to mean a twist or torque in the femur bone and *version* to mean any soft tissue contracture(s) or alterations at the hip. This has produced a great deal of confusion to the student and practitioner in reading both the podiatric and orthopedic

47

articles relative to the hip positioning. An attempt will be made in this text to clarify the terms and to present some continuity of ideas regarding this area.

Antetorsion, as will be defined in this text, is the rotation anteriorly of the head and neck of the femur to the transcondylar axis of the femur relative to the frontal plane. If the femoral head is allowed to be seated in the acetabulum with the greater trochanter positioned most laterally, the transcondylar axis would then be rotated internally in antetorsion (See **Figure 29**).

At birth the antetorsional rotation angle is between 25–40°.[5,27,45,49] This is measured by determining the relationship of the bisection of the head and neck of the femur with a line paralleling the femoral condyles, i.e., transcondylar axis. A measurable angular value is viewed from a proximal–distal or distal–proximal relationship (See **Figure 30A**). The average angulation at birth is between 30–35°. As the child develops, the rotation or twist appears to decrease steadily in the femur. At one year of age, there is a decrease to approximately 25–30°. By age five, 20–25° is the average value, and at the age of 15 years 10–15° is the most frequent torsional angle found. This value of 10–15° is the average adult torsion as well[5,27,45,49] (**Figure 30B**).

Retrotorsion will produce the opposite effect of antetorsion. If the femoral condyles are placed on the frontal plane, a line bisecting the head and neck of the femur is either parallel or posterior to the transcondylar axis (**Figure 31**). By placing the femoral head in the acetabulum with the greater trochanter

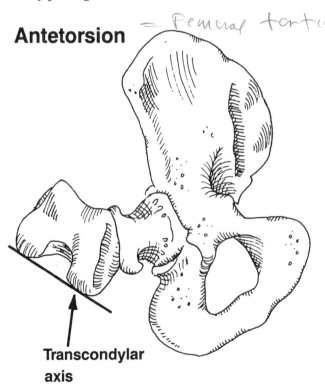

Antetorsion   = Femoral tortion

Transcondylar axis

Figure 29

The head of the femur is seated in the acetabulum with the greater trochanter being most lateral. This is the position assumed with weight-bearing. Note the internal position of the transcondylar axis as a result of antetorsion.

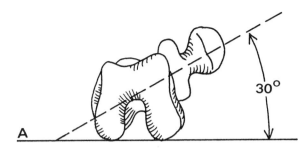

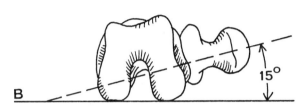

Figure 30   Antetorsion.

(A) The dashed line is passing through and bisecting the head and neck of the femur. A solid line is paralleling the transcondylar axis of the distal femur. The resulting angular value of 30° in this example is average for a newborn. (B) The angular value of 15° represents the average adult torsion in the femur.

= Fem Torsion
AKA
Angle of Declination

Oleg says 10° adult

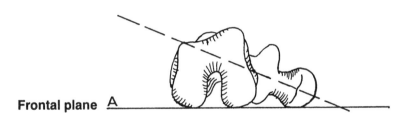

Frontal plane A

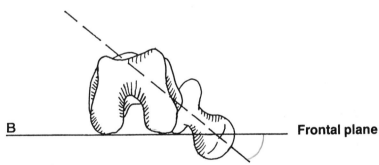

B   **Frontal plane**

Figure 31   Retrotorsion.

(A) The dashed line is bisecting the head and neck of the femur with the solid line paralleling the transcondylar axis of the femur. This example represents a moderate angular relation and should therefore be considered retrotorsion. (B) This example shows a significant angular retrotorsion, which always is considered abnormal.

= Too much change
angle < 10° ex
so now
condyles ex
to FP

positioned most laterally, the transcondylar axis will be externally rotated (**Figure 32**).

As has been shown, the result of torsion within the femur bone will produce an internal or external position of the leg either at rest and/or during ambulation. Of concern is any antetorsional values greater than 35° at birth or the persistence of this torsion beyond the norms expected for a specific age level. An in-toeing gait abnormality will result from this abnormal torsion. Conversely, retrotorsion will produce an out-toeing gait abnormality and is always considered abnormal. The degree of angulation will determine the necessity for concern or correction.[10,21,28,33,36,46]

Clinical Evaluation

To determine the presence of femoral torsion clinically, the utilization of hip range of motion is necessary. Ranges of motion at the hip joint are directly affected not only by the bony attitude but by the ligamentous and muscular influences surrounding this joint. When an examination of this area is undertaken, the inclusion and exclusion of the bony and soft tissue components are necessary to localize the etiological factor(s). The effects of the soft tissue structures on the hip and femoral position will be discussed further in this chapter under the section *Anteversion–Retroversion*.

When one is examining for a true femoral torsional deformity, the hip position should be such that all soft tissue components are reasonably negated. This is accomplished by placing the hip in a flexed position. The child should

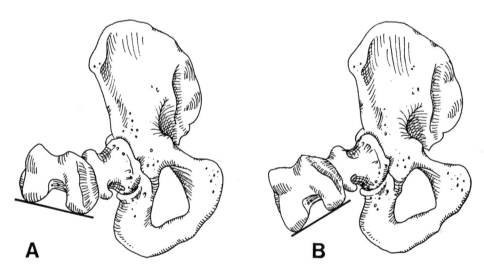

A   **B**

Figure 32

(A) *This diagram represents a normal adult femoral antetorsion when the head of the femur is seated properly in the acetabulum. (B) In this example of retrotorsion the femur is viewed seated in the acetabulum. Note the external position of the transcondylar axis.*

be sitting at the edge of a table with the knees bent at 90° and the hips flexed at 90°. This position will allow ranges of motion to be properly analyzed without the influence of the muscular and ligamentous structures (**Figure 33**). Before actually measuring the ranges of motion, it must be decided which method of measurement will be utilized. Appreciating that many devices and apparatus have been developed and marketed to calculate the amount of motion, with all producing their own inherent errors, this author would like to suggest a more simplified technique to establish the basic data necessary. It is certainly realized that the sophisticated instruments are capable of giving more exacting calculations for research purposes; however, clinically an error of 5–10° on examination would not alter or change the normal course of treatment.[18,21,28,33,35,44,45,53]

This author's proposed method is to have the child seated as in **Figure 33** with the knees flexed over the table. Allow the lower leg to dangle freely straight down. This will reflect a position of zero degrees, or our starting point. Now using the lower leg as a measuring arm, internally and externally rotate the hip joint. The leg is rotated outward or away from the sagittal plane, representing internal rotation at the hip. Inward rotation of the leg produces external rotation of the hip joint. The calculated degree of rotation can be calibrated visually by employing an imaginary protractor behind the lower leg (**Figure 34**). Caution must be maintained to not raise the pelvis off the table. This would produce added motion not representative of the hip joint. To avoid this common error, place your hand across the thigh at the pelvic–thigh juncture and feel for any lifting when measuring the range of motion.

The calculated values of motion should be documented and charted. With

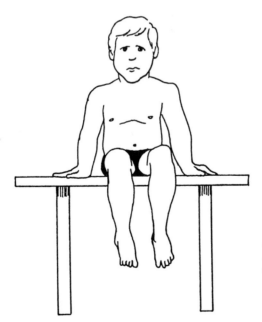

Figure 33

For a proper examination of the hip, have the child seated at the edge of your examination table with the knees and hips flexed. This will relax most all of the soft-tissue structures surrounding the hip joint.

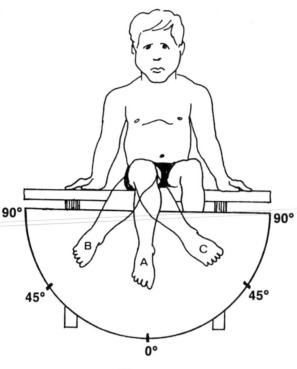

Figure 34

Imagining a protractor present behind the leg to be examined is helpful in determining the actual ranges of motion. Point A represents the starting position and 0° of motion. Point B is with the leg externally positioned but the femur is actually rotating internally at the acetabulum. Point C is showing the leg positioned internally; however, the femur in this case is externally rotated at the acetabulum. Note: Point B is showing 45° of internal rotation at the hip and Point C is showing 45° of external rotation at the hip with the use of the imaginary protractor. Do not become confused with the direction of the lower leg; it is actually positioned in the opposite direction of the femoral rotation.

a little experience in this method of measuring, one can be accurate to within 5–10° of any sophisticated instrument. It is known that the naked eye can discern angular values in increments of between 5–10°, therefore allowing us this ability for measurement.

If the values for internal and external motion are within the broad ranges of normal (described further in this section), then an assumption can be made that no abnormal femoral torsion exists. However, if a unilateral femoral torsional abnormality exists, then a discrepancy in the total range of motion on the affected side would be discernible compared to the opposite side. The range of motion would be excessive in the direction in which the abnormality existed (i.e., greater internal rotation than normal with antetorsion).

Of caution is the bilateral and symmetrical abnormal torsional deformity of the femur. In this situation it becomes imperative that norm values for ranges of motion, both internal and external, be known and the age levels they present be reviewed to determine this bilateral deformity.

Hip Range of Motion

At birth the internal range of motion of the hip in a flexed position is approximately 35–100° with an average of 60°. External range of motion is found to be between 45–110° with an average of approximately 90°. By the time a child reaches the age of 1½–3 years, this range of motion will change. Internal motion will be equal to or greater than the external rotation.[45,49] Before continuing with the natural history of hip motion, let us analyze the present status and cause for the range of motion that exist from birth to age 3. It has been proposed by several authors that the existence of greater external hip motion at birth with the diminution to equality or greater internal motion by age 3 lies in the acetabular position.[8,45,49] When a child begins weight-bearing there, it is felt that the tri-radiate cartilage has a tendency to place the acetabular socket more centrally. Badgley has stated that "adaptive changes of the limb bud from horizontal to vertical, i.e., medial of the axis of the limb, are not complete at birth." He feels that some degree of retention of the fetal position of external rotation is seen commonly after birth.[3] This relative posterior position of the acetabulum places the head–neck-shaft of the femur in a more externally aligned attitude in relationship to the pelvis and frontal plane of the body (**Figure 35**). Internal rotation of the femoral head is limited only to the same degree as would exist if the socket were on the frontal plane. This results in the neutral position being placed more external due to the posterior acetabular position. As a child begins to grow and develop and weight-bearing is initiated, then the pelvic–acetabular–femoral position will alter itself. The acetabulum will align itself on the frontal plane causing the relative range of motion to increase internally comparable to the early nonweight-bearing stage of development. The antetorsion angle will allow an internal positioning of the femur with the femoral head in its neutral position in the acetabulum. With the reduction of the external position of the acetabular–pelvic relationship, there results a greater range of motion internally. For this reason, children in the age level of 1½–3 years present a greater internal motion at the hip in a flexed position. This acetabular–pelvic relationship has been referred to in some of the literature as a *version* deformity.[45] It, however, actually appears to be more of a bony alignment and developmental variant than a true versional abnoramlity as defined in this text.

Now, to continue with the development of the child, the degree of anteversion will progressively decrease reaching adult values between the ages of 8–12 years. Equal internal and external range of motion at the hip is then to be expected. The adult value for antetorsion is between 5–15°. When antetorsion is considered as a singular and an independent entity without any other factors interfering, the range of motion at the hip will be slightly greater internally. This would be considered normal. One must, however, take into account the soft-tissue structures surrounding the hip joint. Though the flexed position of the hip allows the muscular and ligamentous structures to be negated, the actual capsule may present with enough of a variant to affect the joint slightly. Therefore, this aspect cannot be totally eliminated from the picture and should be considered as an effect on the range of motion in cases of equal hip range of motion or a slightly greater external motion.

In addition to the range of motion test, an adjunctive test to help substantiate the degree of femoral torsion has been proposed by Ryder.[41] This

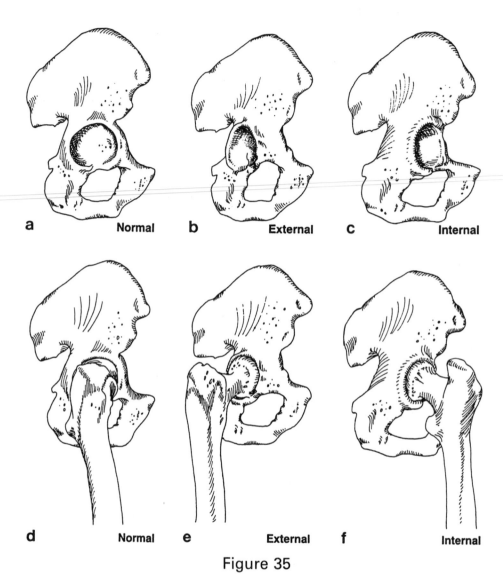

Figure 35

(A) *This lateral view of the pelvis represents a normal acetabular position. The socket is on the frontal plane.* (B) *In this example the acetabular socket is externally positioned to the frontal plane and a commonly found position in infants prior to weight-bearing.* (C) *If an internally positioned acetabular socket exists, it is always considered abnormal and will cause internal rotation of the femur.* (D) *This diagram represents the position of the femur when it is seated in the acetabulum on the frontal plane.* (E) *is the position of the femur with an external acetabular socket, while* (F) *is the position of the femur with an internal acetabular socket.*

maneuver attempts to determine more exactly the actual femoral torsion by clinical means. To perform this test, first place the child at the edge of a table with the knees flexed 90° and the hips extended as shown in **Figure 36**. (This test can also be performed with the hips flexed if desired.) Using the lower leg as the measuring arm, the examiner should imagine a protractor present behind the lower leg (**Figure 37**). Place only the *tips* of your fingers at a point midway between the lateral aspect of the hip region. Apply some finger tip pressure at this lateral position and with the other hand rotate the lower leg internally and externally (**Figure 37**). This rotation will place the head of the femur through its total range of motion in the acetabulum. Under the finger tips should be felt the prominence of the greater trochanter of the femur as it moves from an internal to an external position. To calibrate the degree of torsion, simply find the position in which the most prominent aspect of the greater trochanter is felt most laterally below the finger tips (**Figure 38**). Using the imaginary protractor, estimate the number of degrees of torsion present (**Figure 37**). If one were to find the lower leg externally positioned (with the femur internally rotated), then an antetorsion component is existing. Conversely, if an internal position of the lower leg was found with the femur externally rotated, then retrotorsion would be present (**Figure 39**).

Ryder's test offers many advantages including: substantiation of the presence of antetorsion or retrotorsion; a means to measure consistently the degree of bone torsion and replication for further development and evaluation; and elimination of soft tissue interference around the hip joint. One word of caution: to exclusively use either the total range of motion test or Ryder's test to evaluate a rotational abnormality in the hip is dangerous. Both tests should be performed together using the Ryder's test as a supportive examination for the findings from the total range of motion test. When a discrepancy is found, then both tests should be performed again possibly at another examination time or by another examiner.

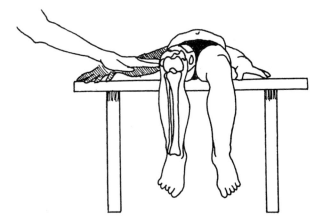

Figure 36

Ryder's test is performed with the child's knees flexed over the edge of the examination table and the examiner's hand placed most laterally and midway between the upper and lower aspects of the hip region. The fingertips should only be used as shown in this diagram.

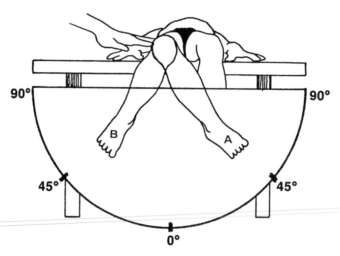

Figure 37

In Ryder's test, the examiner should place one hand at the lateral aspect of the hip region and with the other hand rotate the lower leg through a range of internal and external motion. (A) represents external rotation of the femur and (B) internal rotation. When the examiner feels the greater trochanter directly under his fingertips (most laterally positioned), then an approximate degree of torsion can be determined by calibrating the position of the leg against the imaginary protractor.

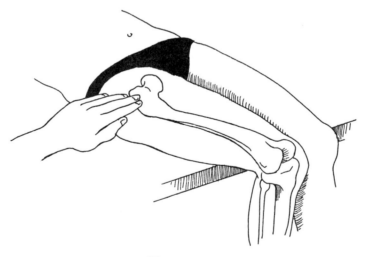

Figure 38

This diagram represents the position of the fingertips as they are feeling the greater trochanter most laterally placed. The head of the femur in this position is seated totally in the acetabulum and assumes the approximate position of weight-bearing.

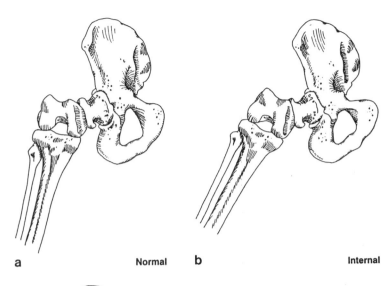

a   **Normal**   b   **Internal**

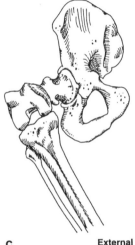

Figure 39

(A) *This sketch represents the head of the femur seated in the acetabulum with a normal adult antetorsion angle of approximately 15°. Note that the position of the lower leg is away from the vertical axis of the pelvis representing the internal rotation of femur with antetorsion. (B) With a high antetorsion angle, a greater internal rotation of the femur will be produced and therefore a greater external position of the lower leg from the axis of the pelvis. (C) Retrotorsion will produce the opposite effect with the femur externally rotated and the leg positioned toward the axis of the pelvis.*

c   **External**

Radiographic Evaluation

In the examination for a femoral torsional abnormality, it is sometimes necessary to incorporate a radiological interpretation as a supportive adjunct to the clinical evaluation. This diagnostic tool is frequently left for the more severe deformities, which may need significant attention. Many techniques for the radiographic determination of a torsional deformity in the hip have been proposed; this author feels that the Ryder and Crane method seems to offer one of the better approaches.[5,23,27,41] This method employs the use of two radiologic projections of the pelvic area to determine an angular value.

The first view is an anteroposterior radiograph of the pelvis. This view will provide the ability to determine the angle of inclination of the femoral head–neck-shaft (**Figure 40**). To expose this view, have the patient lie supine with the hips fully extended and in an assumed neutral position. The x-ray film is then placed under the buttocks and the femur properly positioned with the femoral condyles placed parallel with the table top. The film can now be exposed (**Figure 41**).

The second roentgenogram to be exposed is an oblique–axial view of the femur. To position for this view, flex the hips and knees to 90°. It is then necessary to utilize an apparatus which was developed by Ryder and Crane to place the thighs in a position of 30° of abduction (**Figure 42**). This apparatus has a radiopaque bar which is to parallel the transcondylar axis of the femur. The x-ray plate is placed beneath the buttocks and the exposure is taken vertically with the central ray positioned midway between the hips.

This oblique projection will produce a certain degree of distortion of the true femoral torsion angle; this error is proportional to the degree of true torsion and the angle of inclination. For the determination of true femoral torsion, the use of a triginometric formula is necessary. To avoid the mathe-

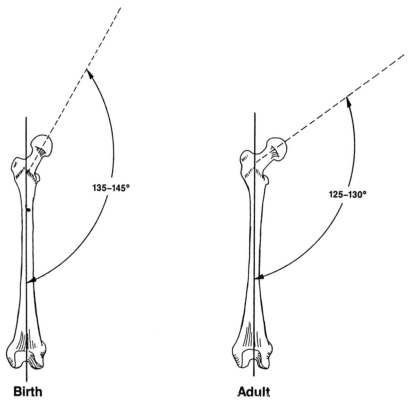

Birth   **Adult**

Figure 40

The angle of inclination of the femoral head–neck-shaft is measured by bisecting the head–neck and bisecting the shaft. The angle formed is referred to as the angle of inclination.

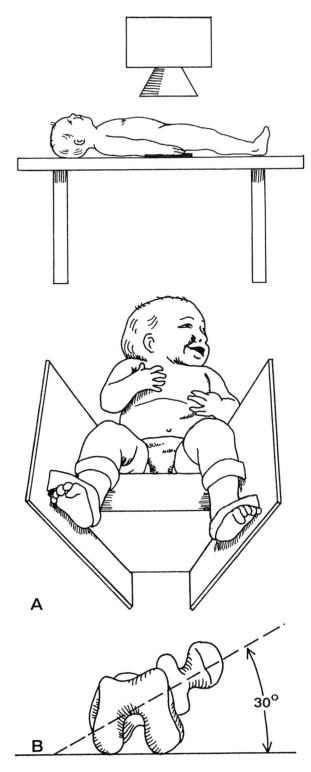

Figure 41

The x-ray film cassette should be placed under the hips and a direct anterior–posterior view is exposed for a proper determination of the angle of inclination of the femur.

Figure 42

(A) This apparatus maintains the thighs in 30° of abduction and has a radiopaque bar paralleling the transcondylar axis. An anterior–posterior radiographic view is taken with the central ray positioned midway between the hips. (B) One can measure from this oblique-AP view the femoral torsional angle by drawing a line bisecting the head–neck and one paralleling the transcondylar axis. This angle is plotted on Table 3 along with the angle of inclination to determine the true femoral torsion angle.

matical calculations, Ryder and Crane have compiled a chart with the calculations compiled (Table 3). Plot the two angular values determined from the two radiographs and read the actual angular value of femoral torsion on the chart. One must be cognizant of the fact that children prior to 6 months of age do not have the presence of a capital femoral epiphysis. It therefore becomes next to impossible to locate an accurate axis for the femoral head–neck region. It is best to wait until the child becomes old enough to allow proper radiographic evaluation.

There are other methods for radiographic interpretation, including fluoroscopy.[49] The author would urge you to review the techniques and methods if this is an area of interest.

Treatment

Because torsional deformities are intrinsic to the bone, and inheritance and ontogeny directly affect the outcome, treatment must be tailored appropriately. It has been stated that the actual structural changes in the bone are the result of the effects of inheritance and will thus resist most external means of treatment.[10,21,30,49,50] Commonly agreed are that many of the treatments proposed for true femoral torsion deformities are directed toward appeasing the parents' concerns rather than truly affecting the bony structure. Over the course of time in which a treatment program is being utilized, the child is also maturing and developing, allowing his normal ontogenic development of the bone to occur. It becomes very difficult for one to assess whether the treatment plan instituted has actually helped and reduced the deformity. The torsional correction may be the result of normal ontogeny. If one were to accept this theory, one would be forced to be extremely selective in proposing any serious treatment program without allowing sufficient time for normal maturation. A child who is injuring himself due to a severe abnormal gait (i.e., unable to negotiate stairs or unable to participate in activities with his peers) should be treated objectively and with serious considerations. On the other hand, if a child is presenting with only a femoral torsion abnormality and is not being hampered in the activities in which he is participating, then treatment should be delayed initially. The parents should be counseled as to the probability of a reduction in the deformity with maturation.

More than 90% of cases with a history of spontaneous correction in other members of the family can be expected to reduce.[46,54] Periodic reevaluation of the problem (approximately every 6–12 months) should be encouraged to determine a regression or progression of the condition. Where there is no significant improvement over a period of 2–5 years, or progression of the deformity is noted, appropriate treatment is necessary and should be encouraged.

The use of bars, splints, twister cables, casts, and the like has little value in the alteration of the actual torque in the femur bone. These means will, however, alter the joint position by changing the balance of the soft tissue and muscular function. This must be cautioned when these treatment methods are

TABLE 3

(from Ryder, C.T. and Crane, L.: Measuring Femoral Anteversion—The Problem and a Method (41))

True angle of femoral torsion

Projected femoral torsion angle

Angle of inclination	0	5	10	15	20	25	30	35	40	45	50	55	60	65	70	75	80	85	90
80	0	3	7	12	16	20	24	29	33	38	43	47	53	59	65	71	77	84	
90	0	4	9	13	17	22	27	31	36	41	46	51	56	62	67	73	79	84	
95	0	5	9	14	18	23	28	32	37	43	47	52	58	63	68	74	79	85	90
100	0	5	10	14	19	24	29	34	39	44	49	54	59	64	69	74	80	85	90
105	0	5	10	15	20	25	30	35	40	45	50	55	60	65	70	75	80	85	90
110	0	5	10	16	21	26	31	36	41	46	51	56	61	66	71	76	80	85	90
115	0	5	11	16	22	27	32	38	43	48	53	57	62	67	72	76	81	85	90
120	0	6	11	17	23	28	34	39	44	49	54	59	63	68	72	77	81	86	90
125	0	6	12	18	24	30	35	41	46	51	56	60	65	69	73	78	82	86	90
130	0	6	13	19	25	31	37	42	47	52	57	62	66	70	74	78	82	86	90
135	0	7	14	20	27	33	38	44	48	54	58	63	67	71	75	79	83	86	90
140	0	7	14	21	28	34	40	46	50	56	60	64	68	72	76	80	83	87	90
145	0	8	16	23	30	36	42	48	53	58	62	66	70	74	77	80	84	87	90
150	0	9	17	25	32	39	45	50	55	60	64	68	72	75	78	81	84	87	90
155	0	10	19	27	35	42	48	54	58	63	67	70	73	77	79	82	85	87	90
160	0	11	22	31	39	46	52	58	62	65	70	73	76	78	81	83	86	88	90
165	0	13	26	36	45	52	57	62	66	70	73	76	78	80	82	84	86	88	90
170	0	18	33	45	53	60	65	69	72	75	77	79	81	83	84	86	87	89	90
175	0	29	48	59	67	71	75	77	79	81	82	84	85	86	87	88	88	89	90
180	0	90	90	90	90	90	90	90	90	90	90	90	90	90	90	90	90	90	90

299

employed. The soft tissue changes can produce serious alterations in function with no real effect on the actual bony deformity. If these treatment devices are inappropriately instituted, they may produce certain deleterious effects not only in the hip joint but also in the knees, legs, and feet. These effects can include: using an excessively wide bar or night splint that will force the hip joint into an abnormal and external rotation; external or internal rotation at the leg producing excessive medial or lateral stresses on the knees, ankles, and feet; medial or lateral knee instability due to the shift in the center of gravity more medially or laterally in the leg; and collapse in the joint structure of the foot and ankles resulting from redirection of the gravitation forces more medially or laterally in the foot and leg. These ill effects encourage one to use extreme care when instituting a treatment program for a femoral torsion deformity. This author feels that it is ludicrous to believe that any treatment device previously mentioned has any significant effect on the femur bone structure and can be supported by the research of Moreland, discussed in Chapter 6 on *Tibio-fibular torsion*.

In an objective review of this condition, it appears that the only type of treatment that will be beneficial and yet conservative is one tailored to protect the limb and foot from secondary changes while the deformity is correcting through its own ontogeny. In-shoe orthotic devices have proven to be beneficial in stopping the compensatory changes that will oftentimes result in the foot and ankle as well as the leg and knees from this type of rotational deformity. The orthotic devices do not alter or change the structural entity in the femur bone; rather, it prevents the adverse effects from the torsional abnormality. If cosmesis is desired in addition to protection, then an out-toeing or in-toeing orthotic device will produce a more acceptable and straighter walking pattern, as well as maintaining the joint congruity in the leg and foot. Orthotic control will allow for ontogeny to progress without altering the soft tissue and joint position. This is not the case with bars, splints, casts, or cables.

On the rare occasion when a child's abnormal torsion deformity persists after a fair period of observation, then surgical correction should be contemplated. Surgery should be considered when the torsion deformity coincides with a significant gait abnormality and/or compensatory changes, and is best considered when the child is at an appropriate age in consultation with a pediatric orthopedist.

Anteversion–Retroversion

In the previous discussion of *Antetorsion–Retrotorsion,* the term *version* was defined as a "change in direction."[13] This is in contradistinction to the "bone twisting" or torsion that had been described previously. A versional component, as described in this text, is actually a positional change in direction secondary to soft-tissue structures surrounding the hip joint. The hip joint is a ball-in-socket joint that allows a large potential range of motion of the whole lower extremity both internally and externally. This degree of motion can alter the actual long axis of the limb and foot in its relationship to the transverse plane. The motion in the hip can be affected by: the shape, direction, and depth of the acetabulum; the capsule and ligaments of the hip; the muscular attachments of the hip; the long muscles that traverse the hip and knee joint attaching further down on the limb; the position of the thigh in reference to the trunk; and abnormalities of the caudal spine may influence the rotation of the thigh.

Described previously were the effects of the position of the acetabulum on the relative hip positioning (**Figure 35**). In some of the literature this entity has been categorized under the heading of *version*.

The acetabular position affects the motion at the hip and is directly related to the attitude of the triradiate cartilage which composes the acetabular socket. In the process of development, there will result a relative position of this socket with the frontal plane of the body. At birth there is a position of a posterior and abducted attitude relative to the frontal plane[45] (**Figure 35**). This position would be referred to as *retroversion*. When the head of the femur is seated in the acetabulum, the limb will be in an external position. Conversely, if the acetabular position was located anterior to the frontal plane, then an internal rotation of the limb would result when placed in neutral position. This would be called *anteversion*. Anteversion, when referring to acetabular position, is a rarity.

The acetabular positioning becomes negligible after a child begins to stand and walk. Standing, as described by Pitkow, provides a stimuli for an infant to internally rotate his hips and thus bring the greater trochanters of the femur into a relatively mid-lateral position.[37] This author feels that the weight-bearing stimuli will forcibly position the acetabular socket most laterally out of necessity for the weight stress to fall into a functionally aligned attitude and position. As a result of this change in the acetabular positioning, the external position and rotation at the hip will decrease proportionately to the degree of realignment of the acetabular socket. It has been stated by Badgley et al. that the intrauterine position of an infant is such that the hips are usually held in a flexed and externally rotated position along with the existence of an acetabular position. This attitude will allow contractures of the soft tissues to develop around the hip joint.[3] Coon et al. have stated that the iliopsoas muscle may be the muscle most often affected to produce an internal positioning. With contractures of this muscle, a limitation in internal rotation would exist.[8]

Once an infant becomes more mobile, these contractions will reduce to the demands needed for proper weight stress in the limbs. A factor that could lead to the continuation of an externally positioned hip would be an abnormal sleeping position. This would result secondarily to the original contractures. In these cases the infant may be either sleeping on his stomach with his legs rotated inwardly or outwardly, or on his back with an external rotation of the limbs. This positioning would continue to promote a preexisting soft-tissue versional deformity. Other factors that should be included in the promotion of a version abnormality are: poor sitting habits, a dislocated hip either partial or total, muscular imbalance, or spasticity. The depth of the acetabular socket will also affect the range of motion. The lips of the acetabulum will cause an abutment with the margins of the femoral neck and can limit the availability of motion.

When development reaches a stage at which the acetabular position no longer is affecting the hip rotation, then the concept of a versional deformity rests in the musculature and/or ligaments surrounding the hip joint. Anatomically there exist ten muscles that function to produce external rotation at the hip joint. Internal rotation is accomplished by only four muscles. Additively the ischiofemoral ligament affects rotation about the hip by limiting internal (medial) rotation while the iliofemoral and pubofemoral ligaments limit external (lateral) rotation. They will only limit motion to the point of their own tension and/or laxity (Table 4).

The existence of an imbalance in the total number of muscles performing the internal and external rotations at the hip may be a cause for a deformity. External rotation would take precedence if the musculature was the only factor affecting the joint position. Pitkow has stated that "external rotation contractures present in infants decrease with growth and are less than 5% present in children over 18–20 months."[37] This can account for the fact that most in-

TABLE 4
Muscles Concerned in Rotation of the Hip Joint

Movement	Muscle
Lateral Rotation	Gluteus maximus
	Obturator internus and gemelli
	Obturator externus
	Quadratus femoris
	Piriformis
	Sartorius
	Adductor magnus
	Adductor longus
	Adductor brevis
Medial Rotation	Iliopsoas
	Tensor Fascia Latae
	Gluteus Medius
	Glueteus Minimus

Int Rot (handwritten annotation next to Medial Rotation)

Ligaments Affecting Rotation of the Hip Joint

Movement	Ligament(s)
Limiting Lateral Rotation	Iliofemoral Pubofemoral
Limiting Medial Rotation	Ischiofemoral

toeing problems existing from an abnormality at the hip (antetorsion) may *not* be recognized or exist until sometime after the age of two years. Combining the aforementioned contractures with acetabular positioning (which does reduce by 1–1½ years), an apparent in-toeing deformity may be obscure until this age level is reached.

Therefore, we now may define retroversion as a condition that will produce an external rotation position around the hip joint when the hip is in an extended posture. This will result from either a posterior positioning of the acetabular socket and/or contractures of the musculature and/or ligaments about the hip. Conversely, anteversion will result in an opposite effect causing an internal rotation position at the hip. Contractures in the musculature and/or ligaments will limit external rotation at the hip joint (Table 4).

On rare occasions the acetabular socket may be anteriorly displaced in its relationship to the frontal plane. This would result in a limitation of external rotation. If existent, this will usually reduce by age one year and not affect the walking child.

Note: Realizing the confusion and difficulty in trying to remember which of these components cause which deformity I recommend that the following be memorized:

- Antetorsion—bone twisting—internal
- Anteversion—soft tissue or acetabular position—internal
- Retrotorsion—bone twisting—external
- Retroversion—soft tissue or acetabular position—external

Clinical Examination

To examine for the presence of a versional deformity in the hip, employ the same maneuvers and procedures as had been described under the section *Clinical Examination—Antetorsion–Retrotorsion* (**Figure 33 and 34**). It becomes paramount that this examination be performed with the hips both flexed and extended with the knees flexed (**Figure 43**). Once numerical values are determined for internal and external range of motion with the hips both flexed and extended, then a determination can be arrived at for a versional (soft-tissue) deformity. The two positions (hips flexed and extended) allow for proper evaluation of the hip range of motion when the hip ligaments and soft tissue are both under tension (hip extended) and relaxed (hip flexed). If on examination one were to find a greater range of motion internally when the hips were flexed than when extended, this could be conclusive of a posterior musculature, soft tissue, and/or ischiofemoral ligament contracture limiting the internal rotation around the hip when extended. Conversely, if the range had greater external motion with the hip in a flexed position opposed to an extended position, an assumption could be made that contractures in the anterior soft tissue and musculature of the hip including the pubofemoral and iliofemoral ligaments were the contributing cause.

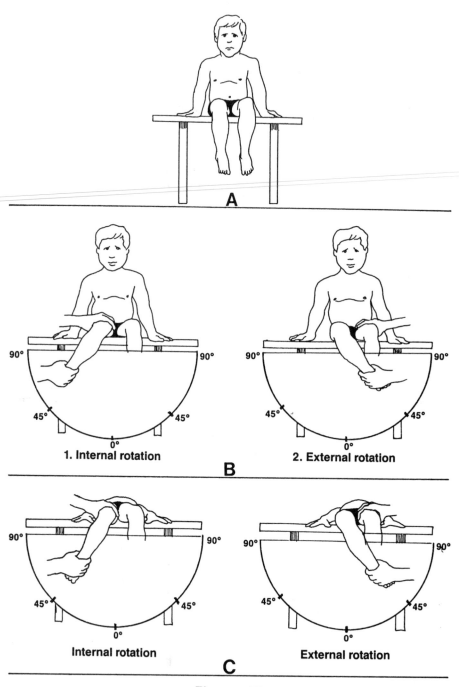

Figure 43

Example: internal range of motion—hip flexed—90°
external range of motion—hip flexed—100°
internal range of motion—hip extended—30°
external range of motion—hip extended—90°

This example exhibits a probable contracture of the posterior musculature and soft tissue including the ischiofemoral ligament. These contractures would produce a limitation in the amount of internal range of motion when the hips are in an extended attitude (retroversion).

A determination must also be made as to the effects of the hamstring muscles on the hip ranges of motion. This is best accomplished by evaluating the total ranges of motion at the hip joint with the knee joints in both a flexed and extended position while the hip is fully flexed. To calculate the total amount of rotation available, use the patellae as a guide to approximate the amount of internal and external motion. The employment of an instrument such as a goniometer can be helpful in this situation. A comparison is made as to whether the knee when flexed or extended had altered the amount of the excursion of the hip joint. Any significant difference in motion between the knee flexed-knee extended attitude, with the hips flexed, would support a muscular involvement of the long muscles of the thigh contributing to an altered joint motion at the hip (Table 5). For example, contracture of the internal rotator muscles of the leg could limit the ability of the thigh to externally rotate at the hip when the knee is in an extended position. Therefore, it becomes obvious that an evaluation for the presence of these contractures is of importance. Failure to include this in your examination would or could easily cause you to arrive at an erroneous or partial conclusion as to the total cause for an abnormal gait.

To conclude, it is important that one examine a child to determine the range of motion with the hips both flexed and extended, and with the knees both flexed and extended, as previously described. This allows proper determination of both ligamentous and muscular involvement and also allows one to differentiate between these two contributing factors. Radiographs will not be any additional help in evaluation of these soft-tissue deformities. They would be helpful for any suspicious bony abnormalities.

Figure 43 (opposite): (A) Position the child so that he is seated over the edge of the examining table with hips flexed and knees flexed. This should be the beginning position for an examination. (B) Place the hip through its range of motion being careful not to go beyond the actual range of motion of the hip. This can be best determined by placing a hand on the same thigh for internal rotation and the opposite thigh for external rotation and feeling when the thigh begins lifting up or off the table. Any range beyond this first lifting up is motion in the lower spine and opposite hip and does not represent the true hip motion. (C) After examining the motion with the hips flexed, have the child lie down extending the hips but with the knees continuing to be flexed. Place the hip through its range of motion and calibrate the total internal and external motion. Note that the examiner's hand is placed on the thighs as in Figure 43 (B) to determine the end range of motion.

TABLE 5
Muscles Affecting Rotation of the Femur on the Tibia

Movement	Muscle
Lateral rotation of the femur on the tibia	Popliteus Semitendinosus Semimembranosus Sartorius Gracilis
Medial rotation of the femur on the tibia	Biceps femoris

Treatment

To attempt to treat soft-tissue contractures of the hip–thigh complex, a program must be developed to attack the specific area(s) involved. In cases where the ligamentous and muscular structures are the sole causative factor, a stretching program for these tissues is necessary. Authors have suggested the use of such devices as twister cables or a Brachman Skate during daily activities for dynamic stretching and a night splint through the sleeping periods for passive stretching.[18,30,33,35,44,49,50] This author would first like to note that twister cables (see **Figure 45**), while doing a fine job of stretching the soft-tissue structure of the hip, will also produce a significant valgus force on the foot and medial stretching of the knee joint during the swing phase of gait. The valgus force will inadvertently cause a stretching of the ligamentous and muscular insertions on the medial aspect of the foot, resulting in a secondary flatfoot deformity. Precautions must certainly be taken to avoid any types of secondary complications when treating a hip abnormality so as not to sacrifice one problem for another. The best approach to avoid these complications is not to use twister cables or to use orthotic control in the shoes when cables or a dynamic walking splint is employed. Type C heel stabilizers work best. Always remember that producing one deformity to compensate or falsely correct another will eventually result in some degree of harm to the child.

Another area to investigate and treat is the sleeping position that these children assume. Sleep comprises approximately one-half to two-thirds of an infant's or young child's life. Positioning during this time can significantly alter a child's structural being and/or sustain an abnormal attitude. Children sleeping with their legs turned inwardly or outwardly or tucked under their chest will require treatment to discourage these positions (**Figure 44**). The use of night splints or bars is extremely beneficial. The more common ones used are the Denise–Browne splint, Fillauer bar, Brachman skate, and the Ganley splint (**Figure 45**). An inexpensive but effective means is to tie the shoes together through the heel area and have the child sleep with them on. This will not allow the legs to rotate abnormally in any one direction. The

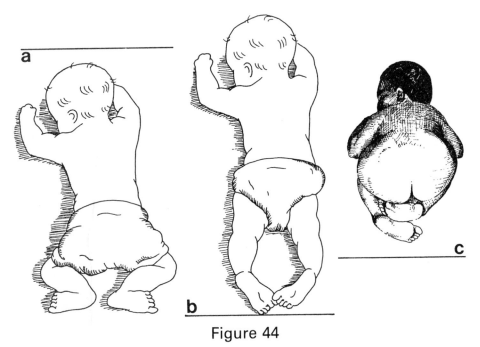

Figure 44

(A) Child sleeping on its stomach with the feet and legs externally rotated. This position will continue to promote any external contractures at the hip if existing. (B) This position will promote or continue to maintain any internal contractures around the hip. This position is not as harmful as (C). (C) A child sleeping on its stomach with the hips flexed, knees flexed, and legs and feet rotated inward will provide changes not only at the hip but at the knees and feet.

bars and night splints also provide effective treatment in the rotation and stretching of the soft-tissue structures of the hip if the child sleeps with the legs and hips in a fully extended attitude. If, however, the extended hip–knee position is not maintained, then this treatment during sleep periods will not produce the proper forces at the level of the hip. If the parents have the child sleep on his back, an extended position at the hips and knees will be achieved, allowing for active stretching to occur at the hip.

A manipulative stretching program can also be instituted by the parents for a small child or infant, and this can be performed 20–30 times each diaper change, holding each time for approximately 10 seconds. To stretch the ischiofemoral ligament and external rotators of the hip, have the parents rotate the legs internally while the hip is in an extended position and the knees are extended (**Figure 46A**). Ask the parents to hold this position with some degree of force for the 10-second period and then release. Remind the parents that the child will probably cry when this is performed but tell them not to become alarmed. If the deformity is due to tight pubofemoral and iliofemoral ligaments and internal rotators of the hip, then an opposite exercise and maneuver should be used, as in **Figure 46B**.

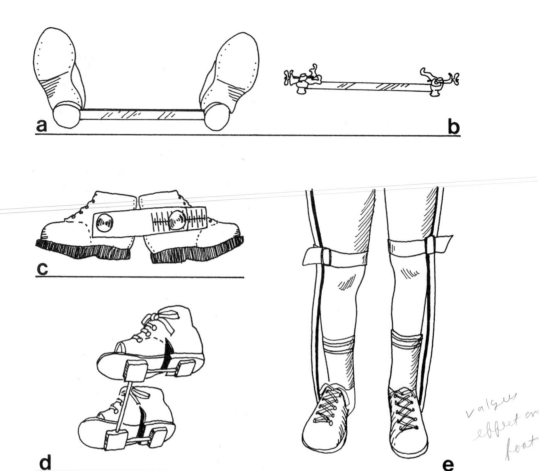

valgus effect on foot

Figure 45

(A) Brachman Skate. *Dynamic splint that can be used both during ambulation and sleep. Somewhat cumbersome for a normal active child.* (B) Fillauer Bar. *There are several types, but the ones with clamps offer the best convenience. This can be removed from the shoes during activities and reattached when the child naps. Probably the most diverse splint and the most widely used.* (C) Counter Splint. *This attaches to the shoe and has several disadvantages: it cannot be removed; it can only correct for internal contractures by turning the feet outward; it cannot independently stretch one side without affecting the other.* (D) Ganley Splint. *Offers an excellent ability to splint independent abnormalities in the foot and maintain good leg position as well. Can only be used during nonambulation and is fixed to the shoes. It does not offer the same degree of independent control of the legs and hips as a Fillauer bar.* (E) Twister cables *are strapped onto the legs with an attachment to the shoes. The amount of tension placed on the cables will affect the degree of external rotational force applied. The torque force is being applied primarily at the distal end (shoe) in dynamic function.*

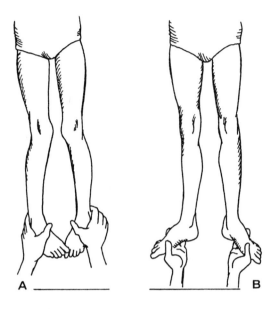

Figure 46

(A) *With the hips fully extended and the legs straight, one can rotate the limbs inward and hold for the count of 10 seconds. This should be performed 20–30 times on the affected limb(s) after each diaper change. This maneuver is performed in cases of a retroversion deformity. (B) Rotating the limbs externally for 10 seconds 20–30 times per diaper change will stretch an antetorsion deformity. Note: These stretching exercises should be coordinated with a night splint to give 24-hour therapy to the deformity.*

If the child is old enough, allow him to sit in the "television position" to stretch the tight posterior structures and the "indian position" for stretching the anterior structures (**Figure 47**). A child using the "television position" with the thighs rotated inwardly or "indian position" with external rotation will usually find this an uncomfortable position at first, but with continued stretching this becomes more acceptable.

If tautness in the hamstring muscles is found to be a contributing cause

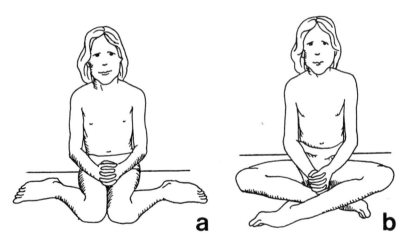

Figure 47

(A) *"Television position" to stretch a retroversion deformity. This position should be avoided and discouraged in children with an anteversion deformity. (B) "Indian position" is used to stretch an anteversion deformity, to be discouraged in a retroversion abnormality.*

for a medial or internal pull of the limb, then stretching is also indicated. Stretching can be accomplished by placing the knees in a fully extended position and raising the leg to resistance at the hip (**Figure 48**). This should be held for approximately 10 seconds and released, and should be performed 30–40 times per day.

When manipulation cannot be employed or followed by the parents, there are manufacturers who supply various types of thigh–calf-leg splints that function in a similar way. A plaster splint can be fabricated to perform a similar task (**Figure 49**). All of these devices will help to maintain a proper position, although they do tend to be cumbersome and awkward.

The key to accomplishing a good result with a treatment program for these types of deformities is to reevaluate the child constantly. Often, the only purpose of the visit is to encourage the parents and reassure them that the treatment is helping. At certain times it may be necessary to change your treatment plan to accommodate the development of the child or the environment in which it is to be used. Continue to stress to the parents that the need for avoidance of improper sitting and sleeping positions is extremely important to accomplish a rapid and proper result.

When dealing with an ambulatory child, it may be necessary to employ an orthotic device to preserve the normal foot structure. Orthotics in themselves do not change the structure of the hip; however, they will prevent compensatory changes from the abnormal stresses imposed on the foot from the rotational abnormality causing abnormal gravitational forces. Additionally, the orthosis may stimulate an inward or outward walking pattern when using, for example, the *gait plate* or the in-toeing or out-toeing heel stabilizer.

With internal rotatory abnormalities, a type D heel stabilizer or a reverse Robert's gait plate can be beneficial in stimulating an outward walking pattern

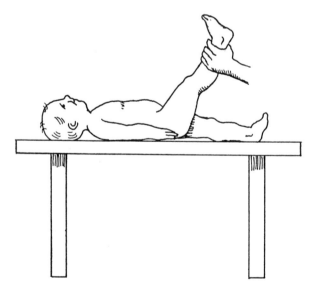

Figure 48

To stretch contractures in the hamstrings, have the child lie flat on the table and raise the affected limb upward with the knee fully extended. Some degree of force must be applied to provide adequate stretch on the muscles.

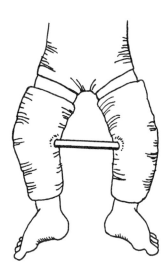

Figure 49

A plaster thigh splint can be constructed by: applying a cylinder leg cast to each leg; rotating the legs either inwardly or outwardly as determined by the deformity; fixing a bar to each cast; splitting the cast; showing the parents how to apply the splint by using an ace wrap to keep it in place.

while still maintaining and protecting the foot structure. The type B, C, or E heel stabilizers and the Whitman, Roberts, or Whitman–Roberts plates are of value in treating the out-toeing child (see Chapter 13). An out-toeing child will have a greater propensity toward an early flatfoot deformity as a result of the medial shift of the center of gravity in the foot (**Figure 50**). Therefore, the maintenance of a good structural position of the joints of the foot is needed by the use of an orthotic device. It is this author's feelings that devices other than those mentioned have little benefit or a place in the treatment of young

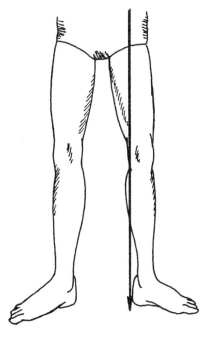

Figure 50

Medial shift of the center of gravity through a limb and foot from an out-toeing deformity will cause considerable stress on the medial joint structures. This can result in a valgus force on the knee and a collapse in the medial ankle and foot structure.

children. Such devices as functional orthoses should be left for the much older child or adolescent when development has reached a level of stability and the ranges of motion in the foot have lessened.

A functional type of orthosis does not provide the proper control and support needed to maintain the laxity found in young children's feet. A device is needed to encompass the foot rigidly enough not to allow further stretching of the ligamentous and musculature structure secondary to any superstructural abnormalities.

Shoe wedging and modifications have proven to be ineffectual in the treatment of these types of rotational abnormalities. They therefore should not be considered in your armamentarium of treatment.

Finally, it must be clearly understood by those employing orthotic therapy for rotational deformities in the hip that their use is solely for protection of the foot. They may provide a more acceptable gait pattern; however, they do not directly affect the causative factor(s). They do not have a direct effect on the hip structures.

In cases where there is existing a spasticity of the musculature surrounding the hip and a resulting rotational abnormality, a surgical intervention may be necessary to alter the resting state of the muscle if stretching was ineffectual. Most frequently, however, soft-tissue contractures causing rotational abnormalities can be treated conservatively and resolved to an acceptable degree.

Hip Disease

There are numerous conditions that may affect the function and development of the hip joint. This section will review several conditions that are more frequently found in a general practice. Included will be congenital dislocations of the hip, pelvic obliquity, osteochondrosis of the hip (Legg–Calvé–Perthes disease), and coxa vara deformity.

Congenital Dysplasia of the Hip

A classification formulated by Haas has been found to be extremely suitable for the discussion of hip dislocation although this author has modified it somewhat[20]:

Classification of Hip Disease

I—Typical
Subluxation
Dislocation
Nondysplastic (dislocatable)

II—Atypical
  Teratologic
    arthrogryposis, etc.
    defective limb bud
III—Isolated cases of unknown etiology
  Traumatic (obstetrical)
  Congenital syphilis
  Little's disease
  Roentgen injury
  Myelodysplasias

Under the classification *typical* hip dysplasia, we find that either the condition of dislocation, partial dislocation, or dislocation may exist primarily at birth. Much speculation and theorization are provided for an etiological explanation in the production of these conditions. There is a known correlation between breech presentations at delivery and a truly dislocated hip. There is felt that the forces imposed with this delivery will cause adduction of the limbs and allow slippage of the femoral head out of the shallowed acetabular socket. This can only occur in the presence of adequate laxity in the joint soft tissues. Another correlative finding for a dislocation is instances in which parents wrap an infant tightly in blankets, forcing the limbs and hip area into a rigid extended attitude. It must be remembered that at birth an infant will present with flexural contractures at the hips and knees secondary to intrauterine positioning. Any degree of force exerted toward the extension position will have the potential to force the femoral head from the acetabular socket. This requires the existence of a predisposing condition as in laxity of the joint tissues. Several authors have agreed that of the many etiologies offered, the single most common factor in causing a dislocation of the hip is premature weight-bearing.[2,3,6,7,17,49,52] Here again, if a predisposing condition exists (joint laxity, shallow acetabular socket, etc.) then any early weight-bearing stress could force the joint out of alignment. The nondysplastic (dislocatable) hip provides an ability for dislocation but is not dislocated at birth. In the case of a subluxed hip, the head of the femur is lying on the rim of the acetabulum and is only partially displaced out of the socket. This hip condition is certainly much closer to a complete dislocation than the nondysplastic type. In each of these cases of the nondysplastic or subluxed hip, careful scrutiny is necessary to detect their presence as they can allude the casual examiner.

The *atypical* hip dysplasia, also referred to as teratologic, will exist in utero and presents with a complete dislocation of the hip joint prior to birth. This type is found in conjunction with other disorders as arthrogryposis multiplex congenita, spina bifida, and myelomeningocele. There are a multitude of disorders that may be associated with a defective limb bud secondary to a genetic predisposition. These disorders will affect the hip structure and position. Radiographically, a malformation of the pelvic area will demonstrate the teratologic abnormalities.

The incidence of hip dislocation is approximately 2 per 1,000 live births in the United States. Other countries have statistics ranging from less than 1/1,000 to as much as 20/1,000 live births. There also exists a prevalence rate of 20% for the right hip and 55% for the left hip. The frequency of both hips is about 25%.[38-40] The statistically higher percentage of incidence of the left hip to the right is being attributed to intrauterine position. The left hip lies posterior and adjacent to the spinal prominence, causing the left hip to lie in an adducted state, thus provoking dislocation. Other noted frequency factors include: greater prevalence in the Caucasian population opposed to Blacks and Chinese; females comprise 65% of the occurrence; and there is between 15–35% incidence in breech and Caesarean section delivery.[3,7,17,20,35,49] The incidence in female breech births is 1 in 35 live births. These incidence factors must be taken into account by the examiner when evaluating newborn infants. A predisposing condition of significant importance in the consideration of a propensity toward dislocation is the presence of generalized ligamentous laxity. The examiner will view hyperextension in the knees, elbows, wrists, fingers, ankles, and feet. The presence of this excessive mobility in these joint areas should arouse significant suspicion of the potential for dislocation or subluxation of the hip joint.

Ramsey has stated that true genetic inheritance seems to only affect 22% of the children presenting with hip dislocations.[39,40] Therefore, other factors must be contributing to the greater incidence of this disorder. Never neglect to view disorders of the feet as signs of hip disease. Jacobs has found that the presence of metatarsus adductus and clubfeet were present in 10–15% of cases presenting with hip dysplasia.[24] Careful evaluation for hip disease in these children presenting with these foot conditions is essential in preventing and avoiding any further hip disorders.

Examination for Hip Dysplasia

When proceeding to examine an infant or child for a hip dysplasia, remember that several factors must be considered. The most important factor is the practitioner's knowledge of what chronological age will elicit a response to a particular sign or test and whether it is considered normal or abnormal. All too commonly we see an examiner report that a specific sign was absent on examination of a 6-month-old infant and the child is therefore considered normal. If the examiner had known that the particular sign reported cannot be elicited positive after 1–2 months, then he would not have been able to have reported a normal finding. A proper history surrounding the birth and postnatal period is extremely necessary prior to any examination. An example of a history that could almost conclude a positive diagnosis for a hip dysplasia may be, "My baby girl was a breech delivery and she seems to not want us to spread her legs apart when we diaper her." The obvious circumstances surrounding this history would be the predilection of the breech delivery and the fact of being a female. We know the incidence rate for a hip dislocation to be

1 in 35 births with this combination. The limitation in abduction is supportive of a more conclusive history. (This will be discussed under *Clinical Examination*.)

This author would caution every examiner to be cognizant that no one sign or test is necessarily conclusive for a hip dysplasia. These signs and tests are meant to alert the practitioner to the potential of its presence. Radiographic examination of the hip is the best conclusive test to confirm any suspicions.

Clinical Examination

Infants, from newborn to 3 months old, will exhibit several signs and produce a number of positive tests supporting a potential for a hip disorder or the presence of a true disorder. As a child matures beyond this age, many of these tests and signs will no longer be discernible or producible.

Limited Hip Abduction Test

A sign frequently used in infant screening for hip dislocation is the *limited hip abduction* test. This test, if positive, will present with an inability for adequate abduction of the hips to occur. Infants are normally expected to abduct between 50–90° from the sagittal plane when performed while the child is on his back (**Figure 51**). If a limitation occurs from a possible hip dislocation, the motion will be less than 40–50° of abduction. This is considered a positive test. There are controversial arguments by some authors regarding the presence or absence of this sign. It has been stated that a hip may be dislocated and not necessarily be limited in its abduction in the early infancy period. This is supported by the fact that true soft-tissue contractures in these early age levels do not exist and therefore do not produce any limitation in the abductory range of motion.[40] To counter this statement, there must be a certain degree of limitation at the hip with it completely dislocated outside the acetabulum. In contradistinction, a dislocatable hip cannot be determined by this method nor the partially subluxed type. One must therefore keep in mind what stage and level of dislocation will provide positive signs or tests and which may not. This is a point supporting the need to exhibit several positive signs along with radiographic analysis to accurately diagnose this condition.

Asymmetry of the Gluteal Folds

In examining an infant for the presence of asymmetry of the folds of the thigh, be certain the anterior as well as the posterior areas of both thighs are examined. The examiner should observe any abnormal deepening of the folds on either side of the thighs and whether the folds differ in number and depth from one side to the other. With any noted difference, a suspicion of a dislocated hip is warranted and further examination required (**Figure 52**).

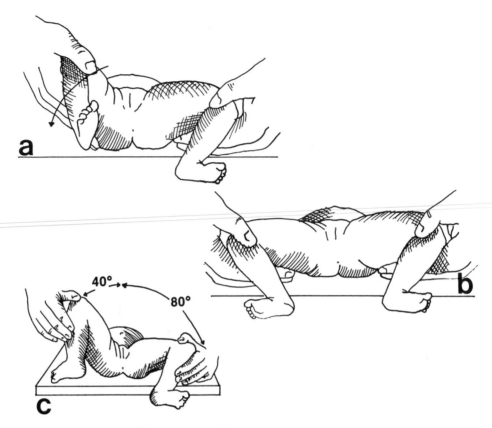

Figure 51   Hip abduction test.

(A) The right hip is being moved into abduction by bringing the femur and knee toward the table top. (B) The right hip is capable of being abducted to a parallel position in this normal child. (C) The left hip in this example is capable of normal abduction while the right hip is limited to only 40° of abduction. This limitation on the right side should warrant further evaluation due to a positive hip abduction test.

Galeazzi's or Allis's Sign

This sign is only discernible in a unilateral hip dislocation. Place the infant on his back and flex the knees and hip as shown in **Figure 53.** Make certain both feet are firmly placed flat on the examining surface. The examiner should view the heights of the knee joint surfaces and determine if any asymmetry exists. If one side is noted to be significantly lower than its counterpart, this is most often the hip with dislocation. This sign is only existent in a truly dislocated hip and will be absent in a dislocatable or mildly subluxed type.

In cases of bilateral dislocations, the knee height would be equal and therefore would not alert the examiner to the presence of a dislocation. In this instance, the examiner must rely on the other signs and tests to help support or reject his suspicions.

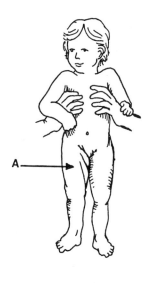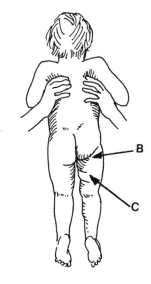

Figure 52 Asymmetric gluteal folds.

(A) Deepening and increased numbers of folds on the right side in comparison to the left reveals asymmetry. (B) An elevated gluteal fold and (C) increased folds in the posterior thigh on the right side are asymmetrical findings suspicious of a possible hip disorder.

Ortolani's Sign

This sign is often used interchangeably with Barlow's test. The two differ markedly in their results and conclusions and should therefore be used and referred to separately.

Ortolani's sign, when positive, demonstrates a truly *dislocated* hip. To elicit this sign, place the infant on his back with hips and knees flexed. Position your thumb at the medial aspect of the thigh with the tip of the thumb pushing into the inguinal area. Your other fingers should be grasping the outer aspect of the thigh at the level of the greater trochanter (**Figure 54**). To determine a positive test, abduct the thigh laterally with your thumb and fingers. Si-

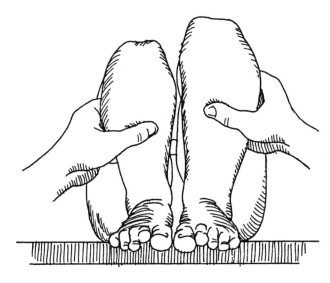

Figure 53   Galeazzi or Allis sign.

This test requires a supine position of the child with the feet firmly placed on the examination table. The height of the flexed knees will help in determining only a unilateral dislocated hip.

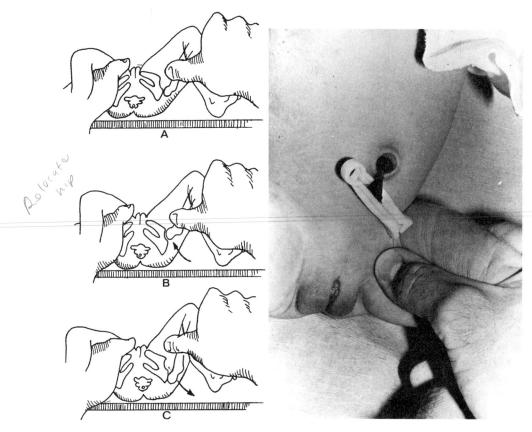

Figure 54   Ortolani's sign.

(A) Place your thumb into the inguinal region with your fingers grasping the outer aspect of the thigh. (B) Move the thigh into abduction while forcing the greater trochanter toward the midline of the body with your finger tips. This will force the head of the femur into the acetabulum and produce a possible "click" or "pop" or just a "giving away" in the hip. (C) Now move the thigh into adduction toward the midline of the body and with your thumb push laterally in the inguinal area. A redislocation of the hip will occur with a second "pop," "click," or "giving away" if the hip is truly dislocated.

multaneously with your finger tips force the greater trochanter toward the midline of the body. In cases of a disloaction, the head of the femur will "pop" back into the acetabulum when this maneuver is performed. Next, adduct the thigh toward the midline of the body. The femoral head will now slip out of the acetabular socket gliding over the posterior rim and another "click" or "pop" will be felt or heard if a dislocated hip does exist. One may either feel or truly hear a "click." More commonly there is felt a slight *giving away* sensation in this area. It is not necessary to actually hear a "click" or "pop" in order for this sign to be positive. If a noticeable sensation of abnormal movement in the joint is felt with both abduction and adduction, then further testing is necessary.

This sign can only be demonstrated in infants up to 4–8 weeks of age. Beyond this age there will exist contractures and adaptive changes that will not allow the relocation of the femoral head back into the acetabulum.

A note of caution: occasionally, an infant may present with an enlarged protruding ligamentum teres (**Figure 55**). If the Ortolani's maneuver or Barlow's test is performed, this ligament may produce a "clicking" sound. The "click" heard or felt occurs only once rather than twice as in a dislocated or dislocatable hip. Other tests and radiographic findings will also be negative with this condition.

Barlow's Test

This test is performed to determine whether a hip can be dislocated even though a normal attitude exists at the time of examination. A dislocatable hip differs markedly from the already dislocated type. This hip normally is in adequate structural position but may have existing a certain degree of capsular and ligamentous laxity. The hip can be dislocated with enough force imposed onto the joint as a result of the instability from the laxity.

To perform this test, place the child and your hands in a similar position as was described under *Ortolani's sign*. This test differs from that of Ortolani's in that an attempt is made to forcibly dislocate the hip joint rather than relocate the hip. This is accomplished by lateral pressure from the thumb with adduction of the thigh toward the midline of the body (**Figure 56**). If laxity does exist in the hip joint, the examiner will feel the femoral head slide out of the

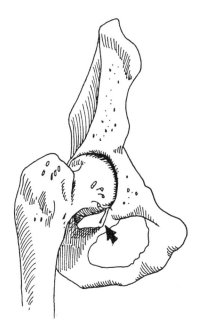

Figure 55

A protruding ligamentum teres may cause a "clicking" sound or sensation with hip abduction and adduction as a result of it snapping over the head of the femur. This is not a condition necessarily causing a hip dysplasia and will only produce one "click" or "pop" when both abduction and adduction of the hip are performed together.

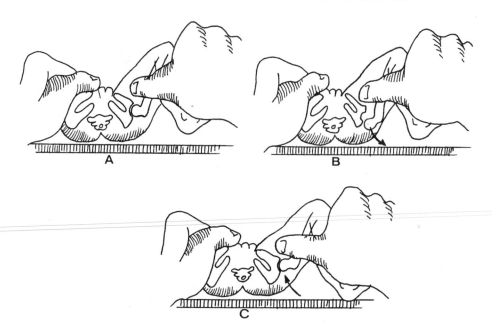

Figure 56   Barlow's test.

(A) The same hand position is used as with the Ortolani's sign; however, this maneuver is used to determine a potentially dislocatable hip, which at rest is in a normal position. (B) With adduction of the thigh toward the midline of the body and the thumb forcing laterally, the head of the femur will dislocate out of the acetabulum in a dislocatable-type hip disorder. A "click," "pop," or a "giving away" will be felt. (C) Abduction of the thigh with pressure of the finger tips over the greater trochanter will relocate the head of femur into the acetabulum and produce a "click," "pop," or "giving away." The hip is now back into a relocated normal position.

acetabulum. A kinesthetic sensation of giving away in the fingers will be noted and a possible audible "pop" or "click." Conversely, when the thigh is abducted, the femoral head will slip back into the acetabulum and will assume a normal joint attitude again.

This test differs from that of Ortolani's in that the hip is actually forced to dislocate in the Barlow test while the Ortolani Sign attempts to reduce the already dislocated hip.

With cases of subluxation of the hip joint, there is neither complete dislocation nor total acetabular seating. The femoral head in this case is seating itself somewhere on the rim of the acetabulum. A positive Barlow test could be elicited in this situation although the joint would not return to a normal position after reduction. This hip would need to be evaluated radiographically to confirm a partial dislocation (subluxation). As in the Ortolani's Sign, the Barlow test cannot be elicited after 4–8 weeks of age due to the soft-tissue contractures and adaptations that do occur.

Telescoping

This test is another that can be performed to help support the presence of a dislocated hip joint. A dislocated hip or an easily dislocatable hip will present with greater ranges of excursion upward and downward than is expected normally. Greater joint laxity will contribute to this. The maneuver is best performed by placing the infant on his back and flexing the knees and hips. Gently but forcibly push the thigh downward toward the table and then pull upward away from the table top (**Figure 57**). Perform this maneuver on both legs and compare the total range of excursion. In a dislocated or easily dislocatable hip, the excursion will be greater on the affected side. This results from the femoral head dislocating out of the joint posteriorly allowing greater downward motion, or being brought back into alignment with acetabular socket as in the case of the already dislocated hip. Equal ranges of excursion will be found on both sides of a bilateral dislocation and therefore give a false–negative result. The telescoping test cannot be elicited after 6–8 weeks of age due to adaptive and soft-tissue changes. *Note:* All the signs and tests described are capable of assisting the examiner to determine the presence of a dislocated or dislocatable hip. Each sign alone is not conclusive for a diagnosis; however, a collection of positive findings of two or more of the signs is more supportive. To finally support or deny a suspected hip dislocation, radiographic evaluation is necessary.

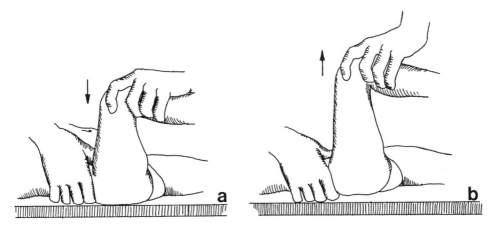

Figure 57   Telescoping.

(A) With the knee and hip flexed, force downward on the thigh and determine the degree of excursion. Compare this to the opposite side. A unilateral dislocatable or dislocated hip will produce greater motion than a normal hip. (B) After forcing downward as in (A) pull the thigh upward and determine the amount of movement. Again compare to the opposite limb for any discrepancy.

Radiographic Evaluation of the Hip

When interpreting radiographs for an infant suspected of a hip dislocation, many indices must be evaluated.

First, a truly dislocatable hip will appear normal radiographically. This is due to the hip only having the propensity toward dislocation without actually being dislocated. Fluoroscopic studies with the hip being maneuvered by Barlow's test will depict the dislocatable quality. This test should be used discretely due to the amount of radiation exposure to the infant. A subluxed or dislocated hip will provide positive radiographic signs discernible by the use of measurement to be described.

When evaluating infants radiographically, remember that the development of the capital femoral epiphysis perceived on x-ray is often delayed in a dislocated hip compared with the opposite normal side. Infants normally will present with the presence of the capital femoral epiphysis by age 3 months and approximately 50% will show its presence at birth.[6]

When interpreting radiographs for a hip dislocation, several indices are relied upon to conclude a diagnosis. Approximately 8–10 different measurements have been proposed for its determination; however, this author will describe four that usually provide adequate information to conclude a diagnosis. These four are: (1) Hilgenreiner's line (Y-line); (2) Perkin's line; (3) Shenton's line; and (4) Acetabular index. All four of these evaluations should be performed to finalize a diagnosis. Do not just accept one positive finding as conclusive.

Hilgenreiner's Line (Y-line)

This line is drawn through the clear areas in the depth of the acetabulum that represent the tri-radiate or "Y" cartilage (**Figure 58**). One then can meas-

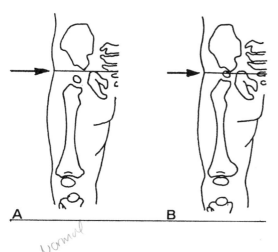

A   B

Figure 58

Hilgenreiner's line (Y line). (A) A Y-line is constructed through the clear area in the depth of the acetabulum. Note the capital femoral epiphysis lies below this line and a distance can be measured from the line to the epiphysis. This example is considered a normal relationship. (B) The capital femoral epiphysis is lying on the Y-line in this example and would be considered abnormal when compared to Figure 58 (A).

ure the distance from the highest point of the femoral neck to the "Y" line. A noted discrepancy in distance of one side to the other would force a suspicion of a dislocation. Unfortunately, this evaluation is only beneficial in a unilateral dislocation. Bilateral dislocations would reflect equal distances, though abnormal.

Perkin's Line

To construct this line, draw a vertical line through the outer edge of the acetabular rim. This will form quadrants with its intersection with Hilgenreiner's or "Y" line (**Figure 59A**). The capital femoral epiphysis needs to be present and should be found in the lower medial quadrant medial to the vertical *Perkin's line*. In cases of hip dislocation, the shallow cartilagenous acetabulum will push the spine-shaped rudimentary neck of the femur or the femoral head upward and/or lateral to Perkin's line (**Figure 59B**). If present this confirms a dislocated hip without the needed asymmetry found only with Hilgenreiner's line.

Shenton's Line

As viewed in **Figure 60A** this is an arc formed by the medial border of the neck of the femur and the superior border of the obturator foramen. In the case of a dislocated hip, there will exist an upward displacement of the femoral head causing the lower border of the neck to not complete the arc (**Figure 60B**). This line is sometimes difficult to evaluate in the newborn but is helpful and conclusive shortly thereafter.

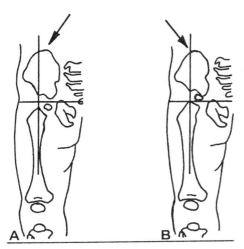

Figure 59   Perkin's line.

(A) A vertical line is drawn along the outer edge of the acetabular rim intersecting with Hilgenreiner's line (Y-line). The capital femoral epiphysis exists in the lower medial quadrant. This is a normal position. (B) The capital femoral epiphysis is located in the upper medial quadrant in this example. This is not normal and is indicative of a dislocated hip.

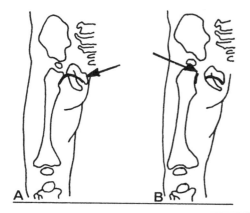

Figure 60   Shenton's line.

(A) Shenton's line is constructed by drawing a line along the superior border of the obturator foramen and continuing along the medial border of the neck of the femur. A normal hip would depict this as one continuous curved line. (B) A dislocated hip will not allow a continuous line to be constructed from the obturator foramen to the medial neck of the femur.

Acetabular Index

This is an angular value that should be calculated when evaluating the hip. To form the angle, first draw a line so that it passes along the ossified outline of the superior portion of the acetabulum. Continue this line until it joins with Hilgenreiner's line (Y-line) previously drawn. The angle formed is the acetabular index (**Figure 61**). The angle value is commonly found to be around 20° in a child 2 years of age. A value of 30° or more in the first year of life is an indicator that an abnormally insecure acetabulum is existing. An acetabular index in excess of 40° is indicative of a true dislocation.

Treatment

It seems to be the agreement and concensus of most authors that treatment of a hip dysplasia before three months of age will usually produce an excellent result. Therefore, the goal of any examiner is to be able to recognize this deformity early enough to institute conservative treatment. The longer the inability for reduction the greater the resulting chances for secondary complications. Children presenting with a hip dislocation or a dislocatable hip in the golden period of treatment prior to 3 months should be double or triple

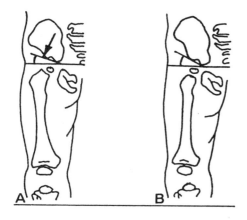

Figure 61   Acetabular index.

(A) A line is needed to be drawn along the superior portion of the acetabulum and intersection with Hilgenreiner's line (Y-line) to form the acetabular angle. A normal angle is usually 20° or less. (B) If the angle is greater than 30° in the first year of life, then an unstable acetabulum is suspected and values greater than 40° are considered a true dislocation.

diapered to maintain an abduction state in the hip area. In so doing there is an allowance for the soft-tissue structures surrounding the hip to contract and stabilize the femoral head into the acetabular socket. In more resistant conditions an abduction splint such as a Frejka pillow splint, polypropylene abduction splint or harnesses may be necessary to properly maintain position. There should be adequate reduction in the deformity both clinically and radiographically when using these splints. If reduction is still not possible after attempts with diapers or splints, then hip spica castings after closed reduction are warranted. Beyond the golden period of 3 months of age, splinting becomes less effectual and necessitates the use of either closed or open reduction with casting to maintain the alignment of the hip joint. This should be performed by a pediatric orthopedist trained in this area.

If a hip dislocation is left untreated, the child will eventually present with a Trendelenburg gait when walking is finally initiated. Often these children will walk later than chronologically expected. Their gait will be of a waddling type with a dropping on the side of the affected hip due to instability and weakness of the hip area (**Figure 62**). Of note is that a Trendelenburg gait

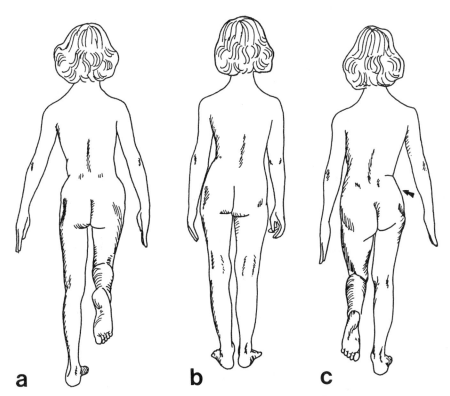

a　　　　　**b**　　　　　**c**

Figure 62　Trendelenburg gait.

(A) The left normal hip can maintain a level position when bearing weight unilaterally. (B) With both feet on the ground, there may be a slight dropping of the affected right hip but not as evident as when the child is asked to bear weight on the right side (C), showing an elevation of the pelvis due to the instability.

(also called a gluteus medius limp) may result from a neurological disorder such as polio and spina bifida, and therefore is not necessarily a pathognomonic sign of a hip dislocation. Also to be included in the production of a Trendelenburg gait are the muscular dystrophies, which weaken the musculature and result in this typical walking pattern.[2,3,6,7,11,17,20,24,29,33,34,38–40,49,50,52]

Congenital Pelvic Obliquity

This condition will mimic a unilateral congenital dislocation of a hip in an infant. Of importance is to not confuse this condition with a true dislocation. Pelvic obliquity is the result of an abduction contracture of the musculature on the opposite hip from the side of suspected dislocation. The dysplasia viewed in a hip with congenital pelvic obliquity is quite different from an actual dislocation of the hip joint. First, in pelvic obliquity the incidence is always unilateral whereas in a dislocation a bilateral involvement will occur frequently. Second, the frequency of occurrence of the male to female ratio is markedly different. Pelvic obliquity produces a 1:3 ratio male to female while in the congenital hip dislocations a 1:6 male to female ratio is encountered.[49,55] Finally, pelvic obliquity is considered a secondarily induced disturbance in the development of the hip. This may be due to faulty fetal positioning and is not considered a true congenital anomaly.

Clinical Examination

Clinically an infant with pelvic obliquity will assume a position in which one leg is drawn up in flexion with abduction and external rotation of the leg and a valgus position of the foot. The other leg will assume an adduction position and an internally rotated position with the foot in a varus attitude. This will be evident with the infant supine but even more apparent when placed in a prone position (**Figure 63A**).

For evaluation, the examiner should bring the legs together and note the presence of tilting of the pelvis toward the abducted side and any apparent shortening of the adducted extremity.

Viewed from a prone position with the legs joined together, the examiner will note asymmetry of the gluteal folds and a concomitant scoliosis of the lumbar spine. Pelvic tilt with an apparent leg length discrepancy on the adducted side will also be observed (**Figure 63**).

To determine the degree of contracture in the abducted hip, first flex the opposite adducted hip. Attempt to bring the affected abducted limb closer to the midline of the body. If a contracture exists on the affected side, there will be an inability by the examiner to adduct the hip and limb toward the midline. The same maneuver should be performed on the opposite adducted hip for comparison. Tests including Ortolani, Barlow, Allis, etc. for hip dislocations should be negative in congenital pelvic obliquity.

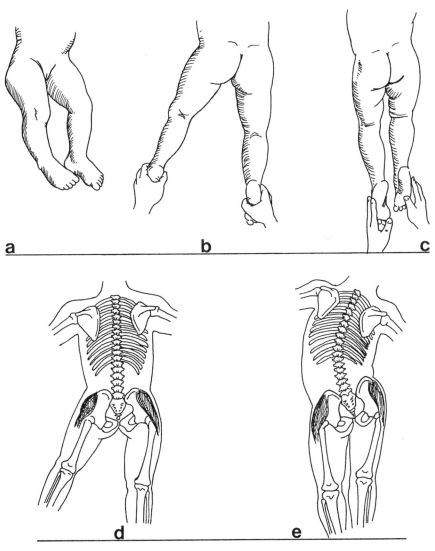

Figure 63   Congenital pelvic obliquity.

(A) *Supine position showing the left leg drawn up in an abducted, externally rotated, and flexed attitude and the foot in a valgus position. The right leg is internally rotated, adducted, and the foot in varus. (B) The left leg is in abduction with contractures of the musculature. (C) With both limbs brought together in a prone position, note the asymmetry of the gluteal folds, obliqueness of the pelvis, and lumbar scoliosis. (D) and (E) represent the contractures on the left side causing the right hip to be elevated and the pelvis to be obliquely positioned.*

Radiographic Examination

If the limbs of a child presenting with pelvic obliquity are joined together and a radiographic exposure of the pelvic area performed, there will be noted an abducted position of one hip and a pelvic tilt toward the abducted side. The adducted side will present with a sloping of the acetabular roof. An upward and lateral displacement of the femur will be viewed. This appearance may cause one to falsely interpret a dysplasia in the adducted hip.

Treatment

The treatmant of congenital pelvic obliquity is usually conservative. Initially, careful observation with stretching of the musculature is advised. Spontaneous regression occurs in the vast majority of cases. This condition becomes more evident and apparent between the ages of 2–6 months. The appearance at this age is due to the infant beginning to extend the legs and reduce their desire to maintain a fetal position. Reevaluation of this condition should be carried out every 3–4 months. There has been a correlation with documentation that with greater degrees of abduction contractures there will be a higher incidence of subluxation in the opposite hip. If a subluxation is suspected, then appropriate splinting or casting is necessary to maintain proper position.

One should avoid any forceful extension and tight binding of the legs together. Diapering should be applied to enhance abduction of the adducted hip, and exercising of the contracted hip is beneficial.

Osteochondrosis of the Hip (Legg–Calvé–Perthes disease)

In 1910 Dr. A. T. Legg, an American, described the disorder of osteochondrosis of the hip. In that same year Dr. G. C. Perthes in Germany and Dr. J. Calvé in France also described this same disorder, and so these three gentlemen have been credited with its description, referred to as *Legg–Calvé–Perthes disease*. This disorder has been described as a self-limiting condition of the femoral head in children. It is characterized by changes believed to result from one or possibly several avascular episodes in the capital femoral epiphysis. The disease seems to affect children between the ages of 3 and 14 with the highest frequency in the 4–8 year-old age group. Boys have a greater predilection and are found to be affected 4–6 times more often than girls. Approximately 10–15% of the cases are bilateral in involvement and children with skeletal maturity significantly below their chronological age are most affected.

Although the etiology is not known, there is speculation that trauma, infection, genetic predisposition, synovial effusion, and vascular occlusion may be the cause for the vascular insult to the hip.[15,16,25,26,31,36,42,47,49,51]

Clinical Examination

The presenting complaint in children with Legg–Calvé–Perthes disease is either pain or a limp, or both. In Legg's original paper he cited that four of the five cases he presented did not relate pain in the area but merely complained of the limping gait. If pain is existent, it most frequently is located in the groin area with referred pain to the distal thigh or knee region. Tenderness in the hip region may be noted along with atrophy of the buttock or thigh musculature. A decrease in the hip range of motion may be noticed particularly with abduction and internal rotation.

A differential diagnosis of rheumatic disease, villonodular synovitis, hypothyroidism, Gaucher's disease, and hemoglobinopathies such as sickle cell disease should be considered.

Radiographic Evaluation

FIRST STAGE (incipient stage)

In this stage radiological findings are similar to those of synovitis. There will be an increase in the joint space and bulging of the capsular shadow. (**Figure 64A**).

SECOND STAGE (avascular stage)

Arrest of the apparent growth in the ossification center will occur. Radiographically this is depicted by a general increase in the density of the epiphysis of the femoral head (**Figure 64B**).

THIRD STAGE (fragmentation stage)

A radiolucent line will appear below the subchondral bone overlying the central segment of the femoral head. This is followed by convolution of the cartilage of the weight-bearing portion of the femoral head along with a flattening in appearance of this area. There will also be viewed a collapse of the ossific nucleus of the femoral head (**Figure 64C**).

FOURTH STAGE (regenerative stage)

In this period, new bone formation is occurring and can be best discerned by serial x-ray views. This stage of repair, regeneration, and remodeling continues to a point where the structure of the femoral head is finally reconstituted (**Figure 64D**). A bone scan can detect an early stage if other symptoms and a history indicates this disorder.

The entire process from Stage One to Stage Four can be completed in as

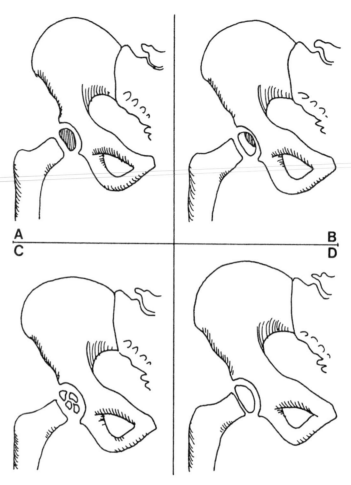

Figure 64

(A) *First Stage (incipient stage) shows increased joint space and capsular bulging with some density of the capital femoral epiphysis.* (B) *Second stage (avascular stage) reveals greater areas of increased density of the capital femoral epiphysis.* (C) *Third stage (fragmentation stage) produces collapse of the femoral head with fragmentation of the cartilaginous area.* (D) *Fourth stage (regenerative stage) will produce repair and regeneration of the head. Depending on the condition of the head and the degree of damage, the repair may be complete or only partially completed. Residual damage will present in the more severe cases.*

little as 18 months or can extend as long as several years. Resulting from the disorder are various degrees of residual deformity. This is primarily dependent on the degree of change that may occur to the femoral head.

Catterall's classification is valuable in determining the potential prognosis of this disorder (Table 6). Most authors agree that the outlook is promising for classifications 1 and 2 while categories 3 and 4 have a reasonably poor prognosis with the association of significant residual deformities. Latent osteoarthritis of the hip joint accounts for the primary concerns during the active stages of Legg–Calvé–Perthes disease. Although the actual percentage of latent deformity varies significantly from author to author, the average is less than 15% of those involved. This percent rises sharply in those cases in groups 3 and 4 of Catterall's classification.

Treatment

As outlined, this disorder is a self-limiting disease. Therefore, treatment should be tailored to allow proper maintenance and seating of the femoral head in the acetabulum. Full ranges of motion must be encouraged. If there are noted any abnormal biomechanics or pathomechanics of the foot, this should be controlled appropriately. These mechanical abnormalities of the foot will and do produce weight stresses on the hip joint that will be detrimental to a favorable prognosis if not controlled. The use of an orthosis to maintain proper structural position of the feet during the period of this disease is extremely beneficial. To properly maintain the hip joint, a need for abduction and internal rotation of this joint is necessary. The purpose for this positioning is to reduce the chance for subluxation of the joint and collapse or extrusion of the femoral head. Regarding the effects of weight-bearing on the joint, the consensus seem to agree that weight-bearing in a splint is beneficial. It has been found that children under the age of 6 presenting with the disease classification of 3 or 4 by Catteralls did poorly either with weight-bearing or nonweight-bearing.[33] Several surgical approaches have been offered to properly maintain coverage of the femoral head.

TABLE 6

Catterall's Classification of Legg–Calvé–Perthes Disease

GROUP I	Anterior portion of the epiphysis is involved with no collapse or sequestrum.
GROUP II	Up to half of the epiphysis is involved but an intact medial and lateral portion prevents collapse.
GROUP III	About three-fourths of the epiphysis is affected. Collapse may occur, in which case a large sequestrum can be seen.
GROUP IV	The entire epiphysis is affected. The poorest results are found in this group.

Congenital Coxa Vara

Coxa vara is defined as a bend in the femur bone that causes the distal end of the bone to be directed toward the midline of the body in excess of what would be considered normal. The head of the femur will usually be seated properly in the acetabulum. **Figure 65** provides the normal developmental changes in the angulation of the femoral neck shaft. Any early increased weight stress from walking along with overactivity of the hip abductor muscles will cause the angular values to gradually decrease with age. A slipped capital femoral epiphysis will also produce a coxa vara deformity. A history of trauma or a metabolic disorder may cause this condition. Careful evaluation is needed to eliminate these secondary etiologies.

The deformity of coxa vara will exist when the angular value of the femoral neck shaft is less than 120°. Values less than 100° are considered to be a significant deformity. It appears that the deformity does not manifest itself until significantly after birth. Most frequently it is not discernible until the child has begun walking.[1,4,9,14,16,19,23,32,49,50]

Clinical Examination

Children with a coxa vara deformity may present with a lurching (Trendelenburg) limp, though it will not be painful (**Figure 62**). Easy fatigability may be noticed by the parents and/or examiner. Examination will reveal a significant genu valgum (knockknees) either unilaterally or bilaterally. In the bilateral case there is usually noted a Trendelenburg gait. A unilateral deformity will present with a limb length shortage on the affected side and the presence of a lumbar lordosis (**Figure 66**).

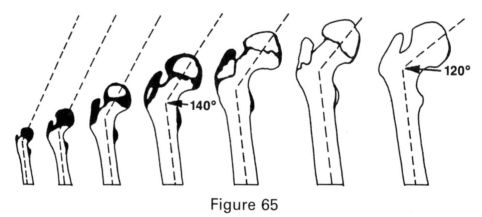

Figure 65

The development of the femur is presented showing a gradual reduction in the angle formed from a bisection of the head–neck and a bisection of the shaft.

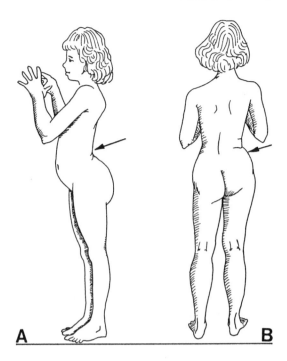

Figure 66

(A) Lumbar lordosis will produce a protrusion of the abdomen with a concavity in the lower part of the back. (B) The affected limb will cause the pelvis to be elevated resulting in a limb shortage.

A   B

Radiographic Evaluation

The neck shaft angle is measured on an anteroposterior view. Values greater than 120° would confirm the nonexistence of a coxa vara deformity (**Figure 67**). A slipped capital femoral epiphysis can be diagnosed either radiographically or in conjunction with a bone scan.

Treatment

Neck shaft values greater than 100° but less than 120° can be best treated with a lift on the affected side and passive hip abduction exercises if contractures are evident. Orthotic control of both feet should be instituted to prevent the imbalancing stress existing on the foot structure. A lift can be incorporated in the orthosis on the affected side or added to the shoe.

The parents should be informed that the genu valgum deformity along with the limping gait will most frequently improve with time and the angulation of the bone should decrease with development.

If the angular value measured on x-ray is 100° or less, and a significant Trendelenburg gait is observed, then a surgical intervention will be necessary. These surgical procedures are directed to alter and change the angular relationship of the femoral neck shaft. Timing of the surgical procedure becomes extremely important and at present is still very much controversial. Most often this is left to be performed after puberty.

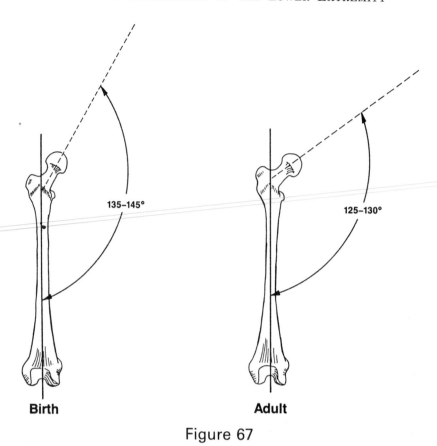

135–145°

125–130°

Birth   **Adult**

Figure 67

The angle of inclination of the femoral head–neck-shaft is measured by bisecting the head–neck and bisecting the shaft. The angle formed is referred to as the angle of inclination.

References

1. Aadalen, R.J., et al: Acute slipped capital femoral epiphysis. *Journal of Bone and Joint Surgery*. Volume 56-A, Number 7, October, 1974.
2. Artz, T.D., et al: Neonatal diagnosis, treatment and related factors of congenital dislocation of the hip. *Clinical Orthopedics and Related Research*. Number 110, July–August, 1975.
3. Badgley, C.E.: Etiology of congenital dislocation of the hip. *Journal of Bone and Joint Surgery*. Volume 31-A, 1949.
4. Barash, H.L., et al: Acute slipped capital femoral epiphysis. *Clinical Orthopedics and Related Research*. Number 79, September, 1971.
5. Budin, E., Chandler, E.: Measurement of the femoral neck anteversion by a direct method. *Radiology* Volume 69, 1957.
6. Campos da Paz, A., et al: Congenital dislocation of the hip in the newborn: A correlation of clinical, roentgenographic and anatomical findings. *Italian Journal of Orthopedic Traumatology*. Volume 2, 1976.

7. Carter, C.O., et al: Genetic and environmental factors in the etiology of congenital dislocation of the hip. *Clinical Orthopedics and Related Research.* Volume 33, March–April, 1964.
8. Coon, V., Donato, G., Houser, C., Bleck, E.E.: Normal ranges of hip motion in infants six weeks, three months and six months of age. *Clinical Orthopedics and Related Research.* Number 110, July–August, 1975.
9. Cordell, L.L.: Slipped capital femoral epiphysis. *Postgraduate Medicine.* Volume 60, Number 4, October, 1976.
10. Crane, L.: Femoral torsion and its relation to toeing-in and toeing-out. *Journal of Bone and Joint Surgery.* Volume 41-A, 1959.
11. Cyvin, K.B.: Unsatisfactory results of early treatment of infants with unstable hips at birth. *Acta Orthopedia Scandinavia* Volume 48, 1977.
12. Davis, E.D.: Congenital genu recurvatum with femoral rotation. *Clinical Orthopedics and Related Research.* Number 110, July–August, 1975.
13. *Dorland's Illustrated Medical Dictionary.* 24th Edition. W.B. Saunders Co., Philadelphia, P.A., 1965.
14. Eisenstein, A.: Biomechanical abnormalities in patients with slipped capital femoral epiphysis and chondrolysis. *Journal of Bone and Joint Surgery.* Volume 58-A, Number 4, June, 1976.
15. Ferguson, A.B.: Recent advances in understanding Legg–Perthes disease. *Orthopedic Survey,* Volume 1, Number 4, 1978.
16. Fields, L.: The limping child. *Journal of American Podiatry Association.* Volume 71, Number 2, February, 1981.
17. Fredensborg, N.: Congenital dislocation of the hip: Results of early diagnosis and treatment in males. *Int. Orthop.* Volume 1, 1977.
18. Ganley, J.V.: Lower extremity examination of the infant. *Journal of American Podiatry Association,* Volume 71, No. 2, February, 1981.
19. Hafezi, F.F.: Recurrent congenital coxa vara associated with primary hypoparathyroidism. *Clinical Orthopedics and Related Research.* Number 79, September, 1971.
20. Haas, J.: *Congenital Dislocation of the Hip.* Charles C. Thomas Co., Springfield, Illinois, 1951.
21. Hensinger, R.N.: Rotational problems of the lower extremity. *Postgraduate Medicine,* Volume 60, Number 4, October, 1976.
22. Hernandez, R., et al: C.T. determination of femoral torsion. *American Journal of Radiology,* Volume 137, 1981.
23. Hirsch, P.J., et al: Slipped capital femoral epiphysis. *Journal of the American Medical Association.* Volume 235, Number 7, February 16, 1976.
24. Jacobs, J.E.: Metatarsus varus and hip dysplasia. *Clinical Orthopedics.* Number 16, J.B. Lippincott Co., Philadelphia, P.A., 1960.
25. Kamhi, E.: Legg–Calvé–Perthes disease. *Postgraduate Medicine,* Volume 60, Number 4, October, 1976.
26. Kamhi, E.: Osteochondritis dissecans in Legg–Calvé–Perthes disease. *Journal Bone and Joint Surgery.* Volume 57-A, Number 4, June, 1975.
27. Kinglsey, P.C., Olmstead, K.O.: The techniques of measurement of antetorsion. *Journal of Bone and Joint Surgery,* Volume 30-A, 1948.
28. Kite, J.: Torsion of the legs in young children. *Clinical Orthopedics.* Number 16, J.B. Lippincott Co., Philadelphia P.A., 1960.
29. Kumar, S.J., et al: The incidence of hip dysplasia with metatarsus adductus. *Clinical Orthopedics,* Volume 164, 1982.
30. LaPorta, G.: Torsional abnormalities. *Archives Podiatric Medicine and Foot Surgery.* Volume 1, 1973–74.
31. Legg, A.T.: An obscure affection of the hip joint. *Boston Medical Surgery Journal,* Number 162, 1910.
32. Letts, R.M., et al: Mirror image coxa vara in identical twins. *Journal of Bone and Joint Surgery.* Volume 57-A, Number 1, January, 1975.

33. MacEwen, G.: Hip and leg problems in children. *Postgraduate Medicine*, Volume 60, Number 4, October, 1976.
34. Mathes, A.L.: The importance of early diagnosis of congenital dislocation of the hip. *International Surgery*, Volume 47, Number 5, May, 1967.
35. McDonough, M.W.: Fetal positioning as a cause of right and left-sided foot and leg disorders. *Journal American Podiatry Association*, Volume 71, Number 2, February, 1981.
36. Morgan, J.P., Sommerville, E.W.: Normal and abnormal growth of the upper extremities of the femur. *Journal of Bone and Joint Surgery*, Volume 42-B, 1960.
37. Pitkow, R.B.: External rotation contracture of the extended hip. *Clinical Orthopedics and Related Research*, Number 110, July–August, 1975.
38. Ramsey, P.L.: Congenital dislocation of the hip associated with central core disease. *Journal of Bone and Joint Surgery*, Volume 57-A, Number 5, July, 1975.
39. Ramsey, P.L., et al: Congenital dislocation of the hip. *Journal of Bone and Joint Surgery*, Volume 58-A, Number 7, October, 1976.
40. Ramsey, P.L.: Congenital hip dislocation. *Postgraduate Medicine*, Volume 60, Number 4, October, 1976.
41. Ryder, C.T., Crane, L.: Measuring femoral anteversion: The problem and a method. *Journal of Bone and Joint Surgery*. Volume 35-A, 1953.
42. Salter, R.B.: Legg–Perthes disease: The scientific basis for the methods of treatment and their indications. *Jefferson Orthopedics Journal*, Volume 7, 1978.
43. Scholtenfeld, M.: Primary care guide to diagnosing and treating the painful hip. *Modern Medicine*, April 30–May 15, 1979.
44. Schuster, R.D.: Intoe and outtoe and its implications. Archives of podiatric medicine and foot surgery, Volume 3, Number 4, 1976.
45. Sgarlato, T.E.: *A Compendium of Podiatric Biomechanics*, California College of Podiatric Medicine, San Francisco, 1971.
46. Shands, A.R., Steele, M.K.: Torsion of the femur. *Journal of Bone and Joint Surgery*, Volume 40-A, 1958.
47. Snyder, C.R.: Legg–Perthes disease in the young hip—Does it necessarily do well? *Journal of Bone and Joint Surgery*, Volume 57-A, Number 6, July, 1975.
48. Statham, L., et al: Early walking patterns of normal children. *Clinical Orthopedics and Related Research*, Number 79, September, 1971.
49. Tachdjian, M.O.: *Pediatric Orthopedics*, Philadelphia, P.A., W.B. Saunders Co., 1972.
50. Tax, H.R.: *Podopediatrics*, Williams and Wilkins Co., Baltimore, Maryland, 1980.
51. Théron, J.: Angeiography in Legg–Calvé–Perthes disease. *Pediatric Radiology*, Volume 135, 1980.
52. Tuell, J.I.: The congenitally malformed–congenital hip disease; Northwest Medicine, Volume 65, Number 3, March, 1966.
53. Valmassy, R.L.: *Lower Extremity Pediatric Examination. Perspectives*, Podiatry Arts Laboratory, Winter, 1981.
54. Weiner, D., Weiner, S.: The management of developmental femoral anteversion: Sham or science? *Orthopedics*, Volume 2, 1979.
55. Weissman, S.L.: Congenital pelvic obliquity. *Clinical Orthopedics*, Number 36, J.B. Lippincott Co., Philadelphia, P.A.

Chapter 5

EXAMINATION OF THE KNEES

*I*n gait, the knee joint passes through a period of flexion and extension to allow proper distribution of gravitational forces and minimize the expenditure of energy (**Figure 68**). At the point of heel strike in the gait cycle, the knee is in full extension and locked. Flexion will begin while the foot is progressing to and through midstance. The purpose of flexion is to allow a deceleration of the leg and a lowering of the arc of upward motion to occur. There exists approximately 15° of flexion during this deceleration period. The knee becomes locked again in extension as it progresses through the propulsive phase of gait. Finally, a second period of flexion occurs at the toe-off phase of gait to allow the foot and leg to pass forward.

Children up to the ages of 3–4 years present with a markedly different mechanism of action at the knee joint. This mechanism is almost the exact reverse of that mechanism described for older children and adults. Statham and Murray have shown through extensive studies this reversal of knee mechanics.[13] Their findings revealed that the knee joint is not in a fully extended and locked position at heel strike as is found in later life. Rather, the knee is in a partially flexed attitude throughout the period of weight acceptance. These researchers also observed that with this flexion attitude the foot did not meet the weight-bearing surface in the typical heel-to-toe pattern. Instead, the foot contacted the ground with a foot-flat attitude at the initiation of weight-bearing. From foot contact to midstance the knee is in extension from its flexed position. The extension does not approach the fully extended position found in the older child or adult. At the propulsive phase the knee will again begin to flex and continue throughout the swing phase, to and including foot flat (**Figure 69**).

A theory that has been proposed to explain this phenomenon is the presence of a backward inclination of the articular surface of the proximal tibia in young children.[13] With this flexion attitude existing in both knees, the opposite supporting limb in these young children will result in a lower pathway for the swinging leg and foot. This explains why one sees the tips of children's shoes worn significantly. Also in the case of new shoes, the extra length of the

Older child and adult

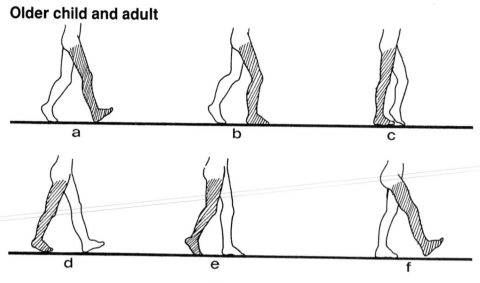

Figure 68

(A) Heel strike—knee extended and locked. (B) Foot-flat—knee begins to flex to allow deceleration and absorb transverse plane motion. (C) End of midstance—knee extends and locks once again in preparation for push off. (D) End of push off—knee begins to flex a second time thus unlocking the knee joint. (E) Swing through—knee flexes even more to allow the foot to pass through without hitting the ground. (F) Heel strike—knee extended and locked.

Young child

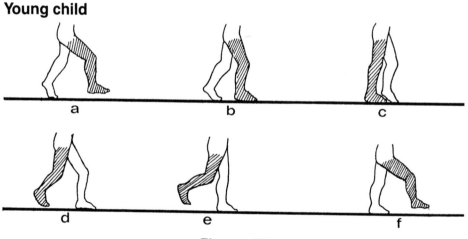

Figure 69

(A) A knee-flexed attitude with the foot parallel to the ground existing prior to contact. (This is opposite of an older child who has the knee extended and the forefoot elevated at heel strike.) (B) Foot-flat contact with the ground and the knee is still flexed. (C) Knee extension occurs just after foot contact and persists thru midstance. (D) The knee again flexes at propulsion. (E) Continued flexion through swing phase. (F) Beginning of foot contact again. A knee-flexed attitude with the foot parallel to the ground existing prior to contact.

shoe will cause the child to trip initially until he is able to adjust his swing to avoid this toe dragging. As the child develops and matures, there is a reversal of this pattern with the presence of a more extended attitude at the knee and thus a lengthening of the supporting limb.

Biomechanics of the Knee

The axis of the knee joint, as well as the common axis of both knees, lies in both the transverse and frontal planes (**Figure 70**). Simply stated, the motion in the knee will occur in the sagittal plane of the body when anatomic position is maintained. Rotatory motion can occur in the transverse plane when the knee is in a flexed and unlocked position. During dorsiflexion and plantarflexion of the knee, there exists a "cork screw" motion, i.e., a rotatory movement of the tibia on the femur. In flexion the tibia is rotated inwardly relative to the femoral condyles. As the knee begins to extend, there is an external rotation of the tibia as it becomes fixed against the femoral condyles. With full extension and "locking" of the joint, the tibia is in complete contact with the femur and no transverse motion will exist. With any degree of flexion at the knee, an unlocking of the joint will occur, allowing transverse plane motion.

Investigators have shown there exists approximately 15° of transverse plane motion in newborns when the knee is examined in full extension.[11,15] They also state that this reduces as the child develops. This author would like to take issue with this observation. The knee joints of newborns are majorally

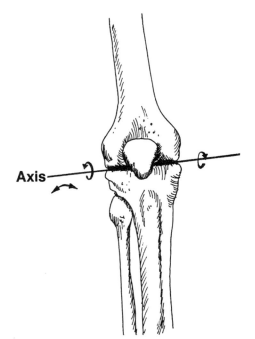

Figure 70

Axis of the knee joint lies on both the transverse and frontal plane allowing for flexion and extension as well as medial–lateral rotation with flexion.

in a contracted attitude due to fetal position. Appreciating that this contracture is in a flexed position, it becomes extremely difficult to attempt full extension of the knee joint to a point of locking without injuring the joint and surrounding tissues. Therefore, this joint can only be examined with partial flexion and not full extension, allowing for transverse plane motion to occur. This then accounts for the approximate 15° of motion noted in the attempted extended knee.

Internal Genicular Position

In order to understand disorders surrounding the knee joint, a thorough appreciation of the anatomy and biomechanics is paramount. A review of the information provided earlier in this chapter is recommended before progressing. As was described, the knee joint will move in a "cork screw" fashion and will lock in a fully extended position. Noted were the findings that children under the ages of 3–4 years present with a completely reversed mechanism of gait from that viewed in the older child or adult. These factors, along with a review of the muscular anatomy of the knee joint (Table 7), will provide an explanation for the deformity this author refers to as *internal genicular position*.

As viewed in Table 7, there is an obvious inequality in the balance of musculature for internal and external motion and stability. This inequality must be taken into account when examining a child for a gait abnormality, particularly an in-toeing deformity. With the addition of the "cork screw" mechanism for locking of the knee and the knowledge that children under 3–4 years walk with a knee flexed attitude, this author would like to explain the mechanics of an etiology for in-toeing called *internal genicular position*. Historically there have been suggestions that soft-tissue alterations exist around the knee joint to cause an in-toeing gait abnormality. Unfortunately, the lack of previous knowledge for the biomechanics of the knee did not allow for a clear understanding. It is realized now that a partially flexed knee will allow transverse plane motion to occur. If an altered neutral position of the knee joint exists, then an altered degree of internal and external range of motion will result throughout gait.

If contractions or contractures of the internal rotator muscles of the tibia are in excess of normal, the resulting neutral position of the knee will be internal during the nonweight-bearing unlocked position of the knee. The cause for these contractures can include: continued internal rotation of the flexed limb during the fetal development; abnormal innervation causing greater contractions to the internal rotation muscles; poor innervation with weakening of the external rotator muscles; continued poor sleeping habits causing the limb to be maintained internally; and spasticity of the internal rotator muscles as in cerebral palsy. With the presence of this positioning after birth, a child may continue to assume an inwardly rotated limb during sleep (**Figure 71**). When sitting, the child may assume the classic "television position" (**Figure**

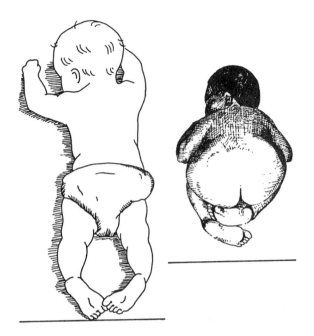

Figure 71

A child may assume an internal leg and foot position either by lying on his stomach with hips extended or with the hips flexed.

72). This positioning allows reduced tension on the internal rotator muscles at the knee and therefore is more comfortable for the child. Parents should be questioned as to these habits when the initial history is obtained.

It is realized from Table 7 that a greater muscle mass is producing internal rotation (five muscles) than external rotation (one-half of a muscle). Therefore, whatever factor(s) may provide these internal rotators a greater advantage would ultimately place the neutral position of the knee in an internal attitude. The fact that children walk with a flexed unlocked knee attitude throughout the swing phase of gait and at heel strike until age 3–4 years, along with the ability of greater muscle strength toward the internal side, can ultimately lead to the production of an in-toeing deformity. If an infant is allowed to maintain an internally positioned neutral state at the knee until walking, one will observe an in-toeing gait characterized by the lower leg rotated inwardly throughout the swing phase and heel strike of gait while the knee joint is maintained in a flexed unlocked position.

When the knee joint is unlocked and motion is allowed in the transverse plane, the tibia is actually rotating in relationship to the distal femur. This internal rotation of the tibia with knee flexion results in the leg and foot being placed in an internal attitude. As the child develops, less flexion exists at the knee and a reversal in the mechanics of the knee joint in gait will result. Prior to this stage of development, the knee will not fully extend throughout gait and a more noticeable inward rotation will present.

This author would like to bring attention to a term frequently used to describe this same condition, i.e., "pseudolack of malleolar torsion." In clarification, malleolar torsion refers to an actual bony twisting of the tibia which

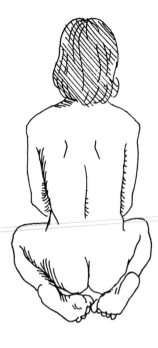

Figure 72

Children sitting in this position ("television position") will continue to promote an internal lower leg or foot deformity.

TABLE 7
Muscular Anatomy of the Knee Joint

Movement	Muscle
Medial rotation of the tibia on the femur	Popliteus Semitendinosus Semimembranosus Sartorius Gracilis
Lateral rotation of the tibia on the femur	Lateral head of biceps femoris
Flexion	Biceps femoris Semitendinosus Semimembranosus Grastrocnemius Plantaris Sartorius Gracilis Popliteus
Extension	Quadriceps femoris

is not involved in the condition presently being described. Pseudolack infers a false absence of this rotational twist in the tibia, which becomes even more confusing. There is no involvement of a torsional component of the tibia in this rotational abnormality nor a false absence of it. This author feels this term should be discarded for one more descriptive of the location of the deformity without reference to a bony component. Therefore, the term *internal genicular position* has been provided for description.

Clinical Examination

The best position for examination of a child for an abnormal genicular position is for the child to be seated at the edge of an examining table with his knees and hips flexed (**Figure 73A**). This places the knee in an unlocked position and reduces the tension of the musculature surrounding the knee joint. Measurements are taken for the range of motion internally and externally, and again when the hips are extended. Hip flexion will cause greater tension on the musculature originating above the hip joint. Use the lower leg and foot as the measuring instrument for the determination of motion. There is no need for instruments to calibrate these measurements. Your own visual comparisons and known normals are sufficient to diagnosis this condition. If you do desire to use a goniometer or other measuring instruments, remember these can be cumbersome, awkward, and inaccurate.

To measure the ranges of motion at the knee on the transverse plane, use an imaginary line which will bisect the foot (**Figure 73**). Start by placing the foot parallel to the sagittal plane (**Figure 73A**). Now grasp the foot and ankle area with one hand and rotate the lower leg and foot using the malleoli as points of force. Rotate the lower leg through its maximum range of motion internally and externally. Using the imaginary bisection line of the foot from its zero point, which is parallel to the sagittal plane, calculate the degree of rotation in both directions. Try to imagine a protractor existing below the foot and use it to approximate the degree of motion (**Figure 73A–C**). Normally the human eye can discern 5–10° increments and this level of accuracy is sufficient to determine any existing abnormality. Assuming tibial torsion to be normal and therefore externally rotated, examination of motion of the lower leg should exhibit greater motion externally than internally. This may approach a 2:1 ratio toward external in normal children or it may be as little as 1:1. If a finding of greater internal range of motion than external occurs, then one can assume that *internal genicular position* is present. If the range of motion internally is greater with hip flexion than extension, one can assume the musculature is playing a significant role. Conversely, if the ranges are great toward internal but unaffected by hip flexion and extension, then the deformity is due more to ligamentous tightness with secondary muscular involvement. An example of *internal genicular position* would be an internal range of motion from 70–100° and external motion of only 0–20° (**Figure 74**).

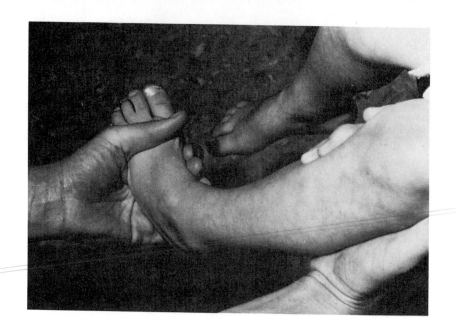

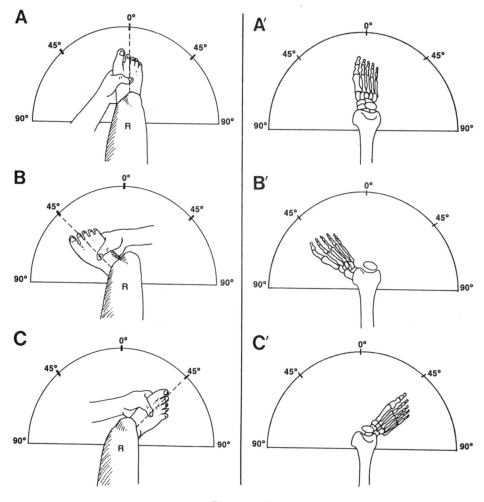

Figure 73

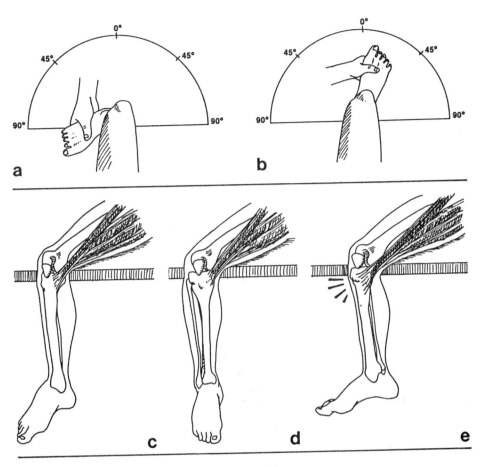

Figure 74

(A) With internal genicular position, the leg will be capable of rotating inward greater than 45–65° and (B) limited in external rotation of 45–95°. (C) A relaxed leg with knee flexed and the presence of internal genicular position due to the contractures of the soft tissue at the medial aspect of the knee. (D) Internal rotation will have little effect on the medial tension. (E) External rotation will be limited due to the contractures of the muscles attached to the medial aspect of the tibia.

Figure 73 (opposite): (A) The knee is flexed and the ankle is at 90° with the bisection of the foot placed on the sagittal plane of the leg representing 0°. The hip should be either flexed or extended for the first measurement and then reversed. (B) Internal rotation of the lower leg at the knee should normally be approximately 45–65°. (C) External rotation should be approximately 45–95°.

A question often asked is whether the ranges of motion internally and externally will change with the gradual extension of the knee joint. It is this author's experience that the proportional difference between the internal and external motion remains constant up to the point of complete extension and locking. After the locking mechanism occurs, then transverse plane motion becomes negligible. In determining the neutral position of the knee joint, total the amount measured internally and externally and divide by 2. Subtract this amount from either the degree of measured motion internally or externally. This will show the approximate neutral knee position. For example, if the internal motion is 90° and the external 10°, the total would be 100°. Dividing by 2 leaves 50° to be subtracted from either range. If subtracted from the internal 90°, the net neutral position would be 40° internally. If subtracted from the 10° external, the same neutral position of 40° internally results. In this example the leg would assume an internally positioned attitude of 40° (neutral position) through swing phase and foot contact when the knee is in a flexed position. When examining for the presence of this deformity, be certain to evaluate both limbs for symmetry or asymmetry.

Treatment

Efforts to treat *internal genicular position* need to be directed to the primary etiology, i.e., muscular and ligamentous contracture and imbalance. Therefore, the mode of treatment suitable for correction is muscular stretching. Several methods are available to stretch the contracted internal rotator muscles at the knee effectively. Most simply, the use of the parents in daily stretching exercises can be minimally effective; parents are instructed to: rotate the leg externally with the knee flexed; hold for the count of 10 seconds once maximum external rotation is achieved with extension; and perform 30–40 repetitions, holding each for 10 seconds 3 to 4 times per day. Unfortunately, when this responsibility is left to the parents, it is usually not followed properly or consistently. Moreover, we appreciate that continuous stretching (i.e., 24 hours a day) will accomplish a more lasting and faster reduction in the deformity. Intermittent periods of stretch cannot physiologically produce a resting state in a lengthened attitude as effectively as can continuous stretch. Therefore, the treatment program comprised of intermittent parental stretching done only a few to several times per day and unable to be performed during sleeping periods is not likely to be effective. A more effective and gratifying treatment is the application of stretch casts. The parents should be properly informed that the purpose for using a long leg cast is to effectively place the involved muscles under a 24-hour stretching program. This usually will relieve their concerns. The application of the cast is best performed with the child on the parent's lap to provide a feeling of security. A three-part cast is applied after an application of cast padding from the toes to the groin area (**Figure 75**). Children with diapers usually benefit by the application of several extra layers of padding in the groin area for absorption. The first part to be applied

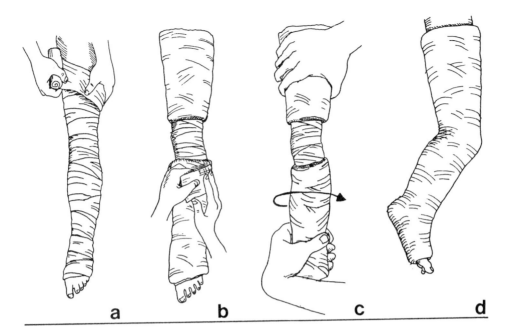

a   b   c   d

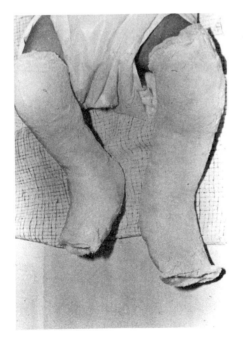

Figure 75

(A) *Webril padding 2–3 layers of thickness with reinforcement around the ankle and lower knee. Added padding at the upper end of the thigh is helpful to absorb moisture, etc. from diapers. (B) Apply the thigh cast first and while drying, apply the lower leg–foot section leaving the knee area exposed. (C) Allow both segments to dry. (D) Rotate the lower leg externally and apply the middle portion of the cast at the knee.*

is a cylinder cast from the groin to just above the knee joint. While this is setting, the second part can be applied. A well molded below-the-knee cast is applied with the ankle held at 90°. (*Note:* If there is a concomitant deformity such as a metatarsus adductus deformity or a muscular inbalance in the foot–leg complex, then a correction can be incorporated into this B.K. cast.) Once the two cast parts have set up and are firm, the final third segment can be applied. Flex the knee joint approximately 30° and rotate the lower leg externally to its maximum resistance. This is best accomplished by grasping the foot at the heel area with one hand and the thigh with the other hand. It should be mentioned that the child may dislike this at this point, but do not become intimidated by this. Realize that with a knee-flexed position, rotation is occurring by the external movement of the tibia on the femur and thus an application of stretch to all the internal rotator muscles. While holding the limb in this position, an assistant may apply the third portion of the cast around the knee joint area. Make sure sufficient overlap occurs to ensure a stable cast.

This author has found plaster still to be the best material to use due to its moldability and ease of application. Other casting materials can be used but caution must be used in application. Too tight or a creased cast may cause significant injury to the child. In using plaster, remind the parents that no weight-bearing should occur for at least 12–18 hours. Weight-bearing can follow this period and surprisingly, the child will be able to function reasonably well. Avoid excessive knee flexion as this will impair ambulation. Have the child wear the cast for a period of one week, and then, without removing the cast, make a circular cut through the cast at the level of the knee joint (**Figure 76**). Rotate the leg externally to its maximum resistance and apply plaster to the area to enforce the cut. Remarkably, you will observe that the lower leg will rotate a significant degree more externally after this one-week period of casting than was possible previously.

After this rotation of the cast, allow the child to ambulate for a period of 1–2 weeks. This becomes age dependent as well as the amount of noted destruction to the cast itself. Remove the cast after this 1–2 week period and determine the range of motion at the knee joint (described under *Clinical Examination*). If external motion is not equal to or greater than the internal motion, then application of a second cast is necessary. This should be employed for another 1–2 week period to complete the stretching program. *Note:* When the cast is removed, some children will be unwilling to walk for a period of 1–2 days. This is due to the awkward feeling and loss of the cast weight. You may find other cases in which the child will walk with a bent knee attitude for a short period of time afterward due to the former cast position. This is not cause for alarm and will resolve itself. The parents should be properly informed of this prior to the occurrence.

After correction is achieved, these children should be periodically examined for any signs of reoccurrence. Another 2-week period of casting may be necessary in cases of reoccurrence. It has been this author's experience that

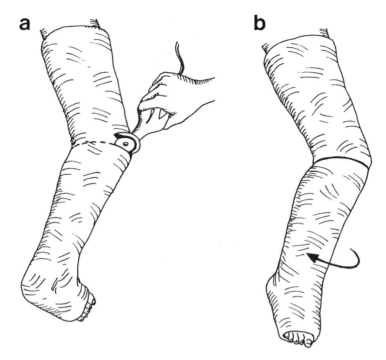

Figure 76

(A) Cut the cast at the knee joint and (B) rotate the lower portion externally. Reinforce the area cut with more plaster and continue for 1–2 weeks.

infrequently is there a reoccurrence noted with follow-ups for periods of 4–7 years.

Following this stretch casting program, the parents should be encouraged not to allow their children to return to sleeping and sitting positions that would promote the recurrence of the muscular contractures. You may advise parents to have their children use small stools, rather than sitting on the floor, and having the child sleep on his side or back would avoid the tendency for the legs to be rotated inwardly. The use of a night splint (i.e., Denis-Browne splint, Fillauer bar, Ganley splint) is beneficial in avoiding improper positions while sleeping. Some will argue that the muscular imbalance occurring around the knee and causing a rotational deformity will resolve by the time the child reaches 4–6 years of age. They therefore state that no treatment is necessary. What is failed to be appreciated with this philosophy is the typical compensatory changes that will result. Compensation is universally accepted as an alteration which ultimately affects a segment of the body involved in an adverse way. Alteration in the foot structure including joint collapse, abnormal patello-femoral position, and hip joint alterations have been indicated as results of compensation for a rotational abnormality. We understand that the body attempts to maintain the center of gravity through a limb with whatever means are available. Therefore, alterations in the various joint segments from hip to foot may occur to position the gravitational center appropriately. The resulting abnormal articular positionings will produce further degenerative changes as the person progresses through life. This will become increasingly more significant in athletes or those very active in strenuous exercises or activities. By the time the child reaches 5–7 years of age, compensatory pronation and collapse in the foot occur secondary to a rotational deformity. The resulting collapse in the foot structure causes an abduction in the foot, and therefore a straighter walking pattern. Unfortunately, sacrificing one body segment to compensate for an abnormality in another segment has a deleterious effect on the future of the compensated segment. We must therefore protect and treat, when possible, the deformities affecting the limb. Orthotic control therapy after casting is advantageous in the ambulatory child to avoid compensation and to attempt to reverse any alteration in the foot structure. This should continue for a period until development and growth assure no reoccurrence of the abnormality of *internal genicular position*. The child also needs to be protected from injuring himself from falls secondary to tripping as a result of an in-toeing deformity.

External Genicular Position

This deformity has not been viewed frequently by this author. In theory it can be conceived as a cause for an out-toeing gait deformity. The anatomy of the knee, as described at the beginning of this chapter, does not lend itself readily to this type of abnormality.

Genu Varum

This condition denotes a bowing at the knee with the distal lower leg being directed toward the midline of the body (**Figure 77**). Concomitant with this condition is an often found varus attitude of the tibia which will actually accentuate the bowing appearance. Ontogenically genu varum is usually self-limiting if it is the result of developmental growth. It may, however, be secondary to other causes including rickets, asymmetric growth disturbances in the epiphyses and Blount's disease (tibia vara).[2,14–16] If developmental, it will exist from birth to approximately age 2–4 years. The reduction in the varum occurs due to epiphyseal stimulation with weight-bearing. The noted bowing in the legs of infants is usually the combination of genu varum, lack of external tibial torsion, and tibia varum. The examiner must take this into account when a diagnosis of bowlegs is decided. Statistically it has been shown that children normally will present with an initial period of genu varum. This eventually corrects itself by age 2–4 years with a progression to a state of genu valgum (discussed further in this chapter).[10–12,14–16]

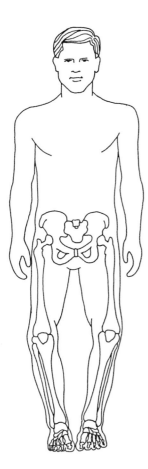

Figure 77

Genu varum is a condition in which the lower leg is directed toward the midline of the body while the knee joint is more laterally placed.

Most important in this condition is the degree of varum present and the length of time it persists. The presence of other conditions that mimic this deformity must also be considered. A differential diagnosis to eliminate the possibility of conditions as rickets, tibia varum (Blount's disease), and asymmetric growth disturbances of the epiphyses is necessary (described in Chapter 6). A family history of bowleggedness is also extremely useful in concluding a prognosis.

Clinical Examination

In examining for genu varum, first allow the child to assume a supine position with the position of the limbs straight forward (**Figure 78A**). While maintaining the patellae parallel to the sagittal plane, approximate the two limbs together until either the medial aspects of the knees or the malleoli touch (**Figure 78A and B**). If genu varum or a combination of genu varum and tibia varum exist, the malleoli will touch first and a certain degree of separation will exist at the knees. To document the degree of deformity, meas-

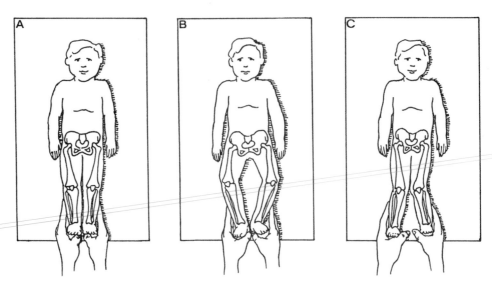

Figure 78   Examination for genu varum or genu valgum.

(A) Have the child supine on the examination table. The absence of any genu varum or genu valgum will allow both legs to touch at the knees and malleoli simultaneously. (B) Genu varum exists when the malleoli touch first and separation exists at the knees. (C) Genu valgum is present when the knees are in contact with each other and there is separation at the malleoli.

ure the amount of separation from the inner aspect of the knee. A separation of greater than 7–8 cm is considered significant. Close periodic monitoring to determine reduction or advancement of the deformity should be performed. If less than 5 cm is measured of separation, then regular examinations should take place to determine the progress.

Radiographically, the transverse plane of the knee joints will be angulated inwardly (medially). The tibia will also be noted to be inwardly angulated in its relationship to femur. The growth center should appear normal with symmetry of both limbs. Alterations in the epiphyses may indicate a pathologic cause and should be pursued appropriately. Asymmetry is almost always an indication of a pathologic condition rather than one of development and needs investigation for possible Blount's disease (tibia vara) or epiphyseal injury.

Treatment

We must first realize that the condition of genu varum is usually observed by the parents or grandparents after the child has begun to walk, even though in most instances it has existed from birth. Reassurance should be offered to the parents as to the normalcy of the cases of symmetrical findings with less than 5 cm of separation at the knee joints. An explanation of normal development with the likely reversal and resolution of this condition will certainly ease the parental concerns. Encourage periodic examinations aproximately every 6–12 months to determine the progression or regression, symmetry or asymmetry, of the deformity. These periodic examinations will allow both the examiner and parents to appreciate the progress. If the condition is due to an epiphyseal injury (determined by asymmetry and/or serial examination), Blount's disease (tibia vara) (determined by radiographic examination—Chapter 6) or rickets (noted by epiphyseal changes, rachitic rosary, and retarded development), then appropriate treatment directed to the etiology and by an appropriate specialist is indicated.

The use of casts or bars is never indicated even though some practitioners often employ them. They become an instrument by the practitioner to appease the parents and buy time for normal development. Unfortunately, they can produce deleterious rather than advantageous results on both the legs and feet. It has been found that a valgusing of the foot will occur with an abnormal genu valgum as a result from bar or cast treatment.[15]

Appreciating that normal development will usually correct this altered limb position, we must further look to understand the effects the positioning will play while normal development occurs. In the foot, a medial downward force will result at the ankle, mid and rearfoot during stance and gait (**Figure 79**). If this force is present for a sufficient time, there will be a collapse in the foot–ankle structure especially if ligamentous and muscular laxity coexist. To avoid this change in the foot, along with changes at the knee and hip joints resulting from the foot collapse, some form of protection should be offered and encouraged throughout the period of developmental reversing of the varus attitude.

The practitioner should be aware that compensatory changes occur from this positional attitude of the limb and will result in structural changes. Both the compensatory and structural changes attempt to maintain proper weight stress in the segments of the limb. Unfortunately, once a developmental alteration as in genu varum corrects itself, the changes and alterations in the surrounding joints and structural segments will most likely not reverse themselves. The reason the body is unable to reverse these changes is because of the added weight stress naturally occurring from a growing child. It becomes inconceivable to imagine that the stretched ligaments holding the bony segments could retighten themselves against the downward weight stresses occurring. This is likened to stretching a piece of elastic material continuously until a point is reached when releasing the elastic no longer allows it to return to its prestretched state. To avoid these compensatory changes, this author strongly suggests the use of orthotic control throughout the period of developmental correction of a moderate or moderately severe deformity. Most effective are orthoses which confine the foot and minimize excessive joint motion with an allowance for better weight stress throughout the entire limb. A type B or C heel stabilizer will encourage proper ankle–foot attitude and not allow bony shifts to occur in the foot (**Figure 80**). Whitman, Roberts', or Whitman–Roberts' plates are also beneficial but do not have as rigid a control (**Figure 81**). Shoe wedging and pads should be avoided as they do not allow proper

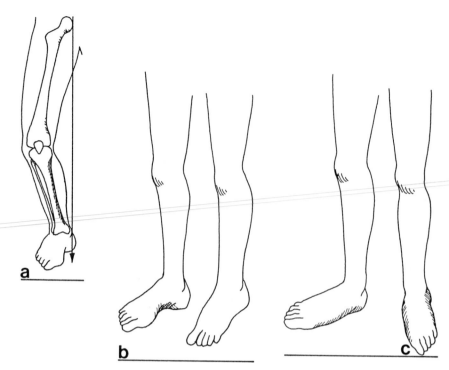

Figure 79

(A) *The arrow is showing the downward force of the center of gravity. With genu varum the force is more medially placed, affecting not only the foot but the knee and hip joints.* (B) *This diagram depicts a normal architecture of a foot without the effects of the abnormal stresses of genu varum.* (C) *Collapse in the foot structure will result from the medial downward force of the center of gravity in a limb with genu varum.*

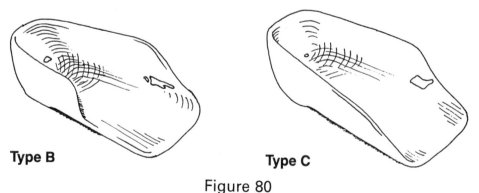

Figure 80

Type B heel stabilizers offer good control of the foot but are not as confining as the type C. A foot that is weak structurally benefits more by a type C.

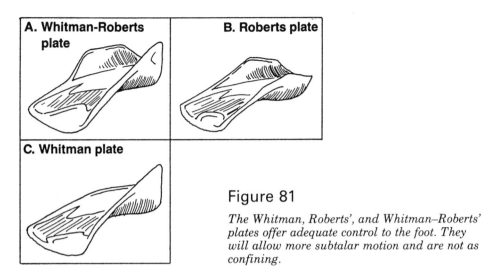

A. Whitman-Roberts plate

B. Roberts plate

C. Whitman plate

Figure 81

The Whitman, Roberts', and Whitman–Roberts' plates offer adequate control to the foot. They will allow more subtalar motion and are not as confining.

control of the foot due to the natural pliability of the shoe counters and gradual wear and breakdown of the shoe.

Genu Valgum

In contradistinction to genu varum, *genu valgum* produces the opposite effect—the so-called "knock-knee" appearance (**Figure 82**). Children present with this attitude between the ages of 2–5 years and normally will correct by the ages of 5–8 years. There are various degrees of genu valgum as was also the case in genu varum. Morley categorized the severity into grades which will be described under *Clinical Examination*.[8] His findings revealed no differences in the incidence with either sex, although there was a correlation regarding the weight of the child and the degree of the deformity.

Secondary to the positioning of the limb in genu valgum, an examiner will oftentimes note a mild degree of in-toeing accompanying this position. This is an attempt to place the center of gravity over the leg and foot in a more advantageous position. These changes in structural positioning will oftentimes lead to muscular fatigue and cramping in the thighs, legs and/or feet. The child or parent may present with this as the chief complaint from this problem.[8,11,14–16]

Clinical Examination

Allow the child to be placed in a supine position either on a table or on a parent's lap. Position the legs in a straightforward attitude with the patellae facing upward (**Figure 78A**). Bring the legs together and note whether the malleoli or knees touch first. With genu valgum the examiner will find that

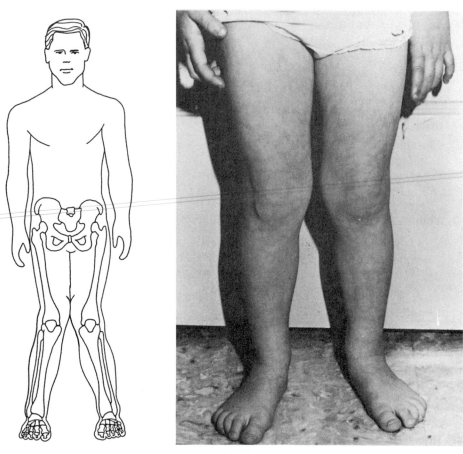

Figure 82

Genu valgum *directs the knees toward each other and will cause the lower legs to be directed laterally away from the sagittal plane of the body.*

the knees will touch first, allowing a certain degree of separation between the malleoli (**Figure 78C**). Moreley's grading system can be used to document the degree of severity.[8] *Grade I* presents with an intermalleolar distance separation of less than 1 inch (2.5 cm). *Grade II* exhibits separation of between 1 and 2 inches (2.5–5 cm), with *Grade III* being between 2 and 3 inches (5–7.5 cm). *Grade IV* is anything greater than 3 inches (7.5 cm). This system of grading will allow the examiner and the parents an ability to follow the improvement, persistence, and advancement of the deformity throughout the observation and evaluation period.

Radiographic evaluation is of little value in developmental genu valgum. It is of benefit to determine epiphyseal injuries contributing to genu valgum as in cases of coxa vara (Chapter 4). With unilateral genu valgum, a careful examination and history for coxa vara must be obtained. Tautness of the iliotibial band is also a cause for valgum at the knee secondary to the lateral pulling on the tibia. In examining for this, attempt to straighten the knee joint by using counterforce at the thigh and lower leg (**Figure 83**). If a prominent iliotibial band or a palpable tightness is noted, then one must consider this entity as part of the etiology.[14-16]

Treatment

Developmental genu valgum need only be treated with protection and proper periodic evaluation. If a *Grade III* or *IV* deformity exist, then concern should be directed to avoidance of any compensatory changes. In-shoe orthotic control is recommended to reduce the tendency for medial collapse in the foot secondary to the medial shift of the gravitational forces. Without this type of control, compensation will occur in the joint structures of not only the foot, but as well to the knees, hip, and possibly lower back. The abnormal weight-bearing stress and stretch on the medial ligamentous and muscular structures of the knee can ultimately cause improper wear of the joint surfaces. Eventually this may lead to degenerative joint arthritis, as documented by Tachdjian.[14]

If an epiphyseal injury or a coxa vara is the causative factor, then proper treatment by an orthopedist is necessary. Protective control of the foot is also of upmost importance in these instances. Tightness of the iliotibial band should be treated by stretching. This can be accomplished by a long leg cast with gradual medial wedging adequately to lengthen the fibers in cases of *Grade III* and *IV* (**Figure 84**). Manipulative stretching can be of benefit in *Grade I* and *II* genu valgum secondary to a taut iliotibial band. With the use of orthotic devices, the medial stress on the knee joint and foot are lessened. This provides for decreased cartilage wear and muscular and ligamentous stretch. Parents must be informed that with this type of control of the leg–foot complex, a mild

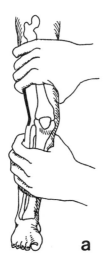 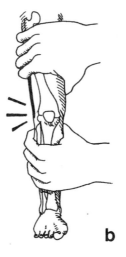

a   b

Figure 83   Tight iliotibial band.

(A) *The examiner should position both hands as shown to determine any tautness in the iliotibial band. (B) Attempting to straighten the knee by bringing the lower leg toward the sagittal plane of the body will stretch the iliotibial band. A palpable or visible tightness indicates a contracture of the band contributing to the genu valgum.*

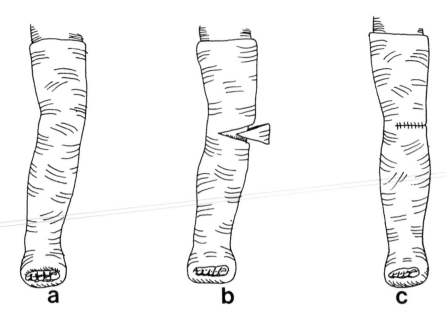

Figure 84   Casting a tight iliotibial band.

(A) A long leg cast is used. The initial cast is applied with a stretch on the iliotibial band. This is left on for approximately 1 week. (B) A wedge can be removed at the knee joint area after one week and reinforced (C). This should be left for 1–2 more weeks. If complete correction is not obtained with removal of the cast, then begin step (A) again and proceed through step (C).

in-toeing gait may result. This is due to a more lateral repositioning of the gravitational center.

Orthoses that work well to maintain proper structural control are Type B and C heel stabilizers, Whitman plates, and Roberts' plates (**Figures 80 and 81**). Shoe wedging and padding, as well as functional type orthoses, do not provide proper and adequate control or support of a child's foot.

Casts, splints, or twister cables are of no value in the developmental type genu valgum and may even cause secondary deleterious abnormalities. Practitioners who claim these splints and apparatus work are actually the victims of normal development. Provided adequate time is allowed for the condition to reverse itself, the implementation of these casts and splints is of no value other than buying this time. Spontaneous correction would in most cases result without treatment. Unfortunately, these treatment devices, having little effect on the genu valgum and its outcome, may in fact cause potential secondary complications due to improper usage or application.

A *Grade IV* genu valgum in excess of 4 inches (10 cm) should be reevaluated more frequently (approximately every 4–6 months). Orthotic control becomes paramount in protection for this degree of abnormality. Persistence of a *Grade IV* condition and/or its existence in adolescence may warrant consideration for surgical intervention by a pediatric orthopedist.

Genu Recurvatum

Genu recurvatum is a condition in which there is a hyperextension of the knee joint. The knee, when fully extended, normally is straight if viewed laterally. A curvature along the limb can exist with the apex of the curve at the knee joint and the convexity of the curve being posteriorly placed (**Figure 85**). Etiologically, the causes can include ligamentous laxity, contractures of the quadricep muscles, weakness of the posterior leg muscles, muscular imbalance as found in neurological conditions, or epiphyseal changes or damage to the distal femur or proximal tibia.[1,3,6,7,9]

Though rare, the condition of a congenitally subluxed or dislocated knee must be differentiated from genu recurvatum. The former has a much more serious prognosis and degree of severity. Arthrogryposis, cerebral palsy, Ehler–Danlos syndrome and myelomeningocele oftentimes may manifest the condition of a dislocated or subluxed knee joint. What is observed is the tibia actually being displaced in an abducted and hyperextended position. Surgical correction is most often needed for proper realignment of the dislocated knee.

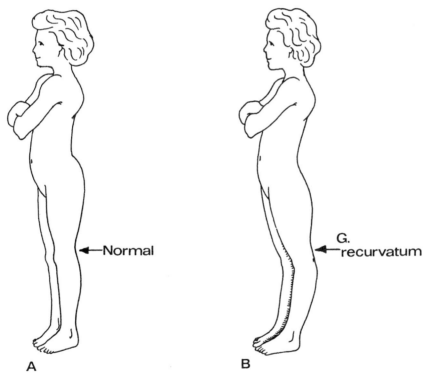

←Normal

G.
←recurvatum

A   B

Figure 85

(A) Normal knee alignment. (B) Genu recurvatum produces a backwards positioning of the knee joint with the apex of the convex curve at this joint.

The examiner needs to be aware that the condition of genu recurvatum can be seen in otherwise normal healthy infants. This can be treated in a less serious fashion than that of a congenital knee dislocation. The treatment usually requires several castings for a period of approximately 6–8 weeks to allow proper stretching of any contractures. It also allows for proper alignment of the femur and tibia at the knee joint. Muscle stregthening and stretching exercises should be instituted to balance the anterior and posterior muscle groups after casting is completed. In cases of persistence, a consideration for muscular realignment and lengthening through surgical intervention may be necessary.

Dislocation of the Patella

There are infrequent occasions when a child will present with a true dislocating patella. If it does occur, it most often will result in a lateral displacement. The predilection for this disorder is toward females approximately 3:1, and there has been found a significantly high frequency of familial tendencies.[4–6]

Several etiological causes have been offered and considered. The most frequent causes are: genu valgum causing the quadriceps to be laterally displaced forcing the patella in this same direction; high degree of antetorsion of the femur or excessive external tibial torsion will produce a rotatory torque at the knee forcing the patella not to tract properly; ligamentous laxity of the medial structures of knee or generalized ligamentous laxity will cause the potential for lateral shifting of the patella due to instability; iliotibial band contractures or altered attachments into the lateral condyle of the tibia may cause displacement particularly during knee flexion; injuries including medial lacerations and lateral displacement-type trauma to the patella will inadvertently cause potential recurrent patella dislocation.[4–6,14]

Clinical Examination

The most common complaint is a feeling of "giving away" of the knee with significant pain followed by swelling and decreasing with each episode. Oftentimes the patient will relate that they have actually fallen down during an episode.

Examination should include determining the presence of one or more of the above mentioned etiologies (genu valgum, antetorsion, external tibial torsion, ligamentous laxity, iliotibial band alterations, and/or injury). An acute attack will present with pain or tenderness along the medial capsular area of the knee and swelling. The *apprehension test* (Fairbank's sign) is useful in determining a dislocating patella. This is accomplished by having the patient lie supine with legs flat and quadriceps relaxed. With one hand, press against the medial border of the patella and force laterally. No reaction by the patient will occur in a nondislocating patella. However, if the patella begins dislocating, the patient will become extremely apprehensive and alarmed and may attempt to stop the examiner.[6]

Radiographically, a tangential view with the knee flexed approximately 30–40° will provide the best position for determination (**Figure 86**). Lateral displacement of the patella will be noted if a dislocation exists.

Treatment

Conservative treatment oftentimes will resolve this condition, particularly in a young child without a chronic history of the problem. Certainly traumatic injury or laceration needs more aggressive care. Exercise and strengthening of the quadriceps muscles with concomitant stretching of the iliotibial band, when necessary, are beneficial. Orthotic control of the foot is effectual in rotating and altering the stress and angle of the knee joint, particularly if genu valgum, external tibial torsion, or antetorsion is existing. The patient should also be discouraged from participating in sports that would impose undue stress on the knees. Surgical correction is indicated in recurrent episodes and should not be delayed due to the patello-femoral arthritis that inadvertently will occur with time.[14]

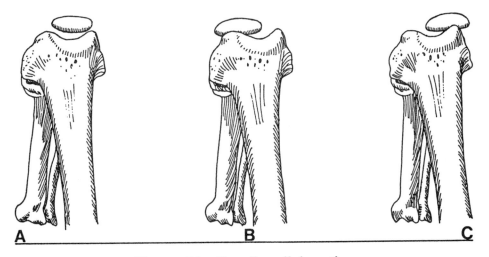

Figure 86   Patellar dislocation.

(A) Normal patello-femoral position in a tangential view. (B) Medially dislocating patella. (C) Laterally dislocating patella.

References

1. Davis, E.D.: Congenital genu recurvatum with femoral rotation. *Clinical Orthopedics and Related Research*, Number 110, July–August, 1975.
2. Fendrich, G.M.: Would you miss the diagnosis of bowlegs. *Modern Medicine*, June 30–July 15, 1979.
3. Finder, J.A.: Congenital hyperextension of the knee. *Journal of Bone and Joint Surgery*, Volume 46-B, 1964.
4. Gallie, W.E.: Habitual dislocation of the patella. *Journal of Bone and Joint Surgery*, Volume 6, 1924.
5. Green W.T.: Recurrent dislocation of the patella. Its surgical correction in the growing child. *Journal of Bone and Joint Surgery*, Volume 47-A, 1965.
6. Hoppenfeld, S.: Physical examination of the knee joint by complaint. *Orthopedic Clinics of North America*, Volume 10, Number 1, January, 1979.
7. Katz, M.P., et al: The etiology and treatment of congenital dislocation of the knee. *Journal of Bone and Joint Surgery*, Volume 49-B, 1967.
8. Morley, A.J.: Knock knees in children. *British Medical Journal*, Volume 2, 1957.
9. Nason, S.S., et al: Congenital subluxation of the knee—An anatomic dissection. *Orthopedics*, Volume 1, 1978.
10. Salenius, P., Vankke, E.: The development of the tibiofemoral angle in children. *Journal of Bone and Joint Surgery*, Volume 57-A, March, 1975.
11. Sgarlato, T.E.: *A Compendium of Podiatric Biomechanics*, California College of Podiatric Medicine, San Francisco, 1971.
12. Sherman, M.: Physiologic bowing of the legs. *Southern Medical Journal*, Volume 53, 1960.
13. Statham, L., et al: Early walking patterns of normal children. *Clinical Orthopedics and Related Research*, Number 79, September, 1971.
14. Tachdjian, M.O.: *Pediatric Orthopedics*, Philadelphia, P.A., W.B. Saunders Co., 1972.
15. Tax, H.R.: *Podopediatrics*, Williams and Wilkins Co., Baltimore, Maryland, 1980.
16. Weiner, D.S.: The natural history of "bow legs" and "knock knees" in childhood. *Orthopedics*, Volume 4, 1981.

Chapter 6

EXAMINATION OF THE LOWER LEG

*T*here are several disorders that may present in the lower leg as causes for gait abnormalities. This book is primarily concerned with reviewing the more common and typical etiologies. The scope here is therefore limited to the rotational and frontal plane deformities of the lower leg and a review of the osteochondroses that may present in this area. The author would encourage the reader to review in other texts tibial and fibular epiphyseal fractures and tumors of the lower leg to provide a well rounded education.

Tibio-Fibular Torsion

"Torsion" has been described as a twist in a bone which will ultimately affect the positional alignment. Investigators have discussed and speculated on the effects of the torsion in the tibia and the fibula for years.[1,2,4,6–11,13–15,18–20,24,25,27–30] Most seem to agree, within certain parameters, that there may exist an abnormal torque in the shaft of the fibula and/or tibia that in turn can affect the gait of a child. There also seems to be an agreement that an infant at birth will present with a certain degree of torsion in either or both the tibia and fibula which will progress normally through a series of stages of torsional rotations to an adult value of normal.

At birth there is found, clinically, minimal torsional rotation in these bones with zero degrees being most frequent. Infants can vary from this by 5–10° internally or externally and still be considered within the normal range. As the child develops, there appears to be a rotation externally with values of 10–15° found by age 1–2 years. Adult values are reached by 5–7 years of 20–30° of external rotation (**Figure 87A**).

Clinicians and investigators have found that values less than those most frequently encountered at a given age level will cause a child to present with an in-toeing gait during ambulation. If a significant reduction from the normal values of external rotation is found, or an internally rotated malleolar position measured from zero degrees (frontal plane) is present, then a more evident malpositioning internally of the limb will be noted. As the child grows older,

125

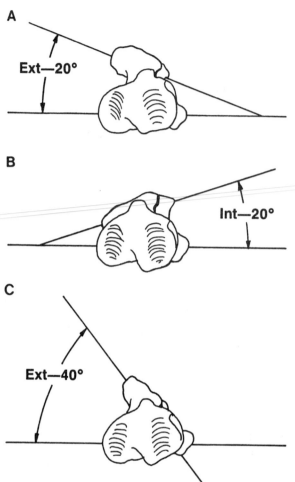

A

Ext—20°

B

Int—20°

C

Ext—40°

Figure 87   Tibial torsion.

(A) *Normal adult values of approximately 20° of external tibial torsion.* (B) *Abnormal internal tibial torsion with the fibular malleolus being anterior to the tibial malleolus.* (C) *Abnormal external tibial torsion exceeding the normal 20–30° expected for an adult value.*

this will either correct itself or there will be less evidence of an in-toeing gait abnormality through adaptation and compensation. If abnormal torsion is persistent, compensatory changes usually will result producing a straighter gait pattern. This may include greater external femoral position, external knee position, and pronation of the foot to achieve this more accepted gait.

Excessive *external* torsion of the lower leg may also exist. In this case the child will present with an out-toeing gait pattern. Oftentimes this is considered a more rare finding, yet is still one that must be considered in an abnormally abducted gait.

The author would like to review anatomically the structure of the fibula so there may be a better appreciation and understanding of the theory behind its effect. The fibula structurally has present four surfaces and borders, which when viewed from proximal to distal actually rotate. The rotation of this bone is external. The fibula also forms the ankle joint mortise which directs the position of the foot by the talar position. In newborns we accept no torsion as being present in the tibia and fibula normally. As the child grows and develops, an external rotation or torque is proposed to occur in these bony components. Both leg bones are to be considered due to the presence of rotation in the fibula as well as the tibia. Though it is often referred to as *tibial torsion*, the fibula is a critical component in the total picture.

The tibia will rotate in development causing the transverse axis of its distal segment to be external to the axis of the proximal segment. The tibial and fibular malleolus will increase or decrease this external position depending on its relative position and rotation. The foot, being locked in the ankle mortise of the tibial and fibular malleolus, follows the direction of the malleolar axis.

Too often tibio-fibular torsion is used exclusively as a diagnosis for an in-toeing or out-toeing gait. Though it may play a role in the overall picture, in itself it may only be a small entity. In order for an abnormal torsion of the tibia and fibula to be a singular cause for in-toeing or out-toeing, it would necessitate being more excessive than is usually and frequently found. More often there are other factors to be considered. Discussed in Chapter 5 was *Internal Genicular Position* which causes a rotation of the lower leg inward during periods when the knee joint is unlocked. The overpowering or contracted musculature causing internal rotation of the leg at the knee area would ultimately place the malleolar axis substantially more inward than would be present in the bony attitude alone (**Figure 88**). If an examiner did not account for this, the measured tibio-fibular torsion would be significantly excessive to

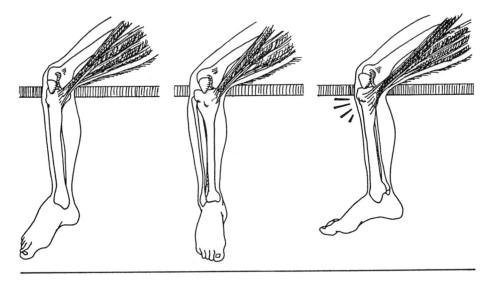

Figure 88

The medial musculature attaching to the tibia will internally rotate the lower leg and secondarily provide an appearance of internal tibio-fibular position. These contractures exist in internal genicular position.

the actual bony torsion, particularly in cases when the child's knee was flexed in examination. Unfortunately, this flexed knee position is the more commonly used position for evaluation than any other method. It has been argued that in using the tibial tuberosity one will negate any knee joint rotational effect. This becomes extremely subjective with the exact placement of the tibial tuberosity. Additionally, the degree of error in placing it exactly on the frontal plane becomes significant and does not ultimately take into account the fibular position. A small amount of rotation proximally will cause a considerable amount of change in direction distally. This principle holds true for any long bone from a metatarsal to a femur.

With excessive external tibio-fibular torsion, several areas must be considered. Congenitally, the tibia and fibula may rotate beyond what is the acceptable norm and cause the child to ambulate in an abducted attitude. More often, however, the cause is an excessive femoral antetorsion or possibly a complication from a poorly managed tibial fracture that caused the external tibio-fibular positioning. With excessive femoral antetorsion, the distal femoral segment is rotated internally when the hip is in its neutral position. This internal position of the femur causes a relative external position of the lower leg and produces an apparently high degree of external tibio-fibular torsion compensatorily. More appropriately, this results in a higher external malleolar axis. Though the torsion may be normal within the bony components of the leg, measurably it would result in an excessive external torsion due to the femur's relative position. This concept must be understood before instituting any type of treatment program.

Clinical Evaluation

Measurement of true tibio-fibular torsion in a child is difficult. One would need to accurately determine an exacting axis for both the proximal and distal segments and angularly relate the two. In cadaveric specimens, pins can be placed through the bony structures to provide analysis of this rotation. Clinically this is virtually impossible and therefore requires a less sophisticated means of determination with the possible usage of radiologic studies. Many instruments have been devised and offered ranging from the very sophisticated as described by Wynn Davis, Khermosh, Levi, and Weissman, to the goniometer and finally the mere use of your hands and eyes to determine the degree of rotation.[10] Unfortunately, most instruments used in an office situation are not sophisticated enough to overcome their inherent errors. They can result in considerable inaccuracies in measurement and are just as well to be forgotten. This author has found, after attempting to try most methods, that the use of your fingers and eyes are as closely accurate as needed for clinical use.

To employ this method, have the child lie supine on a table with his knees fully extended. Attempt to place the femoral condyles and tibia on the frontal plane. Remember, the tibia is locked in position at the knee joint when fully extended. If one finds the tibial tuberosity and the anterior border of the tibia and places it parallel to the sagittal plane of the body, this will be as close to accurate as possible (**Figure 89**). By imagining a protractor behind the ankle, estimate the number of degrees the malleolar axis deviates from 0°. This will give an approximate but reasonably accurate value of tibio-fibular rotation. It has been found that malleolar position is approximately 5° greater than would be found by actual bony measurements in cadavers (**Figure 90**). *Note:* If one measures tibio-fibular torsion with a knee flexed position, soft-tissue rotational factors cannot be eliminated, i.e., *internal genicular position.* Therefore, if a knee flexed position is being used for torsion evaluation, the trans-malleolar axis may be rotated substantially inward and measured as such when the actual torsion is normal in the bony segments. This error would affect the course and mode of treatment.

Radiologically, several methods have been proposed to determine the degree of torsion present in the tibia and fibula. It appears that the method proposed by Hutter and Scott is the one most widely accepted by the investigators and clinicians.[9] This method positions the child so that the knees are flexed over the edge of a table. The feet are placed and positioned on an x-ray cassette with the medial surface of the foot parallel to the sagittal plane and the medial surface of the thigh. The x-ray tube is positioned over the knee with the beam being parallel to the long axis of the tibia. A properly exposed plate will show the malleoli and rear foot clearly. To determine the amount of rotation, draw a line between the medial and lateral tips of the malleoli. A second line is drawn at right angles to the knee joint axis on the film. The intersection of the two lines creates an angle which when subtracted from 90° would give an approximate amount of torsion present (**Figure 91**). This method

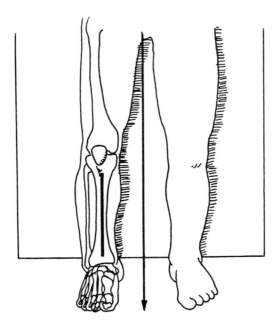

Figure 89

Use the tibial tuberosity and the anterior border of the tibia to place the leg along and parallel to the sagittal plane. This position, with the knee extended and locked, is necessary for an accurate evaluation of tibio-fibular torsion.

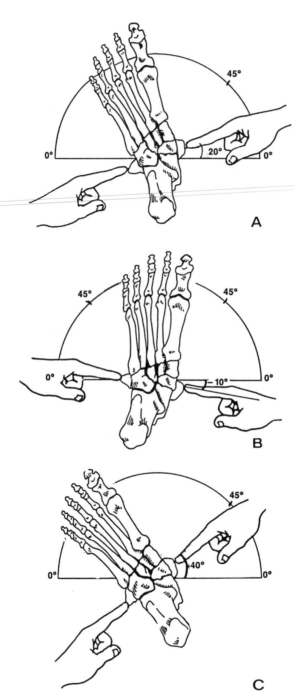

Figure 90

By placing your fingers as shown, you can estimate the approximate number of degrees of rotation inward or outward of the tibio-fibular axis. (A) Normal external tibio-fibular torsion of 20°. (B) Abnormal internal tibio-fibular torsion of (−)10°. (C) Abnormal external tibio-fibular torsion of 40°.

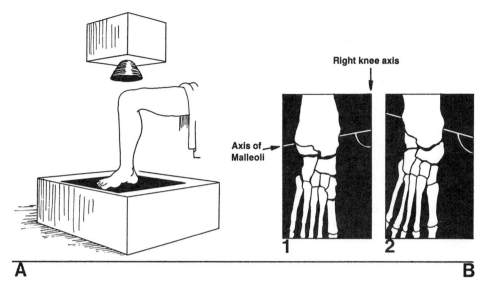

Figure 91

(A) *To determine the tibio-fibular torsion radiographically, place the foot on the film with the medial surface of the foot parallel to the sagittal plane. The x-ray head should be positioned over the knee so the beam will parallel the long axis of the tibia. (B) A line is passed thru the tibio-fibular malleolus and a second line is drawn at right angles to the knee joint axis. The angle created is subtracted from 90° to determine the amount of rotation. (1) shows internal tibio-fibular torsion while (2) represents normal external torsion.*

allows for a considerable degree of error in two respects. First, the knee joint is unlocked and is therefore influenced by the soft tissue surrounding it as in *internal genicular position.* Second, the arbitrary attempt at placing a line at right angles to the knee joint axis is fraught with subjective discretion and therefore error. This author would discourage the use of radiographic interpretation for determination of tibio-fibular torsion.

Treatment

Researchers have shown that to treat and alter a torsion in a long bone is next to impossible and therefore not currently feasible. In a paper by Moreland, it was concluded that forces necessary to be exerted on the epiphyseal structure of the tibia to alter its position was of such magnitude that it was not possible clinically to reproduce in humans.[15] His experimentation utilized rabbit epiphyses to determine torsional changes with castings. He had stated in his conclusion that a rabbit's epiphysis is significantly smaller in diameter than an 8-month-old child and that development in the bone of a rabbit is far more rapid in rate than that of a child. Therefore, to be capable of applying a load force necessary to cause any alteration in the torsion was beyond the clinical capabilities of any methods or devices known and presently being employed. Moreland further stated that a torsional load along the long axis of a bone will produce a rotational modeling only if the epiphysis is fixed and securely held. This would then allow the rotational load to be placed across the growth plate. Unfortunately, the splinting type devices currently in use, i.e., twister cables, rotational castings, etc., are unable to fixate the epiphysis and metaphysis separately to allow the forces to be directed to the epiphyseal plate.

It can be concluded from this study that the treatments being employed presently are not in effect altering the torsion of a bone, but rather rotating and stretching the ligamentous and/or tendinous elements at either or both ends of the bone. In the discussion of *internal genicular position* (Chapter 5) the treatment of stretch castings was utilized to properly align the knee joint area. This author feels that an abnormal external or internal rotation of the knee is being created with the use of rotational casting for tibio-fibular torsional abnormalities. This is due to the forces actually being exerted to the knee joint level. Caution and discouragement should be considered if one is attempting treatment for a true tibio-fibular torsion problem *only*.

Internal Tibio-Fibular Torsion

The proper rationale in treatment of internal tibio-fibular torsion (internal malleolar torsion) is for correction of any surrounding soft-tissue contractions, i.e., internal genicular position, followed by proper control of the foot to avoid compensatory alterations. As mentioned in the section on *internal genicular position*, casting is indicated to properly stretch and maintain a neutral knee joint position. Very often there is a coexistence of a torsional and soft-tissue abnormality. A proper evaluation and determination of the contribution of both is necessary for treatment. Remember, the casting or splinting is only being employed to stretch the soft-tissue abnormalities and is not affecting the actual torsion in the bone.

Orthotic therapy is utilized to not only support and avoid compensation in the joint structures of the foot but to stimulate a more normal walking pattern as well. Gravitational downward forces on a foot in an inwardly positioned attitude will result in collapse of the mid and rearfoot joint architecture to provide a more central position of gravity (**Figure 92**). These changes in architecture are ultimately sacrificing one abnormality for another. The goal in orthotic treatment is to avoid these changes until development and correction of the rotational abnormality can be accomplished. The use of an out-toeing orthosis provides two results: maintains joint alignment of the foot, and stimulates an outward walking pattern. A type D heel stabilizer, Reverse Roberts' plate, or gait plate will all essentially accomplish a similar result (**Figure 93**). The need for a good quality shoe with a stiff counter and flexible sole is important to produce proper function of the orthosis. Shoe wedging is of limited use and value due to its inability to effectively control the foot and

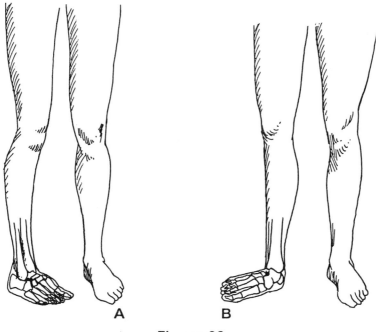

Figure 92

An internal rotational problem will place the center of gravity over the lateral aspect of the foot as in (A). Compensation occurs by collapsing the joint structures of the foot to produce more abduction and therefore a more centrally placed center of gravity (B).

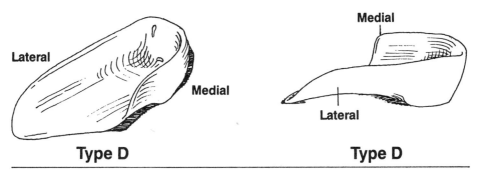

Figure 93

A type D heel stabilizer will forcibly direct the foot outwardly but will support the rearfoot to maintain subtalar position. It works very well in younger children until about the age of 8–10 years. For information on the Reverse Roberts' and gait plates please see Chapter 13 on orthoses.

the fact that it wears down rather quickly. The use of heavy awkward orthopedic type shoes is also of little value and can emotionally affect the child with respect to his appearance and the resulting peer pressures. It should be understood that any type of out-toe wedgings on shoes ultimately gains results from forcibly pronating the foot structure. Thus a collapsed and pronated foot will be the result of treatment of a rotational deformity with wedging and should be avoided at any cost.

External Tibio-Fibular Torsion

When treating an external torsional problem, the desired goal is for protection of the foot and leg structures. With an outward rotation of the leg, the downward force on the limb is medial (**Figure 94**). In time, the medial joint structures of the knee, ankle, and foot can all be affected. The bony torsion cannot be altered, as was mentioned previously, so treatment must be directed toward the correction of any soft-tissue abnormalities and protection of the foot–ankle. In the rare case of *external genicular position*, rotational castings would stretch the contractures and properly align the lower leg.

The foot–ankle is best controlled by the use of an orthotic device to avoid the medial stress not only on the foot–ankle, but on the knee joint as well. Several types are available that will all functionally work well to protect. A type E heel stabilizer will accomplish two goals, i.e., support and control the

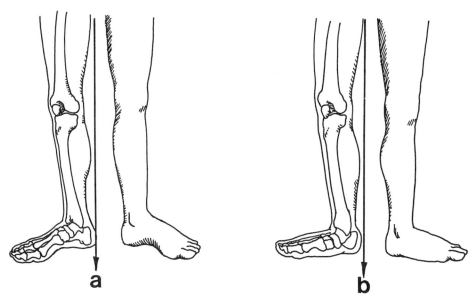

a   b

Figure 94

With an external torsion abnormality the center of gravity will exert its forces medially in the foot–ankle complex as in (A). Over a period of time the joint structures will weaken and collapse as a result of this concentrated stress (B).

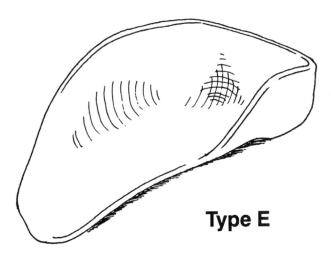

Type E

Figure 95

A Type E heel stabilizer is essentially the mirror image of a Type D. The long medial flange supports and forcibly supinates the foot. This will cause an in-toeing effect in gait. See Chapter 13 for further details on a Type E heel stabilizer as well as the others listed for control of an out-toeing gait problem.

medial side of the foot–ankle and stimulate an in-toeing gait. Others, including the functional, Shaffer plate, pronated orthotic, Whitman and Roberts' plates, will all support but do not stimulate the same degree of in-toeing in gait as does the type E heel stabilizer (**Figure 95**).

Orthotic control for either in-toeing or out-toeing gait abnormalities should be continued for a period of 2–5 years after the deformity has resolved itself. In cases where total resolution is not accomplished, then continued use of orthotic control should be encouraged for proper function and prevention.

Tibia Varum–Tibia Valgum

Tibia varum is a disorder in the long axis of the bone which results in a bowing or varusing toward the midline of the body causing a bowlegged deformity (**Figure 96**). One should use caution when differentiating tibia varum from genu varum. In Chapter 5 genu varum and the etiology and natural history were discussed. It was learned in this section that a child will normally pass through a stage of genu varum in infancy to a stage of genu valgum in early childhood and finally a rectus position in mid-childhood. Genu varum will similarly produce an appearance of bowleggedness as does the condition of *tibia varum*.

In early infancy a child will often present with both a genu varum and a tibia varum. As the child begins ambulation and weight stress is exerted on the knees and lower leg, both of these conditions will improve normally. Cases of persistence of the varus attitude in the tibia beyond the normal stages of development warrant a consideration for a disease process contributing to the cause. These can include rickets, Blount's disease, metaphyseal dysostosis, or asymmetric growth of either the tibial or femoral physes possibly as a consequence of either trauma or sepsis.[3,16,23,28,29] Tibia valgum is a rare finding

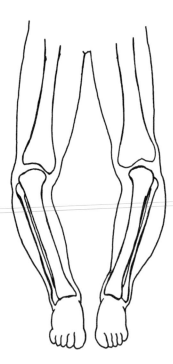

Figure 96

Tibia varum *is the result of abnormal growth caus-ing the lateral portion of the tibia to exceed the me-dial portion.*

and is most frequently the result of injury to the epiphysis or malunion of a tibial fracture.

Rickets

Although rickets has not recently been a prevalent cause for tibia varum, it nonetheless needs consideration if a suspected history is elicited. There are primarily three causes of rickets:

- There is a deficiency in the intake of vitamin D. This cause is unlikely to be very prevalent, since vitamin D is produced whenever a person is in sunlight as well as being a product of many foods. Vitamin D deficiency is usually only seen in the child who has severe malnutrition and has been deprived of sunlight, as could occur, for example, in an inner city ghetto.
- One's body does not incorporate the exogenous vitamin D and it is excreted without absorption. This might be found in cases of sprue syndrome. Diarrhea will cause a rapid loss of fat, and vitamin D is a fat-soluble vitamin. This will result in excretion of the vitamin without absorption.
- An improper supply of the active form of vitamin D to the bones will cause a rachitic syndrome. This may be found in children with renal disease and occasionally in cases of impaired liver function.

Radiographic evaluation will exhibit a widening of the metaphyses of the bones. This will take on the appearance of being mushroom-like. The reason for this appearance is the absence of proper calcification of the osteoid bone, which is formed from the cartilage cells.[3,23]

Treatment is primarily directed to supplementation with vitamin D. Proper control and protection of the limbs are important due to the long-term sequelae of a rachitic deformity, one of which is significant degenerative arthritis.

Blount's Disease (Tibia Vara, Osteochondrosis Deformans Tibiae)

This is an abnormality that is the result of a growth disturbance of the medial aspect of the proximal tibial epiphysis (**Figure 97**). Its occurrence may be either unilateral or bilateral and can affect either males or females. There are two types or stages in which this condition may present, i.e., *infantile* or *adolescent* type. The *infantile type* will present itself somewhere between 12–16 months of life. Characteristic findings are a chubby child who has walked early (7–9 months) and is very active, as related by the parents. The etiology of this disorder may be in the fact that the child had begun walking at an early age. With this early ambulation and weight, there would result an excessive degree of pressure on the physis resulting in secondary destruction. Since the physis may not yet be capable of handling the body weight exerted, the result would be a decrease in growth on the medial aspect from the physis damage.

In the *adolescent type*, the deformity manifests itself some time between 8–13 years of age. The occurrence is usually unilateral although it may present

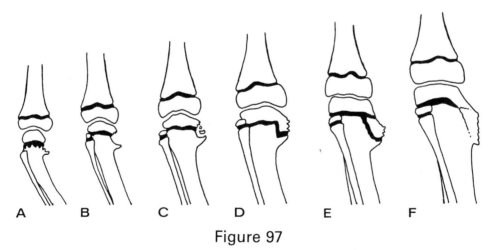

A   B   C   D   E   F

Figure 97

The various stages of Blount's disease is shown from A–F. Eventual loss of the medial epiphyseal growth results in overgrowth of the lateral portion and a varus of the tibia. Early signs are beaking of the metaphyseal area with fragmentation. Fusion (F) is the end result of the medial epiphysis.

bilaterally. This type is much more difficult to treat effectively due to the latent destruction and limited period of remaining growth.[21,28,29]

Heredity, in many cases, is the primary etiology with a familial incidence existing in siblings. When examined clinically, one may be able to palpate a bony beaking on the medial side of the metaphysis of the tibia. This prominence is usually painless but is an important sign in diagnosis. One may also note an internal leg position and pronation in the foot concomitantly. Radiographically, there is seen in the early stages only an irregularity in the physis with possibly some beaking of the physis. As the deformity and stages progress, one notes more beaking and sloping of the physis with an eventual encroachment of the epiphysis onto the metaphysis until it is totally down on the metaphysis as shown in **Figure 97**.

Treatment becomes dependent on the age of the child and degree of deformity. In the early stages one must differentiate from a normal developmental genu varum. When a child completes the transitional stage of normal development from genu varum to genu valgum (2–6 years), one will be able to make the distinction. The obvious persistence of a varus deformity would lead the examiner to investigate the presence of a Blount's disease.

When correctly diagnosed, this condition oftentimes necessitates a tibial osteotomy to relocate and align the leg in severe deformities. Tachdjian finds it advantageous to treat this condition prior to age 8 years or even earlier if one notes a rapid progression of the problem.[28]

The use of orthotic control is important in maintaining the pronated foot and in shifting the gravitational forces away from the medial growth center. Realizing that a chubby child, with a history of early ambulation, has a greater propensity toward this deformity, one should protect and hopefully avoid the medial stress and damage on the physis by controlling the mechanics of the leg–foot with an orthosis. Type B or C heel stabilizers, a Whitman or Roberts' plate are all beneficial in producing proper control.

Osgood–Schlatter Disease

This disorder has evaded researchers in its true etiology. Several theories have been proposed including: vascular damage, traumatic avulsion of the cartilage, systemic disease, endocrinopathy, and structural changes in the tendon insertion. The theory most accepted at present is an avulsion of a portion of the developing ossification center and overlying hyaline cartilage. This fibrocartilagenous growth plate appears to be a structural adaptation to prevent avulsion of the tibial tuberosity away from the anterior tibial metaphysis.[17,28,29]

Radiographically, one sees what appears to be an avulsed area of bone at the tibial tuberosity (**Figure 98**).

Clinically there will be a palpable bump in this area, which is usually painful on compression. The occurrence of this condition is usually in late childhood and early adolescence (10–14 years). It most often has affected males but with the emergence of female athletes, the frequency is equalizing.

Treatment becomes dependent on the age and degree of pain. In younger children advice in avoiding any excessive flexion of the knee is important. For example, if a child was a catcher on a baseball team, it would be advised to switch to a position that would minimize running and bending of the knees. The avoidance of kneeling is also beneficial in relieving irritation to the tibial tuberosity. In cases presenting with a significant protuberance at the tibial tuberosity with impaired activity, a surgical repair of the area may be indicated. This should not be considered until the physis has completely closed.

Oftentimes biomechanical control of the foot–leg structure is extremely advantageous. This reduces the rotation of the tibia and thus reduces the degree of pull of the patellar tendon at its insertion at the tibial tuberosity. This is accomplished by an orthotic device specifically constructed to accomplish this result. Control of the foot–leg should be in conjunction with the other aforementioned suggestions of reduced knee flexion and altered activities.

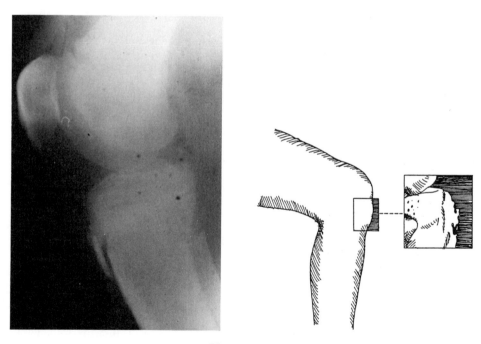

Figure 98

A protuberance at the tibial tuberosity is characteristic of an Osgood–Schlatter's disease. The insert depicts the radiographic appearance with fragmentation and hypertrophic bone.

References

1. Blumel, J., Eggers, G.W.N., Evans, B.: Eight cases of hereditary bilateral medial tibial torsion in four generations. *Journal of Bone and Joint Surgery*, Volume 39-A, 1957.
2. Elftman, H.: Torsion of the lower extremity. *American Journal Physicians Anthropology*, Volume 3, 1945.
3. Fendrick, G.M.: Would you miss the diagnosis of bowlegs? *Modern Medicine*, June 30–July 15, 1979.
4. Ganley, J.V.: Interpretation and management of leg rotation and torsion. Unpublished paper.
5. Graver, H.H.: Cylinder casting: A serial casting technique for rotational and triplane deformities. *J.A.P.A.*, 66:Number 4, April 1976.
6. Haas, M.: A brace for correction of torsion of lower extremities. *Journal of Bone and Joint Surgery*, 40-A:1958.
7. Harris, E.J.: Rotational deformities in infants and young children. Unpublished paper.
8. Hensinger, R.N.: Rotational problems of the lower extremity. *Post-graduate Medicine*, 60:4, October, 1976.
9. Hutter, C.G.: Tibial torsion. *Journal of Bone and Joint Surgery*, 31-A:1949.
10. Khermosh, O.: Tibial torsion in children. *Clinical Orthopaedics and Related Research*, Number 79, September 1971.
11. Kite, J.H.: Torsion of the legs in young children. *Clinical Orthopaedics*, Number 16, 1960.
12. Lichtblau, P.O., Waxman, B.A.: Blount's disease: Review of the literature and description of a new surgical procedure. *Contemp. Orthopedics*, 3:1981.
13. McCollough, N.C., et al: Experimental production of tibial torsion and its clinical relevance. Orthopaedic transactions. *Journal of Bone and Joint Surgery*, Pediatric Orthopaedic Society, 4:1, Spring 1980.
14. McDonough, M.W.: Fetal positioning as a cause of right and left-sided foot and leg disorders. *J.A.P.A.*, 21:2, February 1981.
15. Moreland, M.S.: Morphological effects of torsion applied to growing bone. *Journal of Bone and Joint Surgery*, 62-B:May 1980.
16. Nicholson, J.: Longitudinal osteotomy of the tibia, operative technique. *Journal of Bone and Joint Surgery*, 39-B:1957.
17. Ogden, J.A., Southwick, W.O.: Osgood–Schlatter's disease and tibial tuberosity development. *Clinical Orthopaedics and Related Research*, Number 116, May 1976.
18. Ritter, M.A.: Tibial torsion. *Clinical Orthopaedics and Related Research*, Number 120, October 1976.
19. Rosen, H., Sandick, H.: The measurement of tibio-fibular torsion. *Journal of Bone and Joint Surgery*, 37-A:1955.
20. Schoenhaus, H.D., Poss, K.D.: The clinical and practical aspects in treating torsional problems in children, *Journal of the American Podiatry Association*, 67:Number 9, September 1977.
21. Sevastikoglou, J.A., Eriksson, I.: Familial infantile osteochondrosis deformans tibia. Idiopathic tibia vara. *Acta Orthopedica Scandinavia*, 38:1967.
22. Sgarlato, T.E.: *A Compendium of Podiatric Biomechanics*. California College of Podiatric Medicine, 1971.
23. Sheridan, R.M., Chiroff, R.T., Friedman, E.M.: Operative and non-operative treatment of rachitic lower extremity deformities. *Clinical Orthopaedics and Related Research*, Number 116, May 1976.
24. Staheli, L.T.: Torsional deformities and normal variations in children's lower limbs. *Orthopaedic Transactions (J.B.J.S.)*—Pediatric Orthopaedic Society, 4:Number 1, Spring 1980.

25. Staheli, L.T., Engel, G.M.: Tibial torsion, a new method of assessment and a survey of normal children. *Clinical Orthopaedics and Related Research*, Number 86, 1972.
26. Statham, L., Murray, M.P.: Early walking patterns of normal children. *Clinical Orthopaedics and Related Research*, Number 79, September 1971.
27. Swanson, A.B., Greene, P.W., and Allis, H.D.: Rotational deformities of the lower extremity in children and their significance. *Clinical Orthopedics and Related Research*, 27:1963.
28. Tachdjian, M.O.: *Pediatric Orthopedics*, Volume 2. W.B. Saunders Co., Philadelphia, PA, 1972.
29. Tax, H.R.: *Podopediatrics*. Williams and Wilkins Co., Baltimore, MD, 1980.
30. Weseley, M.S., Barenfeld, P.A., Eisenstein, A.L.: Thoughts on in-toeing and out-toeing: Twenty years' experience with over 5,000 cases and a review of the literature. *Foot and Ankle*, 2:Number 1, 1981.

Chapter 7

EXAMINATION OF THE ANKLE

The podiatric physician should be aware of not only the deformities and abnormalities that arise in the foot and ankle, but also their effects on the superstructure. The contents of this chapter will encompass the more frequent manifestations occurring in the foot–ankle and their relationship to the rest of the limb structure. We realize that an error in the structure or mechanics of the foot will often ultimately cause changes in the lower leg, knees, hips and/or lower back. Conversely, changes in the superstructure (hip, knees, lower leg) will affect the mechanics of the foot. Therefore, careful consideration is paramount in determining the exact etiology and its secondary effects.

Ankle

Several disorders may frequently manifest in the ankle joint area of a child including: aseptic necrosis of the talus, rheumatic disease (i.e., juvenile rheumatoid arthritis and rheumatic fever), osteomyelitis, epiphyseal fractures, tumors, ball and socket ankle joint, and ankle valgus.[3,5,8,10–13]

Aseptic Necrosis of the Talus (Diaz Disease)

This is a rare condition that is often associated with direct trauma to the talus bone. A fall or rapid hyperextension or flexion of the ankle joint may result in sufficient damage to the talus to cause a necrotic destruction to occur. This condition is self limiting. The talus will return to its normal shape and configuration after sufficient time for healing. Protection to the talus with a walking cast or with nonweight-bearing by crutch walking is beneficial during the restructuring period; orthotic control of the foot is advantageous as a follow-up once normal weight-bearing has been regained.[2,7,9,13]

Juvenile Rheumatoid Arthritis (Still's disease)

The manifestation of this disease is frequently found either around the age of 6 years or at the onset of puberty, although it can occur at any time. The knees and ankles are the two most common areas afflicted. The child will commonly present with an antalgic gait resulting from the painful joint(s). Persistent fever and a skin rash with little joint involvement may also occur. The skin rash usually appears as salmon-pink maculae increasing in size and area with the fever and/or trauma. Laboratory tests will aid in confirming the diagnosis. Treatment is best managed by a rheumatologist due to the long-term effects of the disease.

Rheumatic Fever

A history of an upper respiratory tract infection with Group A beta-hemolytic streptococcus along with a poor environmental surrounding is the etiology of this condition. Many times the only manifestation noted is a transient swelling, with or without accompanying pain, of the joints, including the ankles. Frequently a successive pattern is followed of the joints affected. First the knees will be affected, then the ankles. This is followed by the shoulders, wrist, elbows, hips, and feet in successive order. With the subsiding of symptoms in one joint area, there is usually a manifestation in the successive joint area. Early treatment is important to avoid the secondary valvular damage to the heart that may accompany this disease process.

Osteomyelitis

Several types of osteomyelitis may manifest itself in the ankle joint including: pyogenic, tuberculosis, syphilitic, mycotic, and viral. Symptoms often include swelling, erythema, tenderness, and calor of the joints with the possibility of concomitant throbbing pain over the joint site. The medical history, laboratory tests, and radiological findings are needed to help make an accurate diagnosis and follow with proper treatment.

Epiphyseal Fractures

The ankle bones, as well as any other epiphyseal bone in the body, are subject to a classification of fractures referred to as the Salter–Harris Classification.[8] There are five types within this classification. Each type holds its own prognostic results (**Figure 99**).

> *Type 1.* A separation or fracture through the growth plate occurs between the epiphysis and metaphysis. With proper reduction there

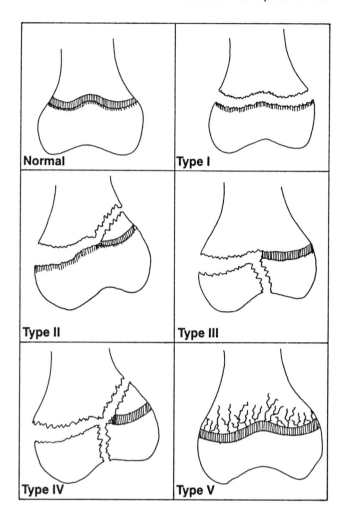

Figure 99

Type I—*Fracture occurs through the epiphyseal plate only. No involvement occurs at the epiphysis or metaphysis.* Type II—*Fracture exists through the epiphyseal plate and through a portion of the metaphysis.* Type III—*The epiphyseal plate and the epiphysis is fractured in this type. The fracture line will pass into the joint space.* Type IV—*A fracture will occur through the epiphyseal plate, metaphysis, and epiphysis extending into the joint space.* Type V—*This type is the result of a compression or crush injury to the epiphysis, metaphysis, and epiphyseal plate.*

will result an excellent prognosis for future growth provided the blood supply to the epiphysis is adequately intact.

Type 2. The fracture line passes through the growth plate and also through a portion of the metaphysis. With adequate closed reduction and a good blood supply to the epiphysis, an excellent prognosis can be anticipated.

Type 3. The fracture line in this type will pass through the growth plate, through the epiphysis and into the joint. Treatment usually requires an open reduction with a fair to good prognosis if proper blood supply is available.

Type 4. This fracture will extend from the joint through the epiphysis, growth plate, and metaphysis. Open reduction with fixation is necessary and sometimes very difficult. The prognosis is usually poor unless a perfect reduction is achieved.

Type 5. This is a crush-type fracture with comminution of the affected structures. This type of injury most often will result in a cessation of growth in the area and a poor prognosis.

The recognition of these fracture types is particularly important in evaluating an injured child. The *Type 1* fracture is probably the most frequently missed on initial screening due to the absence of conclusive radiographic findings with standard views. If a fracture is suspected, a stress view of the area is necessary to determine the separation through the growth center. Without proper reduction and treatment of these fracture types, a significant alteration of the structural and positional function will result.[1,6,8,11]

Tumors

Realizing that several benign and malignant tumors may arise in the bony or soft-tissue structures of the ankle, we refer the reader to a text in which each type is analyzed completely.[8,11,12]

Ball-and-Socket Ankle Joint

A ball-and-socket ankle joint may either result from a congenital anomaly or be acquired from iatrogenic causes. Congenitally, it has been found in short extremities, congenital absence or hypoplasia of the fibula, and in congenital fusions of the rearfoot joints. Iatrogenic causes include surgical fusions of the hindfoot at an early age, which force the ankle joint to adapt to motions previously absorbed in the hindfoot. The ball-and-socket ankle joint has also been experienced in children with insensitive feet as a result of a spinal cord injury or a congenital neurologic defect. This type of joint not only allows for sagittal plane motion (dorsiflexion and plantarflexion) but also transverse and frontal plane movement. This produces a reasonable degree of instability resulting in chronic ankle sprains and arthritic changes. In the congenital type, the talus will usually have a more smooth and rounded dome, in comparison to the acquired type. The acquired variety frequently is accompanied by greater abnormal laxity of the ligaments surrounding the ankle joint. The basic underlying cause for this deformity is a limitation of subtalar joint motion.

This deformity is found infrequently and is usually asymptomatic. The abnormal lateral mobility of the ankle may cause frequent ankle sprains and result in a weakness of the joint. Secondary ankle joint arthritis may ensue in adult life due to the excessive stress on the joint. Fusion of this joint is indicated if these secondary problems manifest themselves.[3,5,11,12]

Ankle Valgus

This condition has been offered as one cause for pes-valgo-planus deformity of the foot. Though rare, this deformity can be considered a secondary etiology

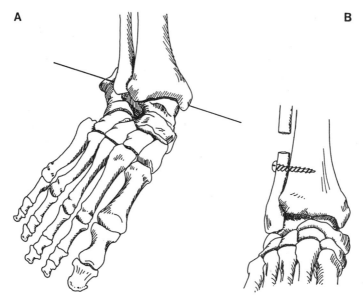

Figure 100

(A) Ankle valgus will result from the fibula, and therefore the lateral malleolus, not being capable of maintaining lateral stability of the ankle due to its shortening. The motion in the ankle will not only allow dorsi and plantarflexion but also eversion and abduction. (B) Correction of the shortened fibula can be accomplished by either a fibula graft to lengthen the bone or as this figure depicts, a fusion of the fibula to the tibia with proper alignment of the ankle mortise.

for pes-valgo-planus. An ankle valgus abnormality will result from either a congenitally short fibula causing elevation of the lateral malleolus, or an acquired form as a result of: a fibular fracture improperly reduced; a segment removed from the fibula for bone grafting; unequal growth of the tibial epiphysis, etc.[4,10,11] If this defect exists, a surgical correction to produce adequate stability to the ankle is necessary. This can be accomplished by grafting new bone into the void or by fusion of the fibula to the tibia in a corrected position (**Figure 100 A and B**).

Equinus

Several types and degrees of equinus may exist in children and adults. A brief highlight of each will better prepare the examiner for a proper distinction. Equinus can be defined as limitation of dorsiflexion of the foot at the ankle joint when the subtalar joint is held in a neutral position. The limitation of dorsiflexion may occur while the knee joint is fully extended, flexed, or both, depending on the cause. Anatomically, the gastrocnemius muscle has its origin above the knee joint while the soleus muscle originates below this joint. To differentiate the effects of these two muscles, the knee joint should be flexed and extended when examining ankle range of motion (**Figure 101**). With the knee joint flexed, the soleus muscle is under physiological tension while the gastrocnemius muscle is in a relaxed loosened state. Conversely, with the knee in an extended position, the gastrocnemius muscle will also assume tension and affect the amount of dorsiflexion at the ankle. With the foot held in a neutral subtalar position with maximum midtarsal pronation, the ankle range of motion should be determined with both a flexed and extended knee joint. Traditionally, greater than 10° of dorsiflexion was considered necessary for normal foot–ankle–leg gait. This is measured from a neutral foot position and the foot–leg at 90° (**Figure 101**). The amount of dorsiflexion necessary is still controversial. More recently there is an acceptance of a minimum of 5–7° for adequate function without significantly affecting the mechanics of the foot and leg motion. Clinically, several conditions may present themselves depending on the severity of the equinus. Toe-walking is frequently seen as a result of limited dorsiflexion. Toe-walking, however, can be a normal aberrant developmental finding without equinus being demonstrable. Compensatory changes will result from an equinus state including subtalar joint pronation, abduction of the entire foot to reduce the need for ankle dorsiflexion, early heel off, genu recurvatum in the more severe cases, and knee flexion during gait to reduce tension on the gastrocnemius muscle.[2,5,6,8,10,11]

Classification of Equinus

CONGENITAL EQUINUS

Congenital Gastrocnemius Equinus:
Clinically, this type will exhibit limitation of dorsiflexion at the ankle when the knee joint is extended. Adequate dorsiflexion will exist with a knee flexed attitude. The congenital gastrocnemius equinus is the result of contracture of the muscle prenatally. This type is probably the one most frequently encountered.

Congenital Soleus Equinus:
Dorsiflexion is limited when the knee joint is flexed. If there is adequate length of the gastrocnemius muscle, the limitation of dorsiflexion will be equal with the knee joint both flexed and extended.

Congenital Gastrocnemius–Soleus Equinus:
This combined contracture will exhibit limitation of dorsiflexion at the ankle with the knee joint both flexed and extended. There is usually an increase in the loss of dorsiflexion when the knee is extended as a result of the tight gastrocnemius. The contracted soleus, however, will allow less than 5–7° of dorsiflexion when the knee is flexed.

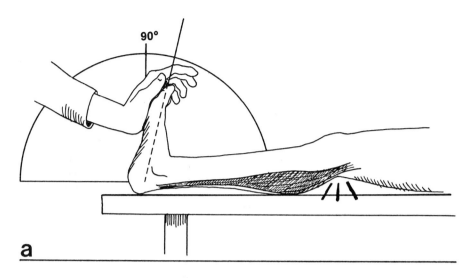

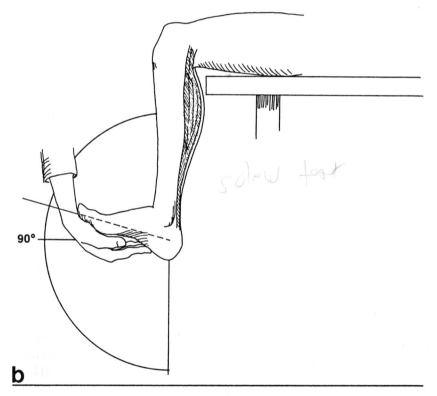

Figure 101

(A) Dorsiflexion with the knee extended will allow evaluation of the gastroc-nemius muscle. 8–15° are considered normal when the foot is held in neutral position. (B) Flexion of the knee will relax the gastrocnemius muscle and allow evaluation of the soleus muscle originating below the knee joint. A discrepancy between the knee flexed and knee extended positions will allow the examiner the ability to determine which muscle group(s) is involved.

Spastic Triceps Surae Equinus:

This type results from a secondary dysfunction as in hyperkinesia from minimal brain damage, diastematomyelia, or spastic paraplegia (cerebral palsy).

The congenital types of equinus outlined will present with a variety of objective findings. These findings will include: a persistent toe-walking gait; genu recurvatum, which will allow the heels to lower themselves to the ground on stance; hypertrophy of the soleus muscle may be noted on palpation; collapse in the subtalar and midtarsal joints of the feet secondary to the muscular contractures; abduction of the entire foot to reduce the need for ankle dorsiflexion; and during gait an early heel-off will be viewed.

The contractures in the musculature are the result of long-standing contractions. The contractures eventually become irreversible when existent for a sufficient period of time. A delay in the maturation of the corticospinal tract in children will cause persistent contractions in these muscles. This most often corrects itself, with the equinus disappearing after approximately 2–5 months. Occasionally, the condition persists up to the ages of 6–8 years. In these cases, proper protection of the feet and legs from the secondary effects of the equinus is very important.

Treatment

Initially, a program of stretching should be attempted to achieve proper motion. The parents should be instructed to hold the foot in a neutral to supinated position and stretch the respective muscle(s) that are contracted. This is accomplished by dorsiflexing the foot and holding for the count of 10 seconds and releasing. Twenty to 30 repetitions several times a day are necessary. It should be stressed to the parents to avoid pronating the foot while performing the exercise. If this occurs, then the motion of dorsiflexion will be at the midtarsal joint of the foot and a stretching of the medial capsule, ligaments, and musculature of the foot will result. A false increase in dorsiflexion will be found due to the pronated foot, allowing the midtarsal and subtalar joints to sublux with lateral joint deviation occurring. One must realize that the sacrificing of one joint or deformity to compensate for another is foolish and should be avoided at all cost.

A second type of treatment that is efficacious is splinting. This will hold the foot–ankle–leg in a neutral 90° position during sleeping periods. This can be manufactured by forming a posterior splint of plaster from the foot to just above the knee joint (**Figure 102A**). The splint can be held in place by an ace wrap and removed during waking hours. If after sufficient time (2–3 months) there is no significant improvement, then the application of a walking cast should be attempted. The cast should be wedged at the anterior of the ankle every two weeks to allow for more dorsiflexion (**Figure 102 B–D**). A second alternative is to remove the cast every two weeks and attempt to apply a new one with greater dorsiflexion. Once adequate dorsiflexion is achieved, the castings can be discontinued. The parents should be instructed to continue with

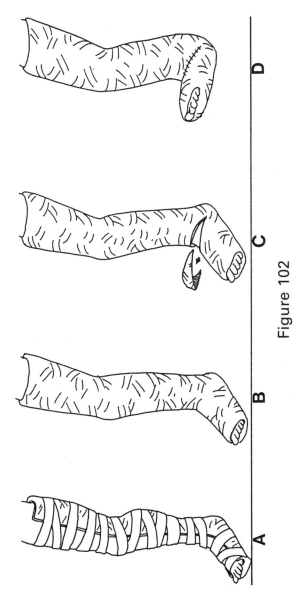

Figure 102

(A) A posterior splint extends above the knee with an ace wrap to stabilize the position. This can be made by applying a full cast and then splitting it and using the posterior segment. This works well during sleeping times to stretch any tight posterior muscles of the lower leg. (B–D) These figures show the presence of an above-the-knee plaster cast with a wedge being removed at the anterior aspect of the ankle to further stretch the posterior muscle groups of the lower leg. Reinforcement after each wedge removal is necessary.

both passive and active stretching of the triceps surae. This is done for several months to avoid recurrence. In children 3–4 years of age or older, stretching can also be accomplished by having them stand with the ball of their foot on the edge of a book at least 2 inches thick (**Figure 103**). Have them lower their heels to the ground and hold for 10 seconds performing this 20–30 times several times a day. Do not allow them to bounce up and down as this will cause the muscle to contract rather than stretch.

When a child has reached the age of 5–7 years and there exists a significant amount of equinus, even after conservative therapy, then surgery may be considered. The congenital gastrocnemius-soleus and soleus equinus are best corrected by the use of a stab slide lengthening of the Achilles tendon (**Figure 104**). This procedure produces minimal scarring, reduces surgical exposure, and provides an earlier recovery and rehabilitation. If, however, the deformity is a congenital gastrocnemius-equinus, then only a lengthening of this muscle is necessary. This can be accomplished by a tongue-in-groove method (**Figure**

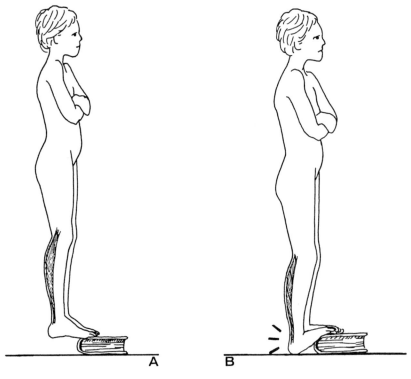

A   B

Figure 103

Stretching of the posterior calf muscles can be accomplished by having the child stand over the edge of a book or step and lower his heels to the ground while keeping his knees straight. One can start with a narrow book or board and move up in thickness as greater stretching occurs.

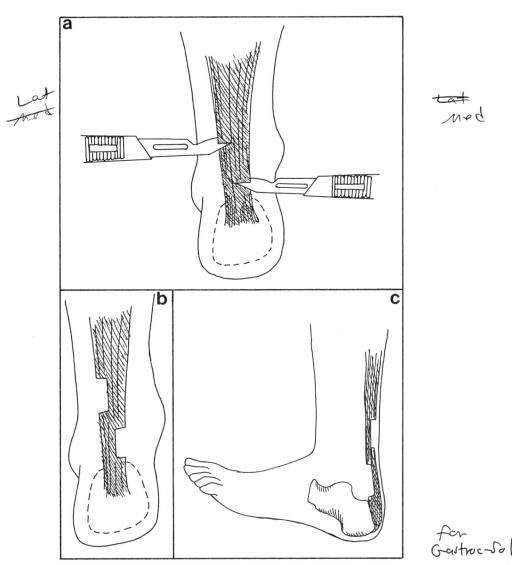

Figure 104   Stab tenotomy of the Achilles tendon.

(A) Using a #15 or #64 blade, a tenotomy of the Achilles tendon can be performed through an initial stab over and lateral to the tendon fibers. Approximately one-half of the tendon is incised. A second incision is then made medially similar to that performed laterally. The two incisions should have approximately 4–8 cm of distance between them to allow adequate lengthening without total separation of the sections. (B) By dorsiflexing the foot, the fibers should glide past one another providing adequate dorsal motion. A void will be noted in the areas where the tendon has separated. (C) This is a side view of the appearance of the tendon after lengthening. The child should be casted for approximately 6–8 weeks in a 90° position with weight-bearing. Vigorous exercise is needed following a cast removal. A calcaneous gait may be noted for several months afterward until sufficient strength is regained. The use of a removal cast may be advantageous in allowing early rehabilitation by passive strengthening with reduction in muscle atrophy.

105). The spastic-type equinus has been best treated by an Achilles tendon advancement into the calcaneus (**Figure 106**).[1,2,4,7–10]

COMPENSATORY EQUINUS (SECONDARY EQUINUS)

Several causes have been cited for pronation in a foot other than equinus. If the foot exists with excessive subtalar and midtarsal motion, then resupination will not occur adequately through the gait cycle. The persisting heel valgus position, which results from the subtalar pronation, will cause a shortening in the actual distance of the origin and insertion of the gastrocnemius-soleus complex. In order for the muscular physiology to continue, it is necessary for the muscle fibers to contract and assume a new resting state. This occurs to maintain proper tonus of the muscles during gait as well as allow for adequate propulsion. When one examines for ankle motion, the foot is normally placed in a neutral to slightly supinated attitude. If a compensatory equinus exists secondary to the pronation in the foot, then limited dorsiflexion will be measured. This is the result of the tight physiologic state of the muscle when the foot is supinated from its valgus pronated position. One must realize that the calcaneus moves through three planes of motion and with supination, the calcaneus becomes more plantarflexed at its posterior aspect. This will cause

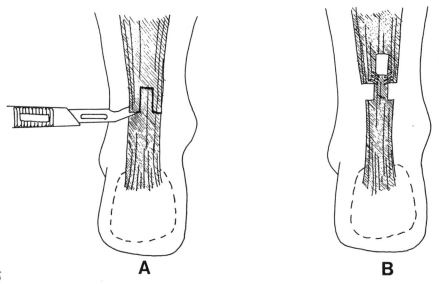

Gastroc equinus

A   **B**

Figure 105   Tongue-in-groove Achilles lengthening.

(A) An incision is made over the area of the myotendinous junction of the Achilles tendon. A tongue-in-groove incision is made at this junction separating any fibers of the soleus from the anterior aspect of the sheath. (B) With dorsiflexion at the ankle, the tongue will slide and the surgeon can decide at what position the tongue should be sutured into the groove. Casting is necessary for approximately 6–8 weeks with vigorous rehabilitation afterward.

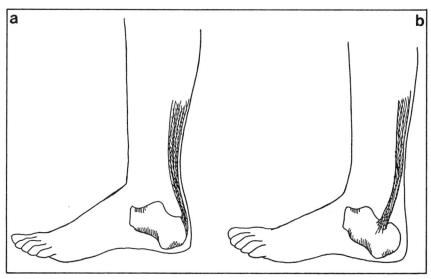

Figure 106   Achilles tendon transfer.

Murphy advancement

(A) In spastic equinus an advancement of the Achilles tendon in the calcaneus will reduce the mechanical pull and the dorsal forces exerted on the foot–ankle. (B) The tendon is inserted in a groove cut in the dorsal-posterior aspect of the calcaneus with a tenodesis resulting. Nonweight-bearing with casting for 6–8 weeks is necessary for adequate fusion of the tendon into the calcaneus.

a lengthening of the distance from the origin to the insertion of the gastroc-soleus complex and will result in greater limitation of ankle–joint dorsiflexion.

Differentiating between compensatory and congenital equinus can be challenging to the practitioner. To arrive at a proper diagnosis, the muscle must first be allowed to be adequately stretched through exercise and orthotic control for the pronation. Within a period of 3–6 months a compensatory equinus will normally resolve while a congenital equinus will continue to persist. When utilizing orthotic control, begin by casting the child in a neutral position and allow him to wear only the neutral shell orthosis without any posting in the heel or forefoot initially. One can then gradually apply a varus heel and forefoot post to allow resupination of the foot. As more resupination occurs, stretching of the Achilles tendon will result (this will only occur in the compensatory type). Each month a varus post should be applied increasingly, as is tolerated. If this is attempted in an adult, there is usually a poor result due to the contractures resulting from the long-standing contracted state of the muscle secondary to the abnormal foot position.

ANKLE EQUINUS (BONE BLOCK EQUINUS)

In ankle equinus there is a loss of dorsiflexion secondary to an abutment of the tibia on the talus. The examiner must differentiate this type of equinus from that of the congenital soleus equinus. Both will clinically present with limited dorsiflexion when the knee is both flexed and extended. Radiologic evaluation is the best method to determine if an ankle equinus exists. This is accomplished by first exposing a normal lateral x-ray of the lower leg and ankle–foot complex. A second x-ray is then taken with the leg bent as far forward to achieve its maximum dorsiflexion. If 15° or more of difference are measured between the superimposition of the tibias, then an assumption of a soleus equinus existing can be made. Less than 15° of difference or the presence of a visible hypertrophic bony block at the tibio–talar interface would imply an ankle equinus (**Figure 107**).

Treatment must be directed to the specific bony abnormality with resolution of the block if possible.

Athletic Equinus

Individuals who actively participate in sports and maintain excellent muscle tone may present with a nonpathologic form of equinus. Normally these individuals will exhibit good foot architecture. In gait, an early heel-off is not uncommon although it would not be considered abnormal. A possible explanation for this phenomenon is in the muscle anatomy. Individuals are born with a specific number of muscle fibrils that do not increase in number with added strength; rather, they increase in the cellular volume of protein. The increased volume reduces the degree of longitudinal elasticity and results in

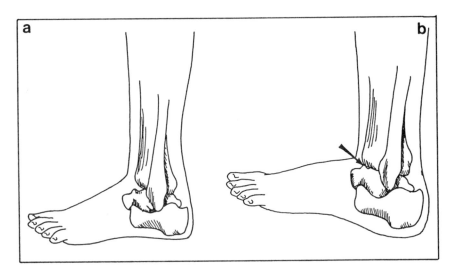

Figure 107

(A) Lateral x-ray view of the foot–ankle will exhibit a bony block over the dorsum of the talus or possibly at the anterior of the tibia. (B) Dorsiflexion will cause an abutment of the hypertrophic area(s) and limit the available motion. Removal of the impingement is necessary in these cases.

a reduction in flexibility. An equinus state will be the resulting condition from this increase. If it becomes necessary to treat this condition, then stretching exercises with the possible use of orthotic control for any secondary structural changes are recommended.[5]

TRANSITIONAL EQUINUS

This form of equinus is the result of a rapid growth in the bony structures of the leg without the muscular components equally lengthening. The gastrocnemius muscle passes over three joint areas—knee, ankle, and subtalar joint—while the soleus muscle passes over two joint areas—ankle and subtalar joint. Any rapid and substantial growth at these bony structures will affect these muscle groups. If the musculature is unable to compensate adequately for the rapidness in bone growth, then a loss in longitudinal flexibility will result. The practitioner must remember this when evaluating a growing child. An inquiry with the parents will usually confirm a recent growth spurt, which will confirm a suspicion of transitional equinus.

A child may exhibit symptoms of leg fatigue and cramping as a result of this muscular tension. Treatment is directed toward proper stretching and adequate structural control of the foot while the body is attempting to equalize the length of the soft tissue.

References

Ankle:
1. Arimoto, H.K., Forrester, D.M.: Classification of ankle fractures: An algorithan. *A.J.R.,* 135:1980.
2. Cavallaro, D.C., Wokasien, R.L., Brown, J.H., Johnston, B.: Osteochondritis dissecans of the talus. *J.A.P.A.,* 69:Number 9, September 1979.
3. Chavnon, G.M., Brotherton, B.J.: The ball and socket ankle joint. *J. Bone & Joint Surg,* 61-B:1979.
4. Griffith, H., Wandtke, J.: Tibiotalar tilt: A new slant. *Skeletal Radiol.,* 6:1981.
5. Jensen, J.K.: Ball and socket ankle joints. *Clin. Orthop.,* Number 85, June 1972.
6. Kleiger, B.: Mechanism of ankle injury. Orthopedic Clinics of North America. 5:Number 1, January 1974.
7. McCullough, C.J., Venugopal, V.: Osteochondritis dissecans of the talus: The natural history. *Clinical Orthopaedics,* 144:1979.
8. Salter, R.B.: *Textbook of Disorders and Injuries of the Musculoskeletal System.* Williams and Wilkins Co., Baltimore, MD, 1970.
9. Scharling, M.: Osteochondritis dissecans of the talus. *Acta. Orthop. Scand.,* 49:1978.
10. Sgarlato, T.E.: *A Compendium of Podiatric Biomechanics.* California College of Podiatric Medicine, 1971.
11. Tachdjian, M.O.: *Pediatric Orthopedics.* W.B. Saunders Co., Philadelphia, PA, 1972.
12. Tax, H.R.: *Podopediatrics.* Williams and Wilkins Co., Baltimore, MD, 1980.
13. Yvars, M.F.: Osteochondral fractures of the dome of the talus. *Clinical Orthopaedics and Related Research,* Number 114, January–February 1976.

Equinus:
1. Banks, H.H., Green, W.T.: The correction of Equinus deformity in cerebral palsy. *J. Bone & Joint Surg.*, 40-A:1958.
2. Hall, J.E., Salter, R.B.: Congenital short tendo calcaneus. *J. Bone & Joint Surg.*, 49-B:1967.
3. Harris, R.I., Beath, M.T.: Hypermobile flatfoot with short tendoachilles. *J. Bone & Joint Surg.*, 30-A:1948.
4. Jay, R.M., Schoenhaus, H.D.: Further insights in the anterior advancement of the tendo achilles. *J.A.P.A.*, 71:Number 2, February 1981.
5. Lichty, T.: Personal communication.
6. Root, M.L.: The congenitally short gastrocnemius. Paper presented by Dr. Merton L. Root.
7. Schoenhaus, H.D., Jay, R.M.: A modified gastrocnemius lengthening. *J.A.P.A.*, 68:Number 1, January 1978.
8. Sgarlato, T.E.: *A Compendium of Podiatric Biomechanics.* California College of Podiatric Medicine, 1971.
9. Smith, S. Personal communication.
10. Tachdjian, M.O.: *Pediatric Orthopedics.* W.B. Saunders Co., Philadelphia, PA, 1972.
11. Tax, H.R.: *Podopediatrics.* William and Wilkins Co., Baltimore, MD, 1980.
12. Tax, H.R., Albright, T.: Metatarsus adducto varus. *J.A.P.A.*, 68:Number 5, May 1978.

Chapter 8

FLATFEET DEFORMITIES

Congenital Talipes Calcaneovalgus

A type of flatfoot deformity that frequently presents at birth is a condition referred to as *Talipes calcaneovalgus*. This deformity can be observed in the newborn infant or may appear shortly thereafter. The incidence of occurrence is approximately 1 in 1,000 births and may be either unilateral or bilateral.[5,6,8–11]

The appearance of the foot is one of excessive dorsiflexion and eversion and limitation of plantarflexion and inversion. Many authors and clinicians feel that a foot capable of dorsiflexing to the point of contact with the anterolateral aspect of the leg is a form of talipes calcaneovalgus (**Figure 108**).[11,31] This author has found through examination of many newborns that it is more often the rule than the exception to find the foot able to touch the anterior of the leg. The critical diagnostic difference between a normal foot and one with talipes calcaneovalgus is the inability to plantarflex and invert the foot adequately. In talipes calcaneovalgus, plantarflexion of the foot at the ankle is usually limited to 90° or less (**Figure 109**). When performing this test, the examiner must be careful not to include the motion available at the midtarsal joints of the foot. To avoid this, grasp the foot at the level of the midtarsal joint when attempting plantarflexion and inversion. Determine the amount of plantarflexion by the angle formed at the ankle while avoiding the use of the distal aspect of the foot (**Figure 110A**).

For an additional finding, stroke the plantar skin of the foot; if talipes calcaneovalgus exists, the infant's foot will dorsiflex and evert. This sign is lost gradually by the time the infant is 4–6 months of age. The podiatrist should be alerted to the difference between the condition of talipes calcaneovalgus and the deformity of calcaneal valgus found in a pes planus deformity. Calcaneal valgus is the everted position of the calcaneus in its relationship to the lower leg (**Figure 111**). It may be the result of a talipes calcaneovalgus or it may exist from other etiologic factors (example: tight Achilles tendon, ligamentous laxity, tarsal coalitions etc.).

159

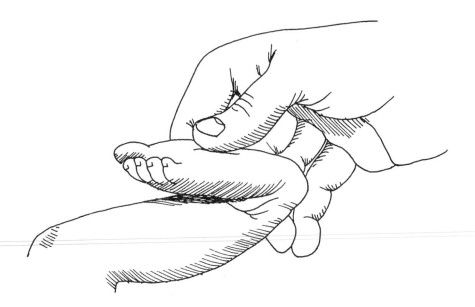

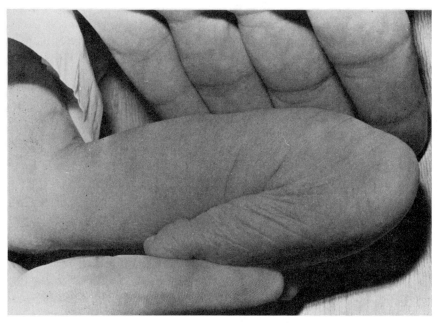

Figure 108

Most newborns have the capability of dorsiflexing the foot on the ankle so that contact occurs at the anterior of the leg. This is considered normal; however, it is also typically found in talipes calcaneovalgus.

Figure 109 (opposite): (A) 15–20° beyond right angle is normal plantarflexory motion at the ankle. (B) In cases of talipes calcaneovalgus, the anterior skin of the ankle will be extremely taut and stretch lines will be observed with plantarflexion. The degree of plantarflexion will usually be limited to 90° or less in talipes calcaneovalgus.

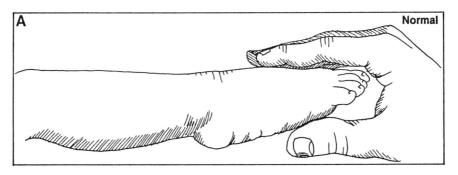

A   Normal

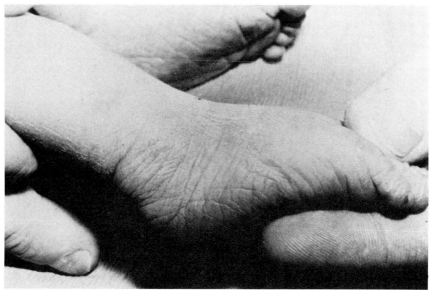

B

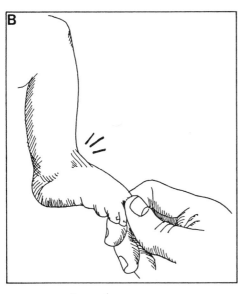

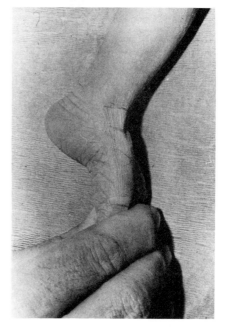

C-V   Figure 109

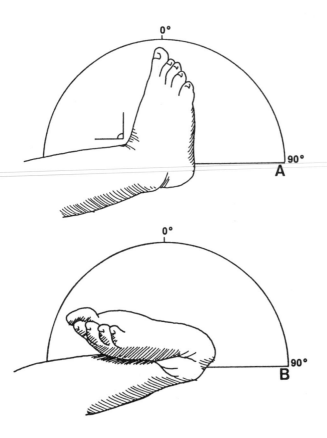

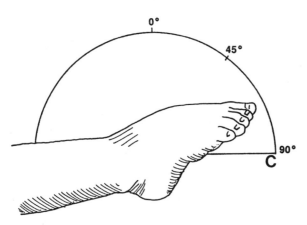

Figure 110

(A) *Imagine a protractor existing laterally behind the ankle. Have the foot placed at 90° to the leg which is the zero or starting point to determine the degree of motion at the ankle. (B) Dorsiflex and (C) plantarflex the foot to quantitatively determine the approximate motions of the foot on the ankle. Limitation of plantarflexion (0° or less) is considered a talipes calcaneovalgus condition.*

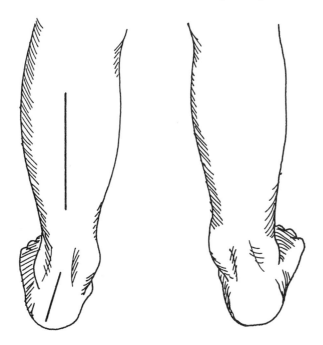

Figure 111 *feel to R F*

*Calcaneal valgus can be the
result of many causes and
should not be synonymously
used for talipes calcaneovalgus. A bisection of the lower
leg and of the calcaneus will
show eversion of the calcaneus in the condition of calcaneal valgus.*

Clinically, talipes calcaneovalgus will exhibit considerable tautness of the soft tissue at the anterior of the ankle with passive plantarflexion. Due to this contracture, the foot assumes a resting position of abduction and eversion ("up and out" position) (**Figure 110B**).

The heel may vary in the degree of valgus from no valgus positioning to one of significant eversion. The skin surfaces about the ankle will show stretching over the tibial aspect with the fibular area revealing creases and folds. The head of the talus will be palpable both medially and plantarly. The forefoot, at the midtarsal joint, will be in an abducted everted position.

Subtalar joint motion is found to be normal. One will find the calcaneus rotating and everting from below the talus with passive range of motion.

Radiographic Findings

When evaluating an infant for talipes calcaneovalgus radiographically, the findings will tend to be consistent and reproducible. For proper positioning of the infant, place the foot in semiweight-bearing and expose a standard dorsoplantar and lateral radiograph. In the presence of talipes calcaneovalgus, the lateral view will display the talus in a plantarflexed position in its relationship to the cuboid bone. The talar head will appear to overlap and project beyond the distal superior area of the calcaneus. The midtarsal cyma line will usually be altered significantly and the talus may be visualized in an equinus attitude. A line bisecting the talus will pass below the middle of the ossification center of the cuboid in talipes calcaneovalgus (**Figure 112**).

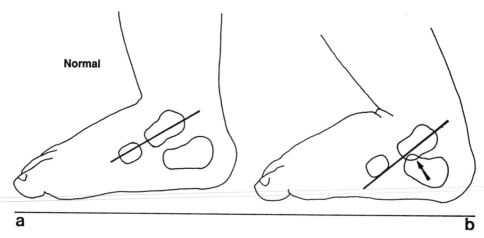

a

b

Figure 112

(A) In a normal foot a bisection line of the talus will also bisect the cuboid or pass above the center point of the cuboid. (B) Talipes calcaneovalgus will exhibit radiographic characteristics of a superimposition of the superior aspect of the calcaneus with the talar head and a bisection line of the talus will pass below the midpoint of the cuboid.

Dorsoplantar radiographic views will also evidence an alteration in the midtarsal cyma line. Subluxation of the head of talus in its relationship to the cartilagenous navicular can be appreciated (**Figure 113**) (*Note:* The navicular is not ossified in the young infant and therefore must be imagined by using the first metatarsal as a guide.) The talocalcaneal angle should be determined. In talipes calcaneovalgus, this angular value is significantly greater than the normal values of 30–40° at birth. (*Note:* When viewing this deformity, remember the talus is actually locked into the ankle joint and acts as an extension of the lower leg. When the foot assumes this calcaneovalgus position, it is the result of the surrounding joints and bony structures moving and deviating away from the talus as a result of the soft-tissue contractures.)

Treatment

When possible, the deformity of talipes calcaneovalgus should be treated as soon after birth to relieve the contracted state. Prognosis will be more favorable, and correction more rapid, if treatment is commenced as early as possible. The milder forms of congenital talipes calcaneovalgus respond well to manipulative exercises with concomitant tape splinting and/or bar therapy. The parents should be shown the manner in which the foot should be plantarflexed and inverted without injuring the child. Instruct them to hold this position for the count of 10 seconds, and then release. This maneuver should be repeated 30 times on each foot after every diaper change (**Figure 114**). This may be followed by applying a J-strap of one-inch adhesive tape to maintain this position between the diaper changes (**Figure 115**). In cases where the skin

Normal

Talips C-V

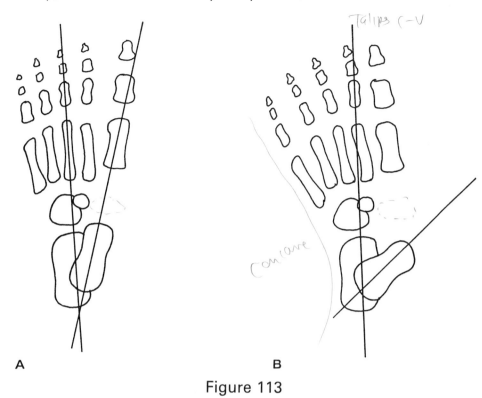

Concave

A   B

Figure 113

(A) Dorsoplantar view of a normal infant's foot will have an alignment of the talus with the first metatarsal and a talocalcaneal angle less than 40°. (B) An increased talocalcaneal angle with abduction of the forefoot is indicative of a talipes calcaneovalgus deformity.

may be irritated by the adhesive tape or the parents may not be cooperative, the use of a night splint (bar) is beneficial to maintain position. The bar should be bent as shown in **Figure 116** to stretch and supinate the foot while preventing it from returning to its abnormal position. The bar should be used 24 hours a day, being removed only for bathing, etc.

Treatment should continue until the child begins weight-bearing. If there appears to be a tendency toward the deformity both clinically and radiographically at this stage of development, an in-shoe orthotic device should be employed (i.e., type B, C, or E heel stabilizers, or Whitman, Roberts' type plates—see Chapter 13).

The moderate to severe cases of talipes calcaneovalgus must be treated more aggressively. These can be distinguished from the mild form by the degree of plantarflexion available at the ankle. (*Note:* This is not to be confused with the rigid vertical talus described later in this chapter.) The mild form will usually plantarflex to 90° at the ankle and possibly a small amount beyond. However, it will have all the other characteristic findings including the talar bisection passing through the lower one-third of the cuboid. The more severe

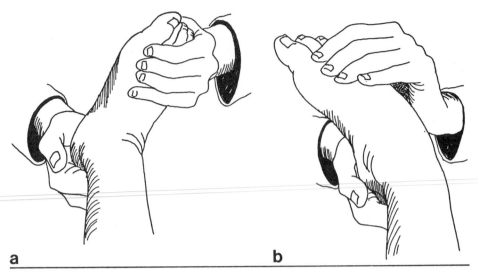

a   b

Figure 114

(A) Position your hands to begin the manipulative exercise for talipes calcaneovalgus. (B) Bring the foot into a plantarflexed inverted position and hold for the count of 10 seconds. This should be performed approximately 30 times with each diaper change.

cases will have greater limitation of plantarflexion and a higher degree of plantar declination of the talar ossification center to the cuboid. The moderate and severe cases must be treated by stretch castings to successfully reduce the deformity.

The procedure for casting is first to prepare the skin by using skin creams or tincture of benzoin to avoid chafing or cracking. Prior to the application of the skin products and the cast, a period of manipulation is recommended to

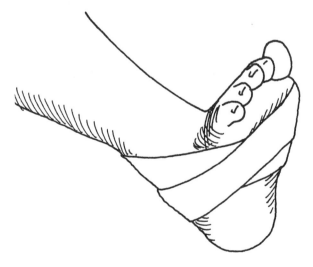

Figure 115

Tape splinting for talipes calcaneovalgus is accomplished by running 1-inch strips from the lateral aspect of the ankle around the plantar of the foot and medially up the inside aspect of the ankle with tension directed into plantarflexion and inversion.

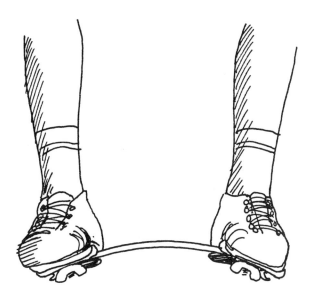

Figure 116

*A night splint should be bent
so the foot will be supinated.
This will provide stretching of
the dorsal contractures over the
anterior of the ankle as well as
limit the ability for eversion.*

reduce the number of casts necessary to reduce the deformity. The foot should be manipulated into a plantarflexed and inverted position forcing the foot to its maximum range of motion without using brutal force. Once this position is achieved it should be held for 10 seconds and released. This should be performed repetitively for approximately 5–10 minutes prior to the application of the cast.

After the period of manipulation, prepare the skin and apply 2–3 layers of padding from above the knees to the tips of the toes. Apply an extra layer or two to the malleolar area, the posterior of the heel, the dorsal area of the toes and the fibular prominence proximally to avoid pressure irritation.

With the advent of many new casting products, the author suggests using whichever is most workable for the patient and the doctor. In the small infant, plaster still is the most acceptable due to its moldability. Since the casts must be changed weekly, plaster seems to be both practical and economically more acceptable. In applying the plaster use either 2- or 3-inch extra fast-setting plaster bandages. Apply the cast above the knee with the knee slightly flexed to avoid slippage of the cast. Smooth the plaster well and avoid wrinkles. Mold it around the heel, ankle, and arch areas. Once applied, the foot is held in its maximum plantarflexed, adducted, inverted position (**Figure 117**). This allows the cartilagenous navicular to realign itself with the head of the talus as well as stretch the soft-tissue contractures. If there is any doubt as to the alignment of the foot after positioning and casting, an x-ray should be obtained to verify the correction.

In cases where an infant is uncooperative or fearful of the noise produced by a cast-cutting saw, the parents can remove the cast prior to the next application. In very young infants, one roll of plaster may be adequate to cover the area. In this case, if the clinician clumps the end of the roll it will leave

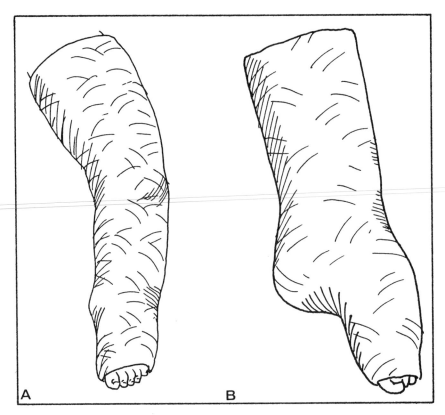

Figure 117   Casting technique for talipes calcaneovalgus.

(A) An above-the-knee plaster cast should be applied to avoid the child kicking the cast off due to the plantarflexion at the ankle. Flexing the knee approximately 30° will provide excellent stability. (B) The foot should be molded into a plantarflexed inverted position to align the fore and rearfoot as well as stretch the dorsal ankle contractures.

a starting point and help facilitate the removal by the parents. Have the parents soak the cast in a tub of warm water with vinegar added for approximately 30 minutes to an hour. Once softened it may gradually be unrolled until completely removed. The parents are instructed to use skin creams afterward to help moisten the drying skin. The removal of the cast should be performed no sooner than the day prior to the next visit.

Cast application may be necessary at weekly intervals for an average period of 2–6 weeks. This becomes totally dependent on the severity and rigidity of the deformity. Once correction has been achieved a maintenance splinting is necessary. The reason for this splinting is to continue to allow the medial soft-tissue structures of the foot–ankle–leg complex to tighten for maintenance of stability. One must realize that stretching the lateral dorsal contractures has no affect on the medial structures unless sufficient time is allowed for retightening to occur medially. The splint that can be used is either the adhesive J-strapping mentioned earlier or the employment of a night splint for a period of 2–8 weeks post casting.

The child should then be followed along until weight-bearing begins. If at this time the foot still exhibits suppleness and laxity on the medial side, even though the lateral dorsal contractures have corrected well, then an in-shoe orthotic device should be fabricated to maintain proper soft-tissue and osseous alignment. Type B, C, or E heel stabilizers, Whitman, Roberts', or Whitman–Roberts plates are most beneficial in controlling the foot structure (Chapter 13). This form of therapy should continue for approximately 4–6 years. A longer period may be necessary in cases of continued laxity and deformity. In some cases orthotic control may be necessary into adult life if the foot structure continues to maintain a pronated attitude. Reexamination and radiographic evaluation of the child should be performed at definite time intervals (6–18 months) until the completion of treatment.

The prognosis is usually good to excellent in infants with congenital talipes calcaneovalgus if treatment is instituted shortly after birth. The parents should be informed, prior to the institution of therapy, of the probable degree of improvement that may be obtained. The prognosis for infants presenting with a definite familial tendency will be more guarded, with the anticipation of continued orthotic control into adulthood. The greater the rigidity of the deformity, the worse the prognosis.

Congenital Talipes Calcaneovarus

This can best be described as an inversion attitude of the entire foot without the equinus deformity seen in talipes equinovarus (clubfoot) (**Figure 118**). On examination, this deformity will be easily reducible and there will be adequate dorsiflexion at the ankle when the foot is manipulated into a corrected position.

The etiology of this deformity appears to be related to intrauterine position rather than a congenital structural abnormality, or the condition may also result from either an imbalance in muscular power or an abnormal innervation of the medial (invertor) musculature causing an abnormal varus contracted state. This foot position has been frequently categorized as a clubfoot deformity although the severity, degree of dysfunction, and total components are greatly lessened.[4,31,32,37]

Treatment

The application of serial casts for a sufficient period of time to reduce the contractures will frequently resolve this condition excellently. By following the standard procedures for application of a cast and preparation of the skin, described under talipes calcaneovalgus, the foot should then be held in a neu-

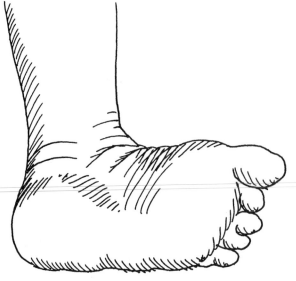

Figure 118

Talipes calcaneovarus will exhibit an inversion of the entire foot. The deformity has been confused with a clubfoot; however, there is no equinus contracture, metatarsus adductus, or rigid contractures indicating any similarity or relationship to a talipes equinovarus.

tral abducted–everted position. Prior to the cast application, the foot should be manipulated into correction for approximately 10 minutes by abducting and everting. The cast should be changed every 5–7 days as necessary until correction is achieved. If an infant can be treated for this condition within the first few months of life, the use of casting may be needed for only 1–3 weeks. This becomes totally dependent on the tautness and reducibility of the deformity. Following casting the foot should be maintained in a well-fitted straight last shoe. Clubfoot shoes are effective but may result in an overcorrection of the condition or a compensatory subtalar pronation as a result. Night splints (bars) are also effective post casting to maintain a good attitude of the foot and also help prevent an abnormal sleeping position, which could force the foot back into its previous abnormal attitude. The splint (bar) should not be bent into a varus attitude as was described for talipes calcaneovalgus as it would only accentuate the deformity. If necessary, the bar can be bent slightly into eversion to help facilitate stretch (**Figure 119**).

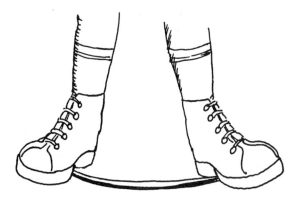

Figure 119

When using a night splint for a talipes calcaneovarus, bend the bar so that a certain degree of eversion is present. This will apply stretch to the medial structures and allow continuous exercising. The arch areas of the shoes should be padded to prevent excessive stress on the arch.

The shoes should be padded in the arch area to avoid excessive pronation. In the older infant an orthosis could be prescribed. The post-cast splinting should be maintained for several months or until the examiner feels sufficient development and a corrected position has been maintained and accomplished satisfactorily. Occasionally it may be necessary to reinstitute treatment if contractures begin to reoccur, although this is infrequent.

Pes Planus (Flatfeet)

Several names have been offered and assigned to describe the deformity of flatfeet. Included are: pes planus, pes valgo planus, pronation syndrome, calcaneal valgus, and talipes calcaneovalgus, to mention a few. The literature contains copious amounts of material written on the etiology, classification, and treatment or nontreatment of this abnormality. Several attempts have been made to properly classify and categorize the varying degrees of this deformity ranging from the mild flexible type flatfoot to the more severe rigid type. None of these classifications seem to adequately encompass the variables encountered clinically. At a point it becomes apparent to those treating children that all the classifications tend to coalesce when applied to clinical practice. The only exception is the deformity of a vertical talus (described further in this chapter), which is truly rigid at birth and is certainly a rare finding.[4,9,11,19,21–23,25,28,30–33]

Any practitioner or investigator will agree that there are varying degrees of collapse and joint alteration in the foot with a pes planus deformity. Let us look first at what areas are changing and being affected. There may be noted a collapse or breech on lateral radiographic examination (weight-bearing) at the talonavicular, navicular-cuneiform, cuneiform-first metatarsal, or a combination of two or more of these joint levels (**Figure 120**). The number of joints affected becomes dependent on the severity of collapse and the amount of deformity in the foot. Dorsoplantar radiographs (weight-bearing) may exhibit widening of the talocalcaneal angle and abduction of the forefoot in its relationship to the talus and calcaneus (**Figure 121A**). These changes may be age dependent or correlated to the degree of laxity in the foot. The etiology will be discussed further in this chapter.

Infants and young children often present with what would be clinically an apparent flatfoot deformity. The arch appears to be flattened to the ground and the heel is in a slight valgus attitude. Radiographs of these children do not, however, exhibit any true structural abnormality. This appearance is the result of a fat pad in the arch or an enlarged abductor muscle belly filling in the natural arch contour. It is also the result of greater joint motion often found in the young child.

The examiner must be cognizant of the absence of the ossification centers in the early development of the child and to appropriately evaluate the foot in view of this fact. The use of the existing ossification centers must be utilized with careful discretion. *Note:* The ossified centers do not actually represent

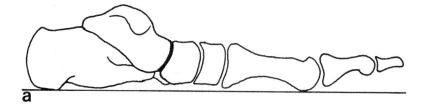

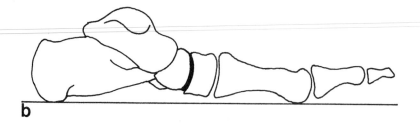

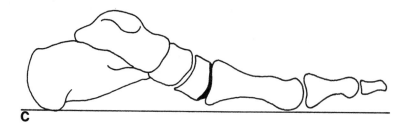

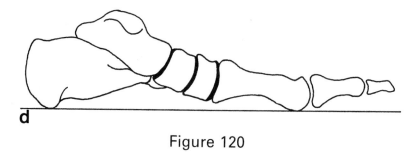

Figure 120

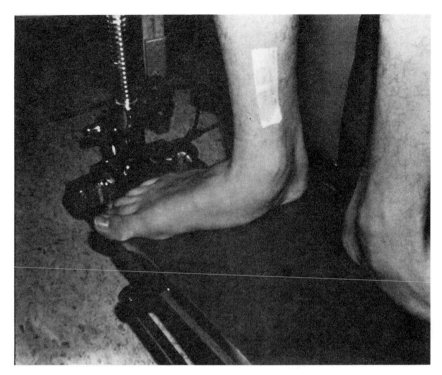

Figure 120 (opposite and above): In a flatfoot deformity, a collapse in the midtarsal joints may be observed on lateral view at the talonavicular (A), navicular-first cuneiform (B), first cuneiform-first metatarsal (C), or a combination as in (D).

the true bony centers nor are they capable of providing an accurate means of comparison when using angular relationships with those centers found in the older child or the mature adult. The clinician should therefore be cautious when evaluating the infant or child so not to be falsely led to an overconcern for a possibly nonexistent deformity.

Etiology

The complexity of causes resulting in a flatfoot deformity becomes bewildering. Several explanations have been proposed and professed through the literature including: ligamentous laxity, varus or valgus deformities in the calcaneus, varus or valgus deformities in the forefoot, compensation for angular or rotational deformities in the legs or feet, improper shoe gear, a weakness in the medial musculature supporting the foot, an abnormal contracture of the lateral muscular attachments to the foot, equinus deformity in the triceps surae complex, tarsal coalitions, and various aberrant neuromuscular disorders causing either weakness or low grade spasticity to distort the foot architecture.[4,9,11,13,20–23,25,26,30–33,38] After careful review of these etiologic factors, there are certain characteristics that are consistent. When viewing a normal foot

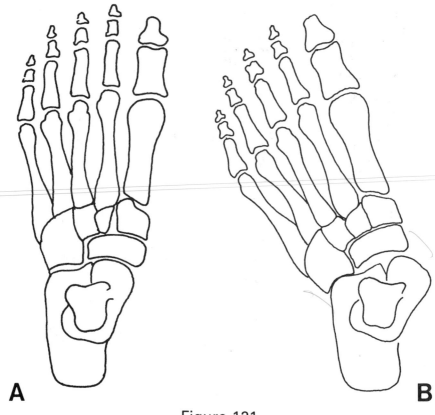

A   B

Figure 121

A dorsal–plantar projection of a normal foot will show alignment of the talus with the navicular and a relatively rectus attitude of the forefoot with rearfoot (A). The flatfoot will exhibit abduction of the forefoot in relation to the rearfoot with the talus appearing to be medially displaced. A loss of continuity of the talonavicular and calcaneocuboid joints will be evident (B).

anatomically, the talus is located over the calcaneus and aligned with the navicular. Approximately 80–90% of the articular cartilage of the talar head is in contact with the navicular surface (**Figure 122**). The calcaneus has a normal inclination from the weight-bearing surface of approximately 15–30° (**Figure 123**). Other normal consistent findings are a natural continuity and curve found through the talonavicular and calcaneocuboid joints both laterally and dorsoplantarly (**Figure 124**). This is referred to as a cyma line. A line passed through the center of the talar neck will pass through the centers of the navicular, first cuneiform, and first metatarsal in a normal foot (**Figure 125**).

A flatfoot deformity will exhibit varying deviations from those normal findings described above. The question that needs to be asked is why has this occurred? We realize the talus is locked into the ankle mortise and therefore

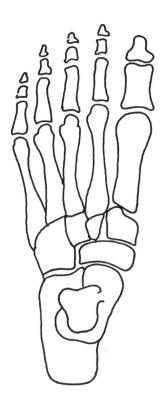

Figure 122

In a normal foot, the talus will be aligned over the calcaneus and the head will be in approximately 80–90% contact with the navicular.

has limited movement. Motion is primarily in one plane, that is, dorsi and plantarflexion with minimal motion in the other two planes. The talus also becomes an extension of the leg due to its locked ankle position. It therefore is affected by the leg's rotatory movements.

The subtalar and midtarsal joints (talonavicular–calcaneocuboid) are therefore the areas affected primarily in a flatfoot deformity. The subtalar joint is held together by several ligaments both between the joint and sur-

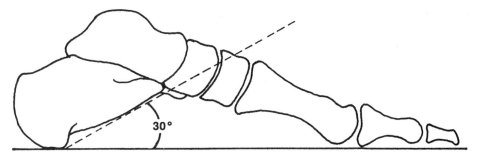

Figure 123

The calcaneal inclination in a normal foot varies from 15–30°. Higher values are found in cavus feet and lower values are found in flatfoot deformities.

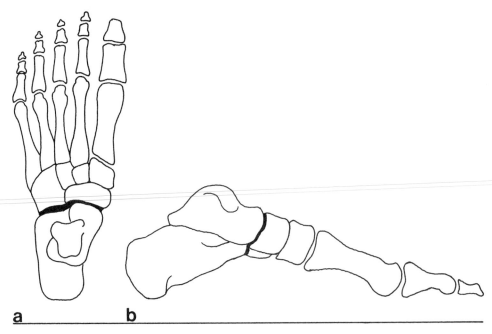

Figure 124   Cyma lines.

(A) Dorsal-plantar projection of a normal foot will have the talonavicular and calca-neocuboid joints aligned transversely and continuously. (B) Lateral projection will also have a continuous alignment of these same two joints. A flatfoot deformity will not have this continuity in either projection.

rounding the joint (**Figure 126**). The medial and lateral ankle ligaments play an adjunctive role in stabilizing the subtalar joint. The midtarsal joints are concomitantly held in alignment with the talus and calcaneus by many of the same ligaments necessary to stabilize the subtalar joint.

When viewing a flatfoot deformity, many consistent findings exist. These include an eversion of the calcaneus, an abduction of the forefoot in relation to the talus, and an apparent medial deviation of talus with plantarflexion. Pronation in a foot has been described as a plantarflexion, inversion, and adduction of the talus in a closed kinetic chain of motion.[25,32] Viewed another way, the calcaneus and forefoot are moving in an everted, dorsiflexed, and abducted attitude away from the talus.

Note: Remember that the talus is locked in the ankle joint mortise and therefore is not necessarily the primary center of movement in pronation.

The flatfoot deformity is better viewed as the calcaneus actually slipping and moving out from beneath the talus rather than the talus moving away from the calcaneus. The reason for this concept is the talus is an extension of the lower leg and is limited in motion. If a buckling of a joint occurs, it is at the subtalar joint not the ankle joint. The calcaneus therefore becomes the free end for movement, not the talus. With the calcaneus moving out from

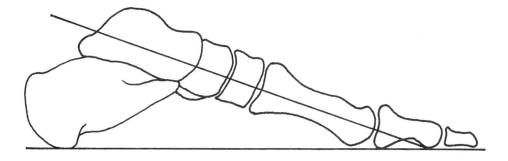

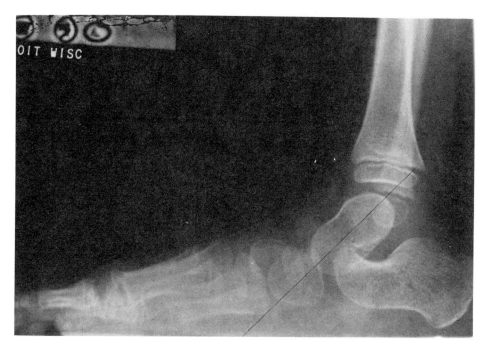

Figure 125

If a line is constructed through the center of the talar head and neck (do not use the body), it should continue distally through the centers of the navicular, first cuneiform, and first metatarsal in a normal foot architecture.

below the talus, there is an everted attitude in its relationship to the lower leg. The forefoot becomes abducted and dorsiflexed relative to the talar head. This is the result of the calcaneus slipping posteriorly, thus relatively forcing the talus anteriorly, plantarly, and medially. Therefore, the primary center of movement in pronation is the calcaneus moving into eversion and moving posteriorly and placing the talus more anterior, medial, and plantar in its relationship to the rest of the foot. The forefoot motion of abduction is due to the relative anterior position of the talus forcing the medial pillar of the foot

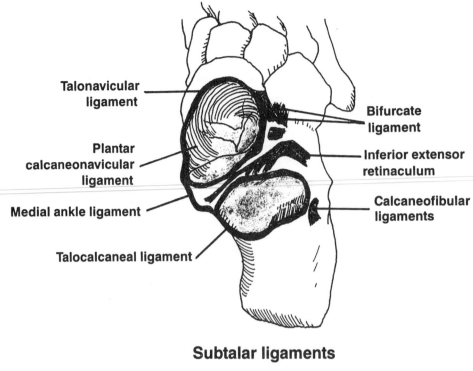

Talonavicular
ligament

Bifurcate
ligament

Plantar
calcaneonavicular
ligament

Inferior extensor
retinaculum

Medial ankle ligament

Calcaneofibular
ligaments

Talocalcaneal ligament

Subtalar ligaments

Figure 126

The subtalar and ankle ligaments together provide stability to the rearfoot. These ligaments will stabilize the talus on the calcaneus as well as provide medial and lateral stability for the talus in the ankle mortise. Loss of congruity or strength of these ligamentous structures will ultimately alter the normal relationships of the bones of the rearfoot, midfoot, and ankle.

(talus, navicular, three cuneiforms, 1st–2nd–3rd metatarsals, and respective toes) forward and therefore in abduction relative to the lateral pillar (calcaneus, cuboid, 4th and 5th metatarsal, and respective toes) that have moved posteriorly (**Figure 127**).

In order for the calcaneus to move from beneath the talus and cause the resulting forefoot conditions, there must exist a sufficient amount of laxity in the sub- and peritalar ligaments with loss of muscular stability. The function of the ligaments is to hold in place the bony structures at each joint level. The musculature primarily causes movement to occur at the joints with secondary stabilization. Therefore, it is more likely that an inheritable trait will cause loss of ligamentous stability due to laxity. Metabolic, dietary, and age-related disorders secondarily affect the strength of the ligaments. Certainly, a nutritional or metabolic imbalance can result in the production of a gradual weakness in the ligaments causing generalized changes in all the joints. An inborn trait, however, allowing for greater laxity is more likely the initiating and

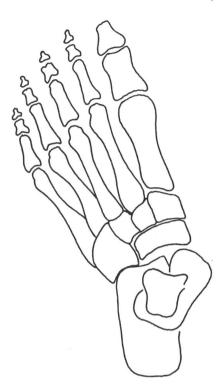

Figure 127

In a flatfoot deformity, the medial pillar of the foot (talus, navicular, three cuneiforms, 1st, 2nd, 3rd metatarsals and their respective toes) is forced distally in relation to the lateral pillar (calcaneus, cuboid, 4th and 5th metatarsals, and toes), which has moved posteriorly. This change forces the forefoot into abduction and the calcaneus posterior to the talus.

affecting cause. The degree of laxity will affect the time frame in which a flatfoot deformity may present. It is known that young children have greater ranges of joint motion that eventually reduce to almost one-half by the time they reach late childhood or early adolescence. If there is persistence of this laxity, then a pronation deformity will progress.

It has been the experience of many practitioners at some point in their careers that an older adult will present with a recent history of one of their feet suddenly collapsing and the arch flattening down significantly. The other foot is most often very normal in appearance. There is usually no history of injury or trauma, nor is there any swelling to indicate the possibility of a spontaneous rupture. One has to ask why this had occurred? A probable explanation is the loss of tensile strength in the ligaments of the sub- and peritalar joints. This comes as the result of continuous stress and the natural process of aging, which will result in a loss of the structural strength of these ligaments. With the loss of this strength, the stability of the foot will be sacrificed. Left untreated, these people will often find that their other foot produces a similar process over a sufficient period of time. With viewing this type of an occurrence, appreciation that a loss of ligamentous stability has to precede the abnormal shift in the sub- and peritalar articulations of the foot, resulting finally in collapse.

To reiterate, ligaments maintain stability and strength between the bony surfaces. It therefore is the ligaments that must eventually give way to allow any movement beyond the normal to occur. The musculature, primarily the posterior and anterior tibial muscles, will play a secondary role in maintaining the joint integrity along the medial side of the foot. Musculature alone cannot provide the needed stability. The ligamentous structures are therefore a crucial entity in the stabilization of the joint structures.[2,9,11,13,22,23,25,31,32,33]

Secondary causes can also exist and include any factors that impose excessive stresses on the foot from the surrounding structures that influence the subtalar and peritalar motion. Rotational deformities, equinus, limb length discrepancies, contractures of the lateral musculature inserting into the foot, and tarsal coalitions are all examples of conditions that will increase the amount of stress on the foot structure. The stress can eventually cause loss to the ligamentous continuity and change the stabilizing strength.

One explanation that has been offered as a cause for flatfeet is an intrinsic varus or valgus abnormality in either the rearfoot or the forefoot. Although these conditions are demonstrable in an adult, I have been unable to demonstrate them satisfactorily in children.

It has been this author's findings that the forefoot and rearfoot will more often be in a rectus attitude when the foot is placed in its "neutral position." (*Neutral position* is found by placing the talar head in line with the navicular and loading the forefoot to its maximally pronated attitude [**Figure 128**].) There may be a variation of 1–2 degrees in either a varus or valgus position, but this is usually attributed to a deviation in error of measurement and not statistically significant.

The young child or toddler will exhibit dorsiflexory range of motion at the ankle of 20–50°, which is between 5 and 35 degrees more than the average adult. This reflects the increase in motion normally found in the joints of children.

With all these normal findings (rectus rear- and forefoot, adequate ankle motion, no apparent rotational or other structural abnormalities), we oftentimes may clinically and radiographically still see a significant flatfoot deformity in these children. An everted calcaneus will be noted on stance with abduction of the forefoot, as well as a medial prominence of the talus (**Figure 129**). Ligamentous laxity becomes the most likely cause of this degree of shift in joint position.

If one views a child just beginning to walk, it becomes evident that there is significant loss of medial and lateral stability of the foot. Once the child begins to develop, the musculature will begin to help stabilize the joints and the ligaments will reduce their laxity and gain greater tensile strength.

If the increase in strength in both the musculature and the ligaments does not occur synchronously with the physical maturation of the child, then the peritalar motion will remain excessive. The excessive motion will cause the foot to continue to maintain a flattened collapsed attitude. The retardation in the development of strength eventually produces a "snowballing effect." That is, as the child becomes older and increases in weight and therefore increases the downward stresses on the limbs, the ligamentous and muscular structures become unable to reverse the collapsed position. This eventually produces a

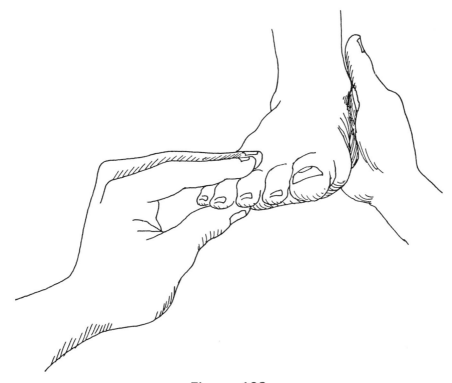

Figure 128

Neutral position of the foot is found by placing the subtalar joint into a position so that the talar head is articulating with navicular maximally. This is a point where there is neither supination or pronation in the subtalar joint. The forefoot is loaded by forcing the 4th and 5th metatarsals dorsally. Care must be taken not to abduct or adduct the forefoot but to just direct pressure dorsally. This is considered maximum pronation of the forefoot and the neutral attitude.

greater degree of joint collapse and deviation as a result of the development of the child.

With the passing of time and the allowance of the foot to continue to function in a collapsed–pronated weight-bearing attitude, the forefoot will eventually assume a varus attitude in its relative relationship to the everted calcaneus (**Figure 130**). This is the result of physiologic shortening of the dorsal and medial muscle insertions in the foot (i.e., tibialis anterior, extensor hallucis longus, extensor digitorum longus and brevis, peroneus brevis), and stretching of the tibialis posterior, flexor muscles, and peroneus longus. In pronation, the three planes of motion occurring are dorsiflexion, eversion, and abduction of the foot in relation to the talus. Therefore, the navicular is actually dorsiflexing over the head of the talus and displacing laterally. Since the navicular, three cuneiforms, and the respective medial three metatarsals and toes are functioning as a unit, the movement of the navicular dorsally on the

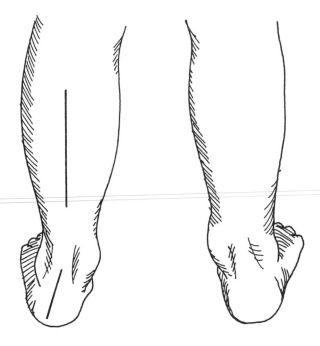

Figure 129

Stance position of a child with a flatfoot deformity will exhibit an eversion of the calcaneus relative to the lower leg and a secondary abduction of the forefoot due to the subtalar and midtarsal joint shifts.

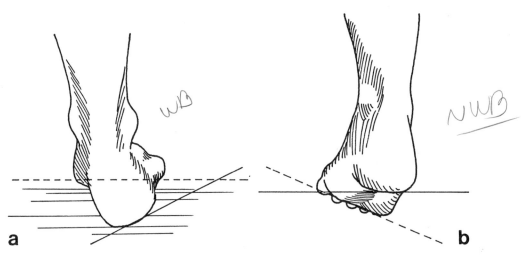

a   **b**

Figure 130

A flatfoot will allow the heel to function in valgus while the forefoot is parallel with the weight-bearing surface (A). If the foot is examined in a nonweight-bearing attitude and the subtalar joint allowed to assume a neutral position (B), the forefoot will take on a varus position due to the medial contractures.

talus will place the medial pillar of the forefoot inverted in its relative relationship to the valgus positioning of the calcaneus (**Figure 130A**). Allowing the foot to function over a period of time in this attitude will result in contractures of the medial musculature to assume this new resting state.

If the foot is placed in its so-called "neutral position" (subtalar joint in neutral position and midtarsal joint maximally pronated), the calcaneus will be forced back under the talus from its functioning everted position. The forefoot, which was functioning parallel to the ground and inverted to the valgused calcaneus in gait, is now forced into "neutral position" and therefore forces the navicular to realign with the talar head. This realignment is directing the forefoot not only to move medially but plantarly as well for the navicular to align itself properly with the talus. The plantarflexion that is to occur may not be possible if there exist contractures in the medial dorsal musculature of the foot. The result would be a varus attitude of the forefoot in its relationship to the calcaneus when viewed as nonweight-bearing. This varus (supinatus) entity is more a compensatory and physiologic change secondary to the joint position in gait than is a primary causal relationship to the flatfoot deformity. This author feels that the conclusion that has been reached regarding the varus position of the forefoot causing a flatfoot condition was extrapolated from examinations performed with retrospective inferences. As was stated earlier in this section, it is a rarity to find forefoot pathology of a varus attitude in young children with a flatfoot deformity. It will only become evident in the long-standing deformity or in those cases of a rigid flatfoot condition.

In the rare cases of a vertical talus, the foot is so severely dislocated at the talonavicular joint, with severe abduction and eversion, that significant contractures in the musculature do not allow reduction of the bony segments through passive movement. This would constitute one of the most severe forms of flatfeet with all others varying to a lesser degree.

Clinical Evaluation

Examination of a child with a flatfoot deformity must cover several areas. The degree of laxity present in the joints becomes one area of primary importance. To evaluate this, dorsiflex and plantarflex the foot at the ankle and determine the total ankle joint range of motion. If excessive dorsiflexion is noted (i.e., the dorsum of the foot is able to reach or touch the anterior of the leg) and plantarflexion is adequate (i.e., ranges greater than 45–90° from 0° [**Figure 131**]), then one must suspect ligamentous laxity. The examiner should also place the foot through its ranges of motion both inverted and everted. If the inversion of the calcaneus reaches or exceeds 90° from its vertical position with the lower leg and/or the eversion exceeding 45°, then a consideration of ligamentous laxity must be assumed. To support this finding of laxity, one can also include other joint changes.

The presence of genu recurvatum, hyperextension of the elbows, hyper-

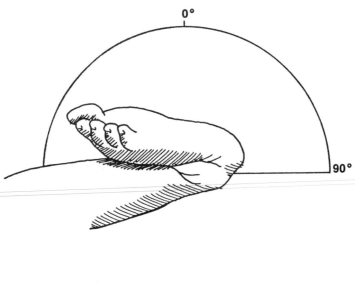

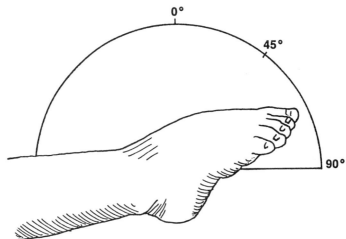

Figure 131

Ranges of excessive motion toward dorsiflexion (top) or greater than 45–90° of plantarflexion (bottom) are indicators of ligamentous laxity. This may be normal in a newborn or an infant 1–3 months old. It will be excessive in children older than 4–6 months.

extension of the metacarpophalangeal joints, and hyperextension of the thumb are all valuable areas for supporting the diagnosis of ligamentous laxity (**Figure 132**). Children possessing this laxity will typically exhibit an everted attitude of the calcaneus on stance, medial talar head prominence, abduction of the forefoot, and a relative internal attitude of the leg secondary to the talar adduction (**Figure 133**).[21,22,31,32]

Radiographically, significant breakdown and collapse are viewed of the

Signs of ligamentous laxity

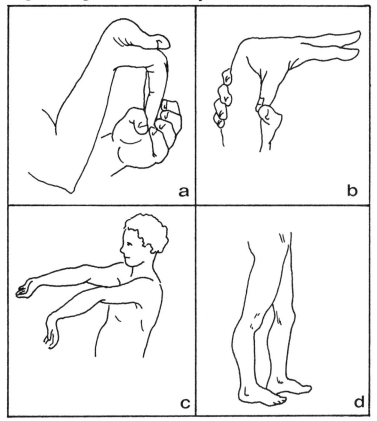

Figure 132

Ligamentous laxity can be tested in other joint areas of the body including (A) hyperextension of the metacarpophalangeal joints, (B) hypermobility of the thumb allowing it to touch or go beyond the arm, (C) hyperextension of the elbows, and (D) genu recurvatum of the knees.

medial joints of the foot with the calcaneus paralleling the weight-bearing surface. This is evaluated with a lateral weight-bearing x-ray. Dorsoplantar radiographs will demonstrate the presence of a high talo-calcaneal angle and an abduction of the forefoot (**Figure 134**). The normal values and proper radiologic interpretation are outlined under the section *Radiological Evaluation*.

Another consideration in the evaluation of the pediatric flatfoot is the medial arch fat pad and/or the presence of a hypertrophic abductor hallucis muscle belly. Both of these entities will produce a clinical appearance of a flatfoot, due to the arch not being visible, without necessarily exhibiting the other typical findings (i.e., calcaneal eversion and talonavicular calcaneo–cuboid joint divergence). For this reason, to accurately diagnose a flatfoot

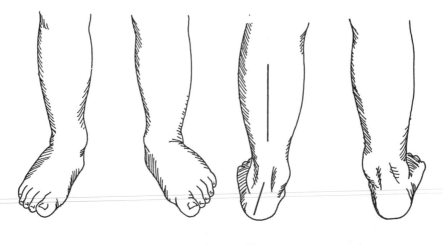

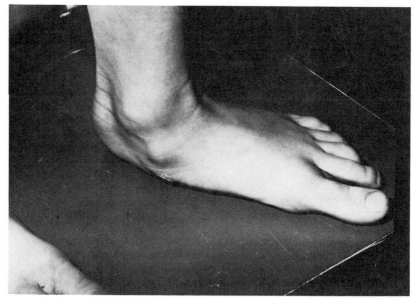

Figure 133

Ligamentous laxity will cause a foot to exhibit eversion of the calcaneus, abduction of the forefoot, and a medial prominence of the talar head. A relative internal rotation of the lower leg in response to the abduction eversion of the calcaneus and forefoot will also be apparent.

deformity a radiologic study becomes paramount. In addition to the radiologic evaluation, a complete biomechanical examination is mandatory to determine not only the components of the foot, but also the structures above the foot which may influence its function (i.e., genu valgum or varum, tibial rotation, femoral rotation, abnormal muscle function, etc.).

The calcaneal position should be determined by first bisecting the calca-

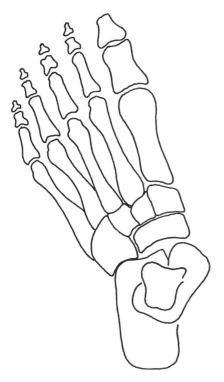

Figure 134

A dorsoplantar radiograph of a ligamentous lax foot will demonstrate a high talocalcaneal angle, abduction of the forefoot, and a medial prominence of the talus.

neus with a line drawn on the skin. A second line bisecting the lower one-third of the leg is also drawn and extended on to the calcaneus (**Figure 135**). With the foot held in its "neutral position" (described previously), one can determine the presence of either a varus or valgus attitude of the calcaneus. If the bisection of the calcaneus is medial to the lower leg bisection, then a varus deformity exists. Conversely, if the bisection is lateral, then a valgus deformity is present. The child should also be examined on stance to determine the amount of excursion through which the calcaneus moves. The amount of valgus or varus can be measured by placing a protractor over the calcaneus.

The calcaneal bisection is then measured from the vertical (90° on the protractor) (**Figure 136**). Normal findings are 1–2° of varus or valgus. Children under the age of 5 years may have a slight degree more of valgus in stance position and still be considered normal. This is due to greater ligamentous laxity.

The forefoot should be examined in its relationship to the calcaneus and its bisection. A line paralleling the plantar surface of the metatarsals, while the foot is in neutral position, can be used to evaluate the degree of varus or valgus (**Figure 137**). This line should normally be at 90° to the bisection of the calcaneus. Variations of 1–2° in either direction are an acceptable normal. This author has found that the greater percentage of children both with or without a flatfoot deformity exhibit a forefoot valgus attitude as a result of a plantarflexion of the first metatarsal. This plantarflexion is the result of the

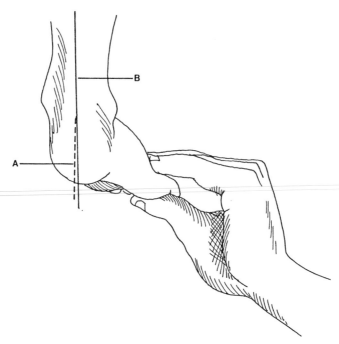

Figure 135   Calcaneal measurement.

Line (A) is drawn as a bisection of the posterior aspect of the calcaneus. Line (B) is a bisection of the lower one-third of the leg and is extended onto the calcaneus to form an angular relationship with the calcaneus. The angle can be measured to determine any varus or valgus deformity.

peroneus longus pulling the metatarsal downward. If sufficient stretching of this tendon occurs as a result of prolonged pronation, then dorsiflexion of the first ray will occur. This eventual dorsiflexion will change the forefoot relationship to the calcaneus from that of valgus to one of rectus or eventually varus positioning.

The amount of change is proportional to the length of time the pronation deformity exists. Therefore, the forefoot position is a secondary result to the rearfoot deformity and not a primary etiologic condition.

Frequently one may examine children who present with a calcaneus in a rather valgused attitude on stance (a positive Helbing's sign, **Figure 138**), with the remainder of the foot appearing very normal both clinically and radiographically. If there are no other contributing deformities, this type of foot would be considered a mild flatfoot deformity. This attitude is the result of subtalar joint laxity allowing the calcaneus to slip from beneath the talus, positioning the calcaneus laterally (valgus). If this foot is left to function in this manner, further breakdown and collapse will result over a sufficient period of time with the combination of any reasonable degree of stress.

A simple test to determine the laxity or rigidity of a flatfoot deformity is to ask the child to raise himself up on the balls of his feet. If a rigid flatfoot

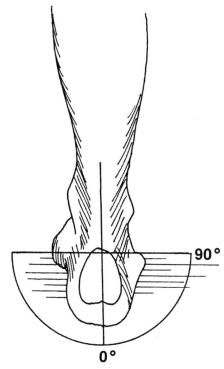

90°

0°

Calcaneal stance position

Figure 136

Placing a protractor so that it lies vertical to the ground will allow a proper determination of calcaneal excursion on stance. Use the bisection line of the calcaneus to determine if the line lies vertical to the ground (0°), or if medial to the line on the protractor, then a varus position exists. Conversely, if it lies lateral to this line, then a valgus attitude is present.

deformity exists, the foot will not resupinate with the heel raising. Instead, one will observe the continued everted valgus attitude of the rearfoot. The nonrigid flatfoot, however, will allow resupination to occur. The calcaneus will move into a varus attitude and the arch area will raise as a result of the lateral rotation of the talus (**Figure 139**). By using this test, one can rule out such conditions as a tarsal coalition, vertical talus, or peroneal spasm. Resupination indicates flexibility, and therefore a foot that can be reduced to a normal attitude and treated appropriately.

The biomechanical examination should also include determination of any superstructural abnormalities (described in the previous chapters), gait analysis, and muscular strength and balance. Rotational deformities, equinus, muscular contractures or weakness, neuromuscular disorders (i.e., spastic or paralytic disease), congenital or teratologic conditions and fractures between the talus and calcaneus must all be considered in the etiologic evaluation as well as their contribution to producing or causing abnormal stress to the foot structure.

Radiological Evaluation

To perform a proper radiographic evaluation of a child, a dorsoplantar and lateral weight-bearing x-ray should be obtained. In children who are not bear-

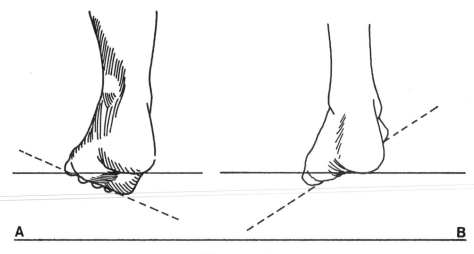

Figure 137

In figure (A) the forefoot is designated by the dotted line and is in a varus relationship to the calcaneal bisection. (B) is an example of a forefoot valgus in which the relationship of the metatarsals are everted in respect to the calcaneal bisection. A normal forefoot will have a 90° relationship with the calcaneus, i.e., no varus or valgus.

ing weight on their feet and legs, a semiweight-bearing position should be utilized. When positioning a nonweight-bearing infant in a semiweight-bearing position, be cautious not to rotate the leg either internally or externally. Rotating it inwardly will result in a falsely pronated foot while outward rotation will produce a supinated foot. Excessive downward force in an attempt to maintain the foot and leg in position may cause a false positioning of the foot as well.

When viewing the radiographs, one must account for the availability of the ossification centers that are age dependent. Prior to 2–3 years of age, the navicular ossification center is not visible. Therefore, to imagine its location

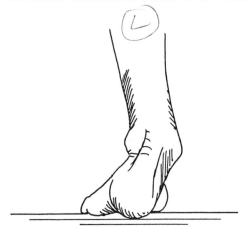

Figure 138

A Helbing's Sign is a curvature in the Achilles tendon secondary to a valgus calcaneal position. The convex side is medial and the concave side lateral.

Resupination test

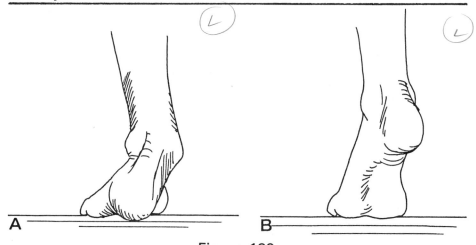

Figure 139

A flexible flatfoot will resupinate from a valgus position (A) when the patient is asked to raise up on the ball of the foot (B). A varusing of the calcaneus with a raising up of the arch area should be noted. In cases where the heel remains in valgus and the arch area does not assume a raised position, then a rigid flatfoot deformity can be considered. Further radiographic study and evaluation is needed to determine the exact etiology.

one must use the first, second, and third metatarsals that are present and the first cuneiform that is present after approximately 1–1½ years of age. It has been found through fetal dissection and radiographic interpretation that the ossification centers do not necessarily represent the actual centers of the respective bones. Therefore, caution should be exercised when extrapolating the interpretations from these radiologic findings.

The talar bisection used on dorsoplantar and lateral views has been one standard reference point or line for interpretation by many authors.[25,33] If used properly and within the norm values suggested, it can be of great assistance in proper interpretation of the radiographic views.

DORSOPLANTAR TALOCALCANEAL ANGLE

To construct this angle, bisect the talar head and neck as shown in **Figure 140**. A second line should be drawn through the long axis of the calcaneus. It becomes necessary to acquire good contrasting x-rays of the hindfoot to properly view the bony structures of the rearfoot. At the convergence of the two lines, an angle is formed and should be measured. At birth 30–40° is considered normal. This reduces to 15–30° by approximately 4–5 years of age. Values beyond this range are indicative of a structural malalignment. When extending the bisection of the talus distally, one would expect the line to fall somewhere within the first metatarsal in a normal foot. This may vary in the presence of

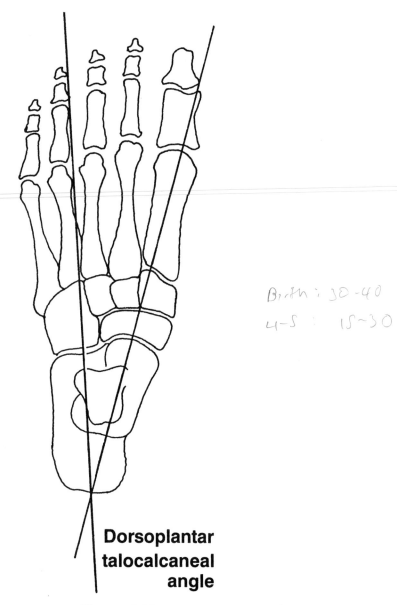

Birth : 30-40
4-5 : 15-30

**Dorsoplantar
talocalcaneal
angle**

Figure 140

metatarsus or forefoot adductus. In this situation the line would be falsely normal even though the rearfoot was diverging from normal (**Figure 141**).

LATERAL TALOCALCANEAL ANGLE

On a lateral weight-bearing radiograph, draw a bisection line through the head–neck of the talus. A second line is then drawn along the inferior surface

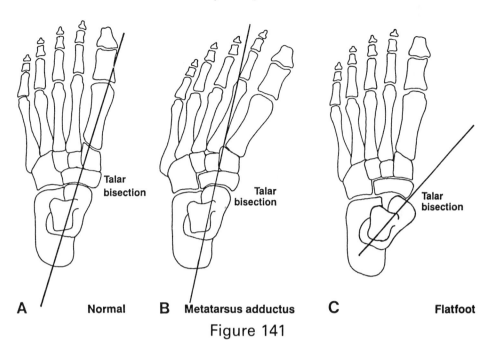

A   **Normal**   B   **Metatarsus adductus**   C   **Flatfoot**

Figure 141

of the calcaneus (**Figure 142**). The two lines will converge to form an angle. At birth the angle will range from 20–50°. When the child reaches 4–6 years of age, the value reduces to 15–35°.

If the line bisecting the talus is extended distally it should pass through the centers of the navicular, first cuneiform, and first metatarsal in a normal foot. The presence of first ray hypermobility may affect this relative position.

CALCANEAL INCLINATION ANGLE

On lateral x-ray, construct a line along the inferior surface of the calcaneus and another line paralleling the weight-bearing surface (**Figure 143**). The

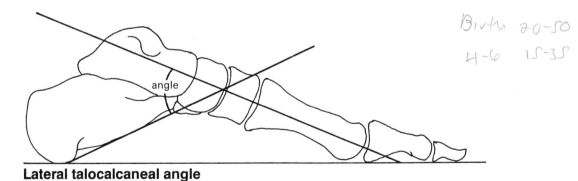

Lateral talocalcaneal angle

Figure 142

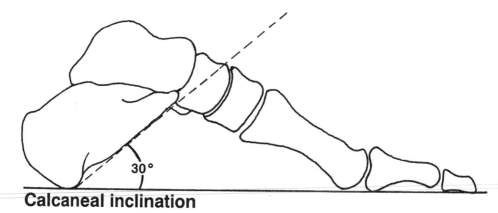

Calcaneal inclination

Figure 143

angle formed should approximate 12–18° in children under one year of age. This will increase in angular value until approximately 6–8 years of age. At this age level the inclination angle is between 15–30°. Values less than this indicate a pronation deformity in the foot, very often secondary to an equinus condition. With an equinus deformity, the posterior of the calcaneus is being pulled dorsally causing the decrease in the angle of inclination, and a collapse in the midtarsal joints is concurrently occurring.

Other measurements and methods can be used including the loss of continuity of the talonavicular–calcaneocuboid joint curvature (Cyma line) and the calcaneal–fifth metatarsal angle (**Figure 144**). These measurements are less consistent and should therefore only be used as supportive documentation, rather than as an initial diagnostic tool.[22,23,25,31–33]

Treatment

A program for treatment should be outlined and tailored to each individual's situation. Rotational deformities contributing to the stress on the foot, ligamentous laxity, familial history, muscular imbalance, equinus, etc., must all be considered and dealt with appropriately and in conjunction with the treatment of the flatfoot deformity.

Treatment should be directed with recognition that contractures and/or laxity in the soft-tissue supporting structures of the foot contributes primarily to its collapse. With early treatment there is hope that the allowance for the soft-tissue structures to assume and maintain proper alignment of the architecture of the foot can be achieved. To accomplish this, one must first treat and correct all contractures present in the soft tissues to allow for the proper positioning of the foot. Stretch-castings should be utilized to resolve any tautness present in the surrounding soft tissue. (See the section on *Talipes calcaneovalgus* for a description of casting method.) Once adequate stretching has been accomplished, the foot should be supported and maintained in proper

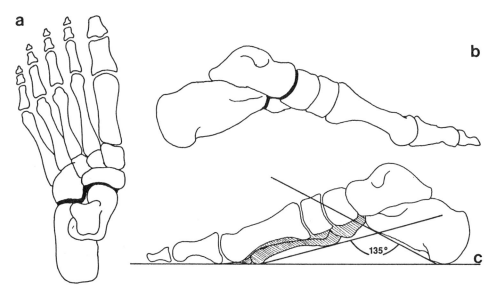

Figure 144

Anterior displacement of the cyma is the result of the calcaneus moving posteriorly, thus forcing the talus distally along with the other bones comprising of the medial pillar of the foot (A). Laterally, the displacement is similarly seen with the talonavicular joint distal to the calcaneocuboid joint (B). The calcaneal-fifth metatarsal angle is also determined from a lateral view. Values greater than 120–135° are considered significant in a flatfoot deformity.

position with an in-shoe orthosis. Children do not require orthotic control prior to standing and walking. This will become necessary and should be considered after weight-bearing is established.

Regarding the type of orthosis to be utilized, this author strongly feels that a device should encompass the foot adequately to maintain position against the flexibility and pliability of a young foot. The material to fabricate the device should be rigid so as not to allow loss of joint congruity and alignment, but sufficiently flexible to not injure the foot. Several types of orthoses have been developed to accomplish this result. Heel stabilizing devices (Types A, B, C, and E) as well as the Whitman, Roberts', and Whitman–Roberts' type devices are beneficial in controlling a flexible flatfoot deformity (**Figure 145**). Functional type orthotic devices should not be used in a young child. Several reasons that govern this opinion include: the inability of a functional orthosis to confine the foot properly; the allowance for transverse plane motion in the foot; and most children do not present with sufficient rearfoot or forefoot varus or valgus deformities to treat in this manner. (See Chapter 13 on Orthotic Devices.)

When a child reaches the age of 8–10 years, there becomes a need to reduce the amount of confinement and the rigidity of the orthosis. This becomes necessary due to the increase in sporting activities and demands of the child along with the concomitant maturation in the bony and soft-tissue struc-

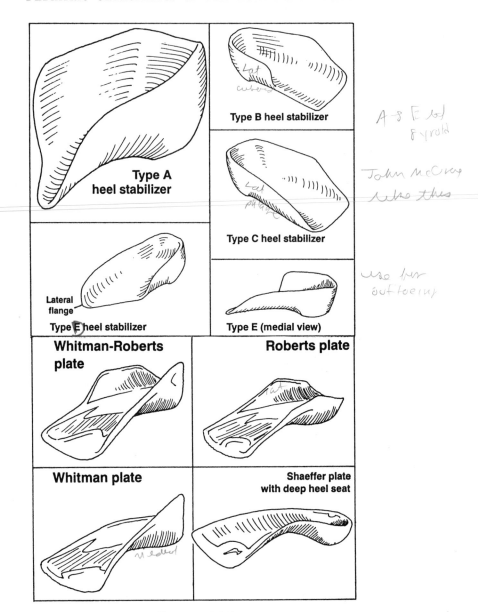

Figure 145

tures and reduction in motion. At this age level a Shaeffer plate type orthosis with a deep heel seat works well to properly support the foot and still allow the necessary flexibility (**Figure 145**). Of great concern by this author is the frequency in which a child is unknowingly placed into a position in an orthosis that will cause persistence of a deformity. It therefore becomes paramount that proper impressions and an appropriate type orthosis be employed to achieve a proper result.

If a functional type orthosis is used, the child is either posted into a varus or valgus deformity. Proper control may not be possible due to the medial–lateral mobility of this young foot. Accepting the premise that a flatfoot is the result of improper ligamentous and muscular stability to maintain joint integrity, then proper maintenance of the foot in a normal attitude is necessary to promote a proper active and resting position for these soft-tissue structures. A neutral subtalar joint with a rectus forefoot to rearfoot relationship is the optimum position. When using a functional type orthosis for children, the desired attitude of a rectus forefoot–rearfoot in development cannot occur when using varus or valgus posting. Additionally, this type of device cannot reduce the medial–lateral instability of joint laxity found in children.

When using an orthosic device to control the foot function in a child, an evaluation every 6 months to one year is necessary to determine any changes in structural position or growth. New orthoses should be fabricated when sufficient growth has occurred in the foot. This can be determined by the length of the orthosis or many times by the complaints from the child. If the tip of the orthosis is significantly behind the metatarsal heads, then refabrication should be considered. Children will often complain of the orthosis hurting them after they have gone along for a period of time without difficulty. This is a key indication for change.

Parents will often ask which type of shoes should be worn with an orthosis. When using the confining type orthotic devices, a flexible or rigid counter shoe can be employed. This author has no objection to canvas shoes being used with these rigid type orthoses since they will control the foot well without causing abnormal instability. Once a less confining device is utilized, then a more stiff counter shoe is advantageous to maintain medial–lateral position. This certainly becomes primarily dependent on the degree of laxity present in the foot.

A question that often arises from practitioners is, when can orthotic control be discontinued safely? Periodic evaluations radiologically will show the progress in the development of the foot. Angular relations of the various bony structures, i.e., talar declination angle, talo-calcaneal angle, calcaneal inclination angle, etc., are all good indicators in the progress of treatment. When normal angular values are reached in conjunction with the clinical appearance of the foot, then the use of an orthosis may be halted. It is advantageous to extend the wear of the orthotic devices for approximately 1–2 years beyond the point of normal finding to maintain the attitude of the foot and ensure greater stability. If normal values and appearance are not achieved adequately, then continuation of the use of the orthosis is necessary.

The parents as well as the patient should be informed of the potential ability for correction of the foot deformity, the possibility of other abnormalities arising, and/or a reoccurrence of the flatfoot condition in later life. It should be explained that this is due to changes in the bodily structures occurring with age and demand. One cannot ensure permanent structural maintenance. If periodic examinations with proper radiographic evaluation are employed, then alterations in the foot structure can be treated early to avoid the secondary problems and complications.

Surgical Correction

An intervention surgically for a flatfoot condition is only necessary when there is an inability to control the foot by an orthotic device. The question is often asked by students and practitioners as to the time to consider surgical correction. It is the opinion of this author that if a foot is; unable to be maintained adequately in an orthosis to allow comfort and the ability to perform the usual everyday activities for that given age level, not properly controlled structurally, causing unreasonable shoe wear even with orthotic control, then surgical consideration for realignment is appropriate. The practitioner should not be fooled into believing that merely because the patient is wearing an orthosis he is being controlled well. A moderate to severe flatfoot condition may force the foot to pronate over and off the orthotic device. This is not properly maintaining the functional position of the foot. One can appreciate that an orthosis will reduce the muscular stretch and stress and provide a degree of relief to the patient, but it is not necessarily providing an adequate structural position to function appropriately.

The goal of surgery is to provide a realignment of the foot sufficient to be controlled with an orthosis. There are surgeons who feel that surgery is indicated for a flatfoot to provide a normal foot structure without the necessity for an external controlling brace, i.e., an orthotic device. This author feels that in most cases of flexible flatfeet, it is the laxity in the ligaments and musculature that offer the foot the ability to move into an abnormal attitude. Therefore, to tighten and stabilize these structures surgically without the potential for stretch and loosening in the future is somewhat unlikely and unrealistic without an orthosis. The goal surgically, therefore, is to provide a foot that can be controlled within an optimal position utilizing an orthotic device and not to expect a normal architecture to be maintained without the control.

Historically, several surgical procedures have been offered to realign the structure of the foot. The procedures most currently being performed will be reviewed and a critique of each given. The goals in flatfoot surgery are to: limit the degree of eversion of the calcaneus; adduct the forefoot; align the talus over the calcaneus; and align the talus and calcaneus with the mid and forefoot. Unfortunately, one procedure is not available to accomplish all these goals for all types of flexible flatfeet. One must tailor the procedure(s) to the areas affected. There is still much to be learned in the etiology of this foot deformity so that more lasting and accurate treatment may be employed.

SUBTALAR ARTHROERESIS

The subtalar arthroeresis has enjoyed a great deal of popularity in recent years by podiatric surgeons. The procedure was first described by J. LeLievre in which a staple over the lateral talocalcaneal joint was used to limit calcaneal eversion.[18,19] The intent was for remodeling to occur over a period of 2–3 years followed by removal of the staple. This procedure was further popularized by Haroldson who began using a bone implant in the sinus tarsi to limit motion.[12] This differs from the Grice procedure which produces a fusion of the subtalar joint.[31]

More recently, two types of procedures are being utilized: the use of a silastic cone or plug in the sinus tarsi, or a polypropylene peg in the sinus tarsi to limit anterior displacement of the talus on the calcaneus (**Figure 146**). These procedures have merit in preventing subtalar valgusing but provide virtually no correction or change in any midtarsal or forefoot alterations. Therefore, it has selected usage in those mild to moderate flexible flatfeet with minimal to no midtarsal joint changes. Its ability to limit calcaneal eversion is advantageous in combination with other procedures for the total correction of the more complicated flatfoot conditions.

The disadvantages to this procedure are: the loss of viability of a bone plug, if used, with resulting loss of correction; the continued presence of a foreign material (silastic and polypropelene) with possible rejection; the finite longevity of the materials used causing the need for replacement in the future; and the need to change its size with the growth of the child. To date, there has been no conclusive evidence to support the theory that the use of a subtalar arthroeresis will eventually alter the subtalar joint architecture to be capable of maintaining its corrected structural position without the continued use of the implant. Advantages to this procedure are the nondestruction of joints, avoidance of joint fusions, no limitation in bone growth, and the ability to be reversed with removal of the implant.

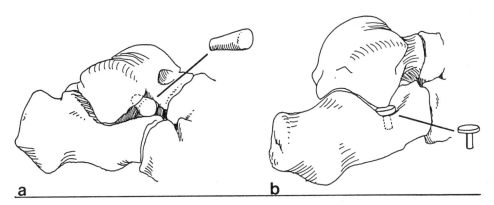

a   b

Figure 146

Two current methods used to limit subtalar motion by a subtalar arthroeresis are the silastic plug (A) which is positioned in the sinus tarsi and the silastic or polypropylene peg (B) which is implanted in the floor of the sinus tarsi. These will limit talar motion distally and plantarly. The procedure is performed through a lateral approach over the sinus tarsi and will produce minimal surgical trauma with rapid ambulation.

HOKE AND MILLER PROCEDURE

These two procedures primarily are concerned with collapse at the navicular–cuneiform and cuneiform–metatarsal joints. The end result is a fusion of the medial midtarsal joints to reduce sag (**Figure 147**). Unfortunately, these two procedures alone do not provide an adequate long-term maintenance of the foot position. Compensatory motion will often occur either proximal or distal to these fused joint segments in the future. This can eventually produce arthritic changes due to excessive stress and deviated joint positioning. If these procedures are considered in the correction of a flatfoot, they should be combined with another procedure to properly align the other segments of the foot. The procedures are inadequate independently and should be avoided as a singular procedure.

SOFT-TISSUE SUSPENSION PROCEDURES

Several procedures can be described under this heading: joint desmoplasty, tendon transfers (Young suspension, Lowman, Kidner, McGlamry), and tendon releases (Achilles lengthening, peroneal lengthening) (**Figures 148–154**). It has been generally found by most foot surgeons that these procedures independently do not withstand the stresses of time. These procedures are particularly inefficient in cases of ligamentous laxity or significant forefoot abduction. The more mild or moderate flatfoot may benefit by tendon transfers and tendon shortening in conjunction with orthopedic control. When these tendon transfers, lengthenings, and shortening are combined with other osseous stabilizing procedures, the results have been proven satisfactory (an example—Evans flatfoot procedure combined with a Young tendon suspension (**Figure 154**)). It is this author's feeling that a combination of procedures is necessary to stabilize both the medial and lateral columns of the foot to maintain stability and correction over a long term.

ARTHRODESIS OF THE REARFOOT

Fusion of one, two, or all three of the joints in the rearfoot is only considered in those feet not amenable to other forms of treatment (**Figure 155**). The severe valgused foot either laxed or rigid (peroneal spastic flatfoot, tarsal coalitions, vertical talus) may need to be fused to provide either stability or reduction in motion to avoid pain. The consideration for fusion should only be contemplated in the adolescent or adult. The younger child (under age 10–12 years) should be treated in a more conservative manner. A complication of an early rearfoot fusion is a ball-in-socket ankle joint causing chronic instability. Knee and ankle joint changes will also result from loss of subtalar joint motion. Traditionally, all three joints of the rearfoot are fused (i.e., talocalcaneal, talonavicular, and calcaneocuboid joints) to maintain stability. Occasionally it may only be necessary to fuse one or two of the joints; however, this is rare and not as stable as the classic triple arthrodesis.

Miller Fusion

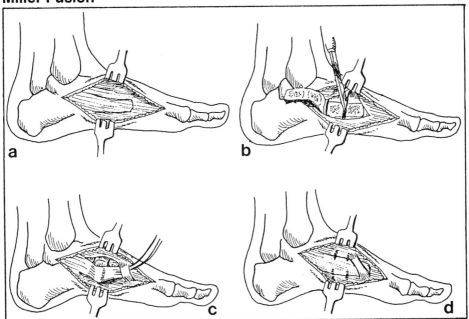

a

b

c

d

Hoke Fusion

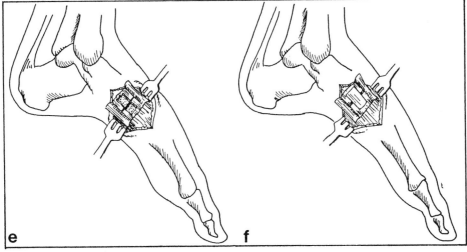

e

f

Figure 147

Miller Fusion. *A flap of the medial periosteum and capsule over the navicular and first cuneiform is first made (A). A portion of the medial eminence of the navicular and first cuneiform is removed along with the periosteum and capsule to be incorporated in the fusion. One can extend this to include the base of the first metatarsal when necessary. Denuding, and when needed, a wedging of the naviculocuneiform and the first cuneiform–first metatarsal joints should be performed (B). A sling is made with the distal periosteum-capsule (C) and the flap pulled through. The foot should be supinated into position and the periosteal-capsular flap sutured under tension. Wire fixation can be employed when greater stability is warranted. Hoke Fusion. This procedure fuses the navicular-first cuneiform and the second cuneiform. After removal of the articular cartilage of the distal surface of the navicular proximal surface of the first cuneiform, and the medial surface of the 2nd cuneiform, a trough is cut to accept a bone graft (E). The use of a graft from either the tibia, pelvis, calcaneus, or bone bank bone can be used to fuse the area (F).*

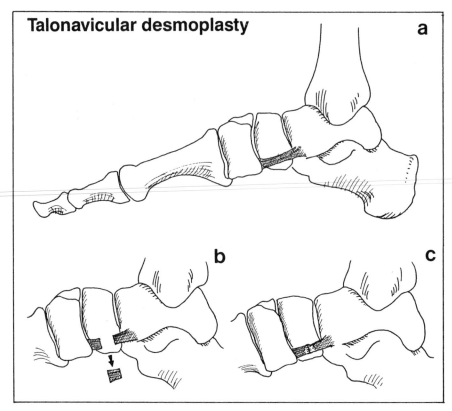

Talonavicular desmoplasty

Figure 148

A talonavicular desmoplasty is the removal of a wedge of the medial capsule and spring ligament to provide medial stability. The spring ligament (A) needs to be identified after the capsule is wedged and removed medially. A wedge is then removed (B) to allow proper tightening. More can be removed after the foot is supinated and the proper tension is determined. Suturing the spring ligament and the medial capsule (C) is performed under adequate tension.

EVANS' FLATFOOT PROCEDURE

This procedure was first described by Dillwyn Evans in the early 1970s.[7] The concept behind this procedure is the medial and lateral column theory of the foot. The foot is viewed with the medial column comprised of the talus, navicular, three cuneiforms, first three metatarsals, and their respective toes. The lateral column is comprised of the calcaneus, cuboid, 4th and 5th metatarsals, and their respective toes. A flatfoot can be visualized as a lengthening of the medial column or a shortening of the lateral column. The lengthened medial column occurs from the anterior shift of the talus forcing the forefoot in abduction. The principle of the Evans' procedure is to regain equal lengths of the columns by lengthening the lateral column. When performed, it adducts the forefoot and simultaneously supinates the rearfoot. The surgery is per-

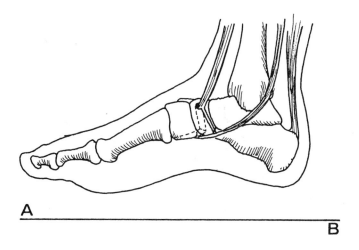

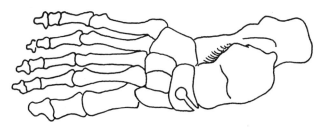

Figure 149

A Young suspension *requires a keyhole-type cut into the navicular (A) with a transpositionalization of the tibialis anterior into the keyhole (B). Either a total tendon or a split tendon transfer can be performed to accomplish a result.*

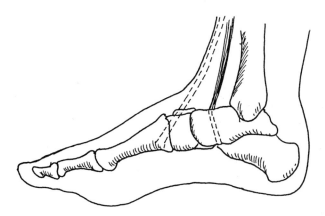

Figure 150

The Lowman procedure *transposes the tibialis anterior tendon into the space between the talonavicular joint. The joint, however, is completely denuded of its cartilage or wedged prior to the insertion of the tendon and it is then fixated for a fusion. This fusion along with the pull of the tendon under tension helps to support the foot.*

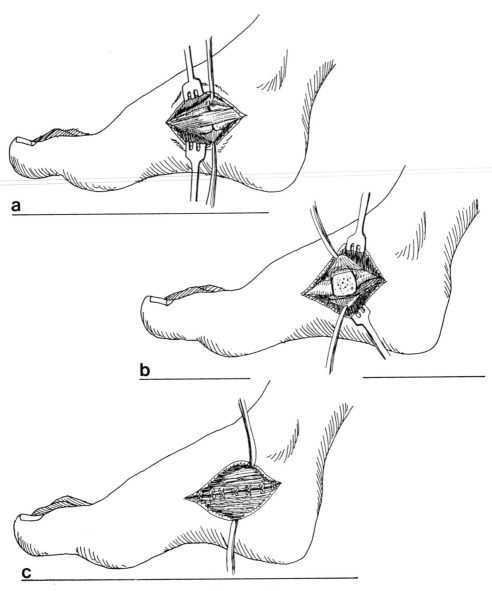

Figure 151

The Kidner procedure *removes the medial eminence of the navicular and when presence
an os tibiale externum accessory bone. A reattachment of the posterior tibial tendon under
tension is also performed to create medial stability. (A) A medial approach is used to
visualize the talonavicular joint. (B) Removal of the medial eminence of the navicular
(removal of any accessory bones should be performed at this stage). (C) Suturing of the
periosteal-capsular and tendinous structures under tension with the foot held in a supinated attitude is finally accomplished.*

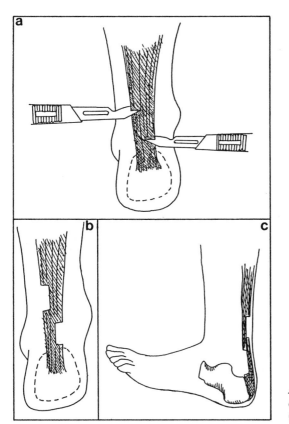

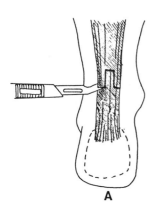

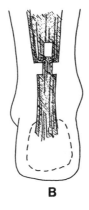

Gastro _ Sdee

Figure 152

An Achilles lengthening can be accomplished by a stab tenotomy (A)(B)(C).

percutanous

Figure 153

A tongue-in-groove lengthening in cases of a short gastrocnemius shortage can also be used for reduction (A)(B).

Gastroc equin

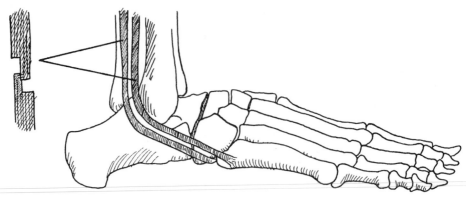

Figure 154

Peroneal lengthenings should be performed when noticeable contractures are evident and resupination is being limited by these contractures. Z-plasty or slide lengthenings should be performed at the lower one-third of the leg and above the ankle joint.

formed by placing a bone graft in an osteotomy at the lateral aspect of the calcaneus to accomplish the lengthening (**Figure 156**).

Children above the ages of 8–9 years provide the best group for this form of correction. This procedure may be combined with a medial desmoplasty, tendon transfers, and shortenings, etc. to provide greater stability in a ligamentous lax condition or in the severely valgused foot needing medial column stability.

Advantages to the procedure are: it does not destroy any joint surfaces as in fusions; it does not impair growth of the foot; and it does not use foreign materials with a finite longevity.[1,3,7,11,12,14–17,19,20,24,26,27,29–31,34–36]

Congenital Vertical Talus (Congenital Convex Pes Valgus)

Congenital vertical talus is a reasonably rare occurrence, more commonly found in boys. This deformity exists at birth and should be recognized and treated as early as possible. The etiology of this deformity is unknown; however, several theories have been proposed. Neurological disorders and intrauterine influences have been suggested as causes, but this does not adequately explain the increased incidence of other congenital aberrations observed commonly in children with this deformity. Conditions of arthrogryposis multiplex congenita, cerebral palsy, myelomeningocele, neurofibromatosis, spina bifida, congenital scoliosis, and congenital hip dysplasias have been found concomitantly with congenital vertical talus.[1,3,7,8–13]

myofibroblast

Anatomic Findings

The gross appearance exhibits the rearfoot fixed in an attitude of moderate equinus and the mid and forefoot dorsiflexed relative to the rearfoot. There

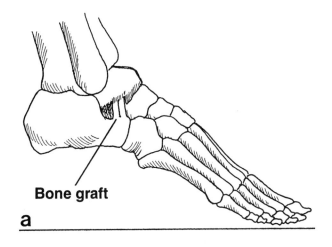

Bone graft

a

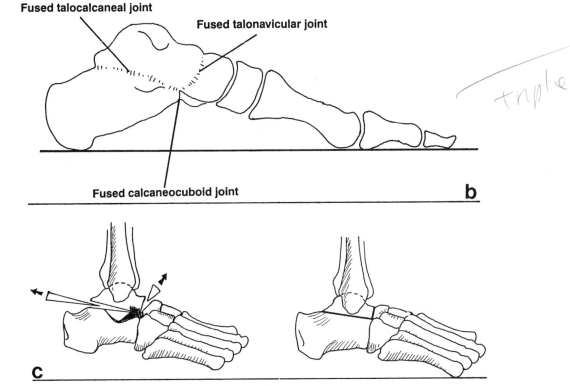

Fused talocalcaneal joint

Fused talonavicular joint

triple

Fused calcaneocuboid joint

b

c

Figure 155

Various fusions may be employed to stabilize the rearfoot. A fusion of the subtalar joint only (Grice procedure) is often used in the younger child with a flexible flatfoot (A). A triple fusion (triple arthrodesis) is performed at the talonavicular, talocalcaneal, and calcaneocuboid joints (B). When necessary, wedges may need to be removed to appropriately align the foot correctly (C).

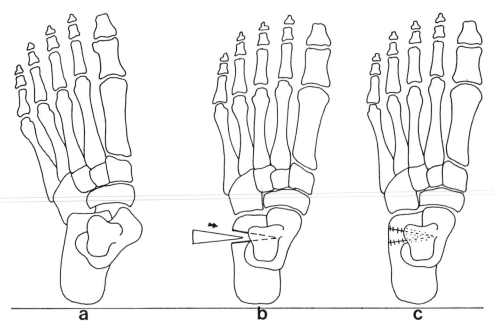

Figure 156

The Evan's flatfoot procedure is performed to achieve an equal length in the medial and lateral columns of the foot. A flatfoot has a lengthening of the medial column with abduction of the forefoot (A). By the use of a bone graft laterally in the calcaneus, the lateral pillar of the foot can be lengthened to resupinate the foot and adduct the forefoot. The calcaneus will also reduce its ability to go into valgus on stance due to the supination effect (B). The graft will be absorbed with the body replacing it with healthy normal bone and a good alignment (C).

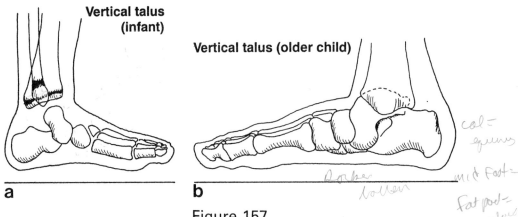

Figure 157

(A) The ossification center of the talus will be severely plantarflexed and almost parallel with the long axis of the tibia in a congenital vertical talus. (B) When the navicular becomes ossified, the articular surface of the talar head is viewed more dorsal and lateral than normally found. A depression will also be noted on the dorsal aspect of the talus in which the navicular has been articulating.

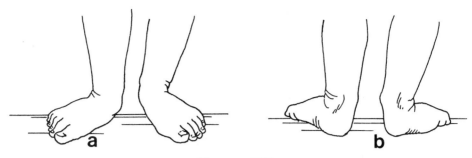

Figure 158

Note that a congenital vertical talus deformity will have similar characteristics to a talipes calcaneovalgus on stance when viewed clinically. An everted calcaneus with an inverted position of the ankle is commonly found. This deformity, however, is rigid and fixed and will not reduce as with a talipes calcaneovalgus deformity.

are contractures of all the soft tissues of the dorsum of the midfoot. Excessive mobility dorsally with an inability to align the midfoot with the rearfoot when plantarflexed and supinated is typically found.

Soft-tissue findings are an anterior subluxation of the peroneus brevis and peroneus longus and hypoplasia of the peroneal groove of the lateral malleolus. The Achilles tendon is often contracted along with the posterior ankle capsule. The extensor tendons on the dorsum of the foot are contracted with the forefoot abducted and dorsiflexed.

The posterior tibial tendon will lie anterior and dorsal to the axis of the forefoot. Frequently there is a partial or complete absence of the intrinsic muscles of the foot. The capsule of the anterior part of the ankle and the anterior talonavicular portion of the detoid ligament is usually contracted. The calcaneonavicular (spring) ligament will be thinned and nonsupportive of the neck of the talus.

The osseous and joint findings include the navicular being dislocated dorsally and rotated nearly 90° from its normal position. The navicular will rest in an abnormal despression on the dorsal surface of the neck of the talus. Articular cartilage of the talus will be present on the dorsal and lateral sides of the head (**Figure 157**). A talocalcaneal subluxation occurs wherein the os calcis is rotated into eversion and the talus is rotated plantarward and medially. There is hypoplasia of the subtalar facets due to lack of articular contact. This deformity will present with the so called "rocker bottom" appearance (**Figure 158**). A rigid deformed appearance as described is almost pathopneumonic of a vertical talus in an infant.

A second type of vertical talus that is more severe than the foot described above is one in which there is concomitant subluxation of the calcaneocuboid joint in addition to the deformities mentioned. This type foot responds poorly to treatment and results in a poorer prognosis than the foot without subluxation of this joint.

Radiographically, the disturbed talonavicular relationship cannot be accurately discerned during the first 2 or 3 years of life. This is due to the absence of the ossification center of the navicular bone.

By the age of 3 years, the navicular can be identified in its dislocated position on the anteriosuperior surface of the neck of the talus (**Figure 159**). Despite the fact that the navicular cannot be recognized, the gross abnormality of the hindfoot can be readily identified radiologically with the vertical attitude of the talus in relation to the tibia.

A congenital vertical talus differs from talipes calcaneovalgus in many respects and should not be confused. Talipes calcaneovalgus is a reducible deformity without dorsal displacement of the navicular, and a normal angular relation of the talus with the tibia.[1-13]

Treatment

Historically, a variety of therapeutic approaches have been proposed. What have been found consistently are: conservative measures usually fail; the talonavicular joint must be reduced and maintained; a posterior release of the ankle and foot must nearly always be performed; and the bone structures primarily involved in the deformity must be held in the corrected position by some means until they become stable. Stretch castings after sufficient manipulation are beneficial in gaining reduced tension in the skin and soft tissues. This will provide a far better correction and easier skin closure.

Several surgical approaches have been described that are dependent on the severity of the deformity and subluxation of the calcaneocuboid joint. The naviculectomy still holds the greatest promise for adequate reduction and adaptive articular changes. Beyond the age of 5–6 years the reducible surgical corrections become less effective and carry a poorer prognosis. It then becomes beneficial to wait until the child is 10 years of age or older to perform a triple arthrodesis with proper wedge correction. It is not advisable to perform the arthrodesis before this age due to the complicating sequelae that often follow at this earlier age, including the ball-in-socket ankle joint.[2,4,6,7,12]

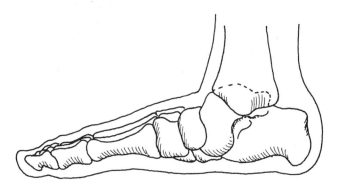

Figure 159

A dislocated navicular positioned on the dorsum of the talus is able to be visualized radiographically after a child is beyond 2½–3 years of age.

Tarsal Coalitions (Peroneal Spastic Flatfoot)

Tarsal coalitions have been known for well over 200 years though only in the past 50–60 years has it been related to the peroneal spastic flatfoot. The various coalitions that may exist to produce this form of flatfoot are: calcaneonavicular bar, talocalcaneal bar at either the posterior middle or anterior facets, and osteochondral fractures of the talar head causing a fusion.

The manifestations of a peroneal spastic flatfoot caused by a congenital tarsal coalition are: limitation of motion in the major tarsal joints or even rigidity; valgus deformity of varying degrees; pain after strain of the foot; contracture or spasm of the peroneus longus and brevis; and congenital anomalies of the major tarsal bones and changes in the tarsal joints.

Several types of coalitions may exist, including the complete or incomplete fusion, the osseous (synostosis), cartilagenous (synchondrosis) or fibrous (syndesmosis) coalitions. In young children tarsal coalitions may not be visible, even though existent on radiographs. The coalition being cartilagenous in the youngster will often ossify later during development. This ossification, and its radiographic evidence, may not occur until the age of 9–11 years. Other radiographic findings may include osteophytic lipping at the talonavicular joint (talar beaking), especially on the dorsum of the talus and diminished articular spacing of the subtalar joint (**Figure 160**). The osteophytes along the dorsal margin of the talonavicular joint (talar beaking) develop more frequently and

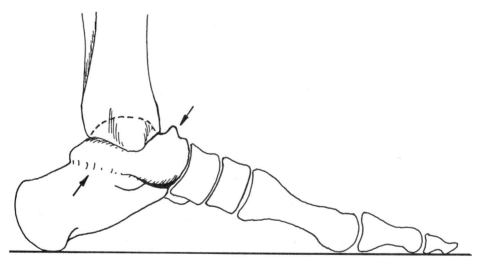

Figure 160

Talar beaking is a common finding in tarsal coalitions, particularly the talocalcaneal type. It is not necessarily pathoneumonic but is supportive in conjuction with other clinical findings. Loss of subtalar joint space is additionally a characteristic sign of a coalition; however, it is not conclusive.

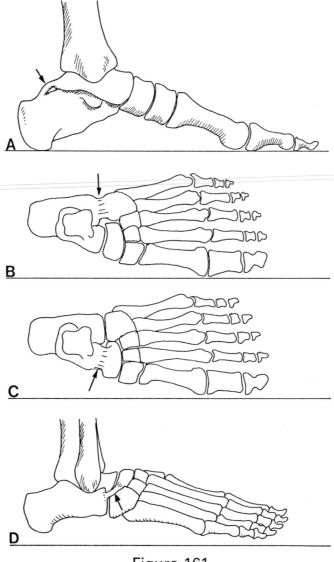

Figure 161

(A) Talar process—calcaneus bar. (B) Calcaneocuboid bar. (C) Talonavicular bar. (D) Calcaneonavicular bar.

earlier in patients with talocalcaneal coalitions than in those with calcaneonavicular bars.

Frequently recognized is the absence of severe calcaneal valgusing on stance along with minimal collapse in the longitudinal arch in the talocalcaneal coalition.

Occasionally one may find a child presenting with a varus (inversion) deformity of the foot as a result of a calcaneonavicular coalition. The resulting spasm in the tibialis anterior and posterior muscles may be the result of an incomplete fusion. The severe varus is an attempt to avoid pressure at the approaching ends of the bar or as a result of splinting in the case of a separation of a cartilagenous bar. Other less frequent bridges may be at the posterior talar process fusing with the dorsum of the calcaneus, calcaneo–cuboid fusion, talonavicular fusion, and cuboid–navicular fusion (**Figure 161**).

When evaluating for a tarsal coalition, a complete radiographic study including tomography is necessary. Computerized axial tomography (CAT) scans are now more useful in determining coalitions that are difficult to discern by other radiographic means.[1-14]

Treatment

If a calcaneonavicular coalition is diagnosed early (prior to bone fusion during childhood or the early adolescent age period), then an attempt at manipulation under anesthesia with immobilization in a below-the-knee walking cast for 6 weeks can be considered. After cast removal, the use of a heel stabilizer type C with the foot being captured in an impression of slight varus should be employed. If the pain persists, then surgical intervention is necessary to relieve the symptoms.

With a calcaneonavicular bar excision, the interposing of the extensor digitorm brevis muscle will usually offer an excellent chance of abolishing the symptoms and restoring mobility to the foot without future restrictions in activity if there exists no radiologic evidence of arthritic changes. This radiographic evidence includes talar beaking and narrowing of the subtalar joint. Calcaneonavicular bars used beyond 13–14 years of age will most likely not respond to excisional correction. A long-standing calcaneonavicular or a talocalcaneal bar will require an arthrodesis of the talocalcaneal, talonavicular, and calcaneocuboid joint to resolve the symptomatology. Although it has been attempted, the talocalcaneal bar in either the anterior, middle, or posterior facets cannot be excised with a good prognosis. Therefore, if a talocalcaneal coalition exists a fusion will be indicated at the appropriate age (beyond 12 years old).[3,4,14]

References

Calcaneovalgus and Pes Planus:
1. Beck, E.L., McGlamry, E.D.: Modified young tendosuspension technique for flexible flatfoot. Analysis of rationale and results: A preliminary report on 20 operations. *Journal American Podiatry Association,* 63:November 1973.
2. Basmajian, J.V., Stecko, G.: The role of muscles in arch support of the foot. *Journal Bone and Joint Surgery,* 45-A:1963.
3. Bratberg, J.J., Scheer, G.E.: Extra-articular arthrodesis of the subtalar joint: A clinical study and review. *Clinical Orthopaedics,* Number 126, 1977.

4. Brocone, D.: Congenital malformations. *Practitioner,* 131:30, 1933.

5. Cohen, L.: Congenital calcaneovalgus. Lecture presented at Illinois College of Podiatric Medicine, November 1974.

6. Cohen, L., Cohen, M.: Congenital calcaneovalgus. *Journal American Podiatry Association,* 66:Number 10, October 1976.

7. Evans, D.: Calcaneo-valgus deformity. *Journal Bone and Joint Surgery,* 57-B:August 1975.

8. Ferciot, C.F.: Calcaneovalgus foot in the newborn and its relation to developmental flatfoot. *Clinical Orthopedics,* Number 85, 1972.

9. Ferciot, C.F.: The etiology of developmental flatfoot. *Clinical Orthopaedics,* Number 85, 1972.

10. Ganley, J.V.: Calcaneovalgus deformity in infants. *Journal American Podiatry Association,* 65:May 1975.

11. Gionnestras, N.J.: Recognition and treatment of flatfeet in infancy. *Clinical Orthopaedics and Related Research,* Number 70, May–June 1970.

12. Haroldson, N.A.: The arthroereisis procedure for correction of flexible flatfoot in childhood. Lecture, Fourth Annual Northlake Surgical Seminar, December 1975.

13. Henceroth, W.D., Deyerle, W.M.: The Acquired Unilateral Flatfoot in the Adult: Some Causative Factors. Foot and Ankle. Volume 2. Number 5. 1982.

14. Johnson, B.: The Sustentaculum Tali Procedure. Lecture, Fourth Annual Northlake Surgical Seminar, December 1975.

15. Koutsogiannis, E.: Treatment of mobile flatfoot by displacement osteotomy of the calcaneus. *Journal Bone and Joint Surgery* 53(B):96–100, February 1961.

16. Lanham, R.H.: Arthroeresis update. *Journal American Podiatry Association,* 71:Number 12, December 1981.

17. Lanham, R.H.: Indications and complications of arthroeresis in hypermobile flatfoot. *Journal American Podiatry Association,* 69:Number 3, March 1979.

18. LeLievre, J.: Current concepts and correction in the valgus foot. *Clinical Orthopedics,* 7:43–55, May–June 1970.

19. LeLievre, J.: Current concepts and correction in the valgus foot. Parts I and II. *Clinical Orthopaedics,* Number 70, May–June 1970.

20. Mitchell, G.P.: Spasmodic flatfoot. *Clinical Orthopaedics & Related Research,* Number 70, May–June 1970.

21. Reinherz, R.D., Reinherz, H.R.: A pedal variant of ehler-danlos syndrome with osseous adaptation. *Journal American Podiatry Association,* 70:Number 11, November 1980.

22. Schuster, R.O.: Flexible flatfoot in childhood and adolescence. *Northlake Surgical Seminar,* December 1974.

23. Schuster, R.O., Port, M.: Abnormal pronation in children. *Journal American Podiatry Association,* 67:Number 9, September 1977.

24. Selakovich, W.G.: Medial arch support by operation—sustentarculum tali procedure. *Orthop. Clin. N.A.,* 4:117–44 January 1973.

25. Sgarlato, T.E.: A compendium of podiatric biomechanics. *California College of Podiatric Medicine,* 1971.

26. Sgarlato, T.E., Morgan, J., Shane, H.S., Frenkenberg, A.: Tendo achilles lengthening and its effect on foot disorders. *J.A.P.A.,* 65:41–49, January 1975.

27. Silver, C.M., Simons, S.D., Spindell, E., Litchman, H.M., Scala, M.: Calcaneal osteotomy for valgus and varus deformities of the foot in cerebral palsy. *Journal of Bone and Joint Surgery,* 49(A):232–246, March 1976.

28. Steward, S.F.: Human gait and the human foot. An ethnological study of flatfoot. *Clinical Orthopaedics,* Number 70, May–June 1970.

29. Subotnick, S.I.: The subtalar joint lateral extra-articular arthroereisis. A follow-up report. *J.A.P.A.,* 67:157–171, March 1977.

30. Sullivan, J.A., Miller, W.A.: The relationship of the accessory navicular to the development of the flatfoot. *Clinical Orthopaedics,* Number 144, 1979.

31. Tachdjian, M.D.: *Pediatric Orthopedics.* W.B. Saunders Company, Philadelphia, PA, 1972.
32. Tax, H.R.: *Podopediatrics.* Williams and Wilkins Co., Baltimore, MD, 1980.
33. Tax, H.R.: Flexible flatfoot in children. *J.A.P.A.,* 67:Number 9, September 1977.
34. Weseley, M.S., Barenfeld, P.A.: Mechanism of the Dwyer calcaneal osteotomy. *Clinical Orthopedics,* 70:137–140, May–June 1970.
35. Williams, P.F., Menelaus, M.B.: Triple arthrodesis by inlay grafting—A method suitable for the undeformed or valgus foot. *Journal of Bone and Joint Surgery,* 59B, 1977.
36. Wilson, F.C. Jr., Fay, G.F., LaMotte, P., Williams, J.C.: Triple arthrodesis. *Journal of Bone and Joint Surgery* 47(A):340–348, March 1965.
37. Wynne-Davies, R.: Family studies on the cause of congenital clubfoot. *Journal of Bone and Joint Surgery,* 46-B, 1964.
38. Yale, J.F.: Growth center injuries of the foot. *Arch. of Pod. Med. and Foot Surg.,* Vol. I, Number 2, October 1973.

Tarsal Coalitions:

1. Badgley, C.E.: Coalition of the calcaneus and the navicular. *Arch. Surg.,* 15:1927.
2. Cavallaro, D.C., Hadden, H.R.: An unusual case of tarsal coalition. *J.A.P.A.,* 68:Number 2, February 1978.
3. Conway, J.J., Cowell, H.R.: Tarsal coalitions: Clinical significance and roentgenographic demonstration. *Radiology,* 92:1969.
4. Cowell, H.R.: Talocalcaneal coalition and new causes of peroneal spastic flatfoot. *Clinical Orthopaedics,* Number 85, June 1972.
5. Harris, B.A.: Anomalous structures in the human foot. *Anat. Rec.,* 121:1955.
6. Harris, R.I.: Retrospect: Peroneal spastic flatfoot (rigid valgus foot). *Journal of Bone and Joint Surgery,* 47-A:1965.
7. Harris, R.I.: Rigid valgus root due to talocalcaneal bridge. *Journal of Bone and Joint Surgery,* 37-A:1955.
8. Harris, R.I., Beath, T.: Etiology of peroneal spastic flatfoot. *Journal of Bone and Joint Surgery,* 30-B:1948.
9. Outland, T., Murphy, I.D.: The patho-mechanics of perioneal spastic flatfoot. *Clinical Orthopedics,* 16:1960.
10. Salter, R.B.: *Textbook of Disorders and Injuries of the Musculoskeletal System.* Williams and Wilkins Co., Baltimore, MD, 1970.
11. Schrieber, R.R.: Talonavicular synostosis. *Journal of Bone and Joint Surgery,* 45-A:1963.
12. Tachdjian, M.O.: *Pediatric Orthopedics.* W.B. Saunders Co., Philadelphia, PA, 1972.
13. Tax, H.R.: *Podopediatrics.* Williams and Wilkins Co., Baltimore, MD, 1980.
14. Tsoutsouris, G.V., Ditmars, J.J., Crovo, R.T.: Coalition of the talocalcaneal articulation. *J.A.P.A.,* 68:Number 2, February 1978.

Vertical Talus:

1. Bowlus, T.H., Dobas, D.C.: Congenital vertical talus. *J.A.M.A.,* 67:Number 9, September 1977.
2. Buchanan, J.R., Greer, R.B.: Pathomechanics and treatment of the vertical talus foot. *Orthopaedic Review,* 10:1981.
3. Clark, M.W., D'Ambrosia, R.D., Ferguson, A.B.: Congenital vertical talus. *Journal of Bone and Joint Surgery,* 59-A:June 1977.
4. Coleman, S.S., Stelling, F.H., Jarrett, J.: Pathomechanics and treatment of congenital vertical talus. *Clinical Orthopaedics,* Number 70, May–June 1970.
5. Drennau, J.C., Sharrard, W.J.: The pathological anatomy of convex pes valgus. *Journal of Bone and Joint Surgery,* 53-B:1971.

6. Fiton, J.M., Nevelos, A.B.: The treatment of congenital vertical talus. *Journal of Bone and Joint Surgery,* 61-B:1979.
7. Herndon, C.H., Heyman, C.H.: Problems in the recognition and treatment of congenital convex pes valgus. *Journal of Bone and Joint Surgery,* 45-A:1963.
8. Mead, N.C., Anast, G.: Vertical talus (congenital talonavicular dislocation). *Clinical Orthopaedics,* 21:1961.
9. Patterson, W.R., Fitz, D.A., Smith, W.S.: The pathologic anatomy of congenital pes valgus. *Journal of Bone and Joint Surgery,* 50-A:1968.
10. Searfoss, R., Bendana, A., King, G., Miller, G.: Vertical talus of unusual etiology. *Journal of Bone and Joint Surgery,* 57-A:April 1975.
11. Specht, E.E.: Congenital paralytic vertical talus. *Journal of Bone and Joint Surgery,* 57-A:September 1975.
12. Tachdjian, M.O.: *Pediatric Orthopedics.* W.B. Saunders Company, Philadelphia, PA, 1972.
13. Tax, H.R.: *Podopediatrics.* William and Wilkins Company, Baltimore, MD, 1980.

Chapter 9

CAVUS FOOT AND CLUBFOOT DEFORMITIES

Pes Cavus (Cavus Foot)

*F*irst described in 1743 by André, *pes cavus* has accumulated several confusing and conflicting theories about its exact etiology, mode of development, and method of treatment. The pathology of the cavus foot can be classified into two types—neuromuscular, and idiopathic. Several neuromuscular disorders can contribute to this foot deformity, including: disorders of the cerebral cortex (hysteria); spinocerebellar tract (Frederick's ataxia); pyramidal or extrapyramidal systems (cerebral palsy); anterior horn cells of the spinal column (poliomyelitis); peripheral nerve root or lumbosacral spinal nerve root disorders (Charcot–Marie–Tooth disease, interstitial hypertrophic neuritis); and muscular dystrophy, hyperinnervation of muscles, muscular imbalance.[1,2,13,14]

The idiopathic type of cavus foot does not exhibit underlying pathology even with electromyographic and nerve conduction studies. As much as 34–40% of cavus feet are considered idiopathic in nature. Several theories have been proposed as to the causative factors for the idiopathic type including: measles, scarlet fever, diptheria, etc. causing a discrepancy in muscular and bone growth; genetic factors (familial incidence); weakness of the extrinsic musculature (extensor digitorm longus, tibialis anterior, gastroc-soleus, peroneals); weakness of the intrinsic musculature of the foot; combination of weakness of the extrinsic and intrinsic musculature.[1,5,13,14]

One can classify cavus feet into several categories. First, the *anterior cavus* exhibits a plantarflexion of the forefoot in relation to the rearfoot and occurs at the tarso-metatarsal or midtarsal joint level. Two subclassifications for an anterior cavus are: the *local type* which is a plantarflexion of the first ray (1st metatarsal and medial cuneiform); and the *total type* which is a plantarflexion of the entire forefoot. The second major classification type is the *posterior cavus* located in the subtalar joint region. This results in a significant increase in the inclination of the calcaneus in its relation to the talus. The third type, and most frequent, is a combination of both the anterior and posterior cavus referred to as global type (**Figure 162**).

These types of cavus feet can further be classified into: *positional cavus* which is nonosseous in nature and therefore will disappear on weight-bearing. This can eventually lead to a more rigid type with the allowance of sufficient time and proper conditions; *structural cavus* is osseous in nature in the more rigid form; the *semi type,* which is transitional from the positional to the structural. This type will exhibit soft-tissue and osseous deformities together. A cavus foot will exhibit several typical deformities including dropping of the forefoot, varus of the calcaneus, increased inclination of the calcaneus, limited ankle dorsiflexion, contracture of the plantar fascial tissue, and varying degrees of clawing of the toes which will be dependent on the type and severity.

Most typically this foot type has an insidious history, appearing gradually at any age from 3 years onward. It can become sufficiently troublesome by the age of 7–10 years to cause concern. And, depending on the exact etiology, this condition may not even begin to appear until adulthood.

Radiographic Evaluation

Radiologic measurements are beneficial in determining the location and degree of deformity. Lateral views (weight-bearing when possible) will provide information for several determinations. The calcaneal inclination angle is determined on the lateral x-ray by a line drawn along the inferior surface of the calcaneus and a line paralleling the weight-bearing surface (**Figure 163**). Values above 30–35° indicate a significant rearfoot cavus. When measured during weight-bearing, it is considered the rigid type. If a line is passed through the middle of the first metatarsal, it will intersect with the line drawn from the inferior surface of the calcaneus (**Figure 164**). The angle formed at its intersection (the calcaneal–first metatarsal angle) should be between 135–145° in the young child. If this angular value is greater than 150°, it would be considered an indicator for a pronated foot. Values less than 130° would indicate a developing cavus foot condition. To determine whether the deformity is positional or osseous and at what joint level, weight-bearing and nonweight-bearing x-rays are necessary. On lateral view, a line drawn through the middle of the talus will intersect with the mid-first metatarsal line (**Figure 165**). The point of intersection will indicate the apex of the deformity. The angle created by the intersection will increase markedly in the nonweight-bearing view if there exists a more positional than structural deformity. Dorsal plantar x-rays will allow a determination of any forefoot pathology and should be evaluated in conjunction with the lateral views.

Treatment

Treatment should be directed toward the apex of the area of deformity. Several conservative and surgical procedures have been offered to correct this

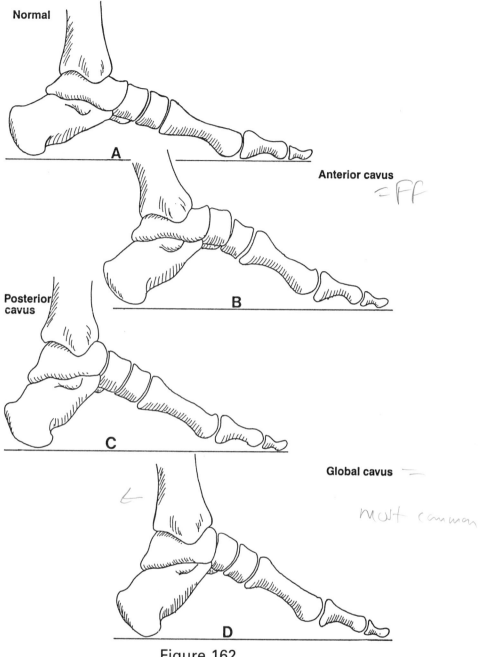

Normal

A

Anterior cavus

= FF

B

Posterior cavus

C

Global cavus —

Most common

D

Figure 162

A pes cavus deformity can occur solely in the forefoot (anterior type) producing a plantarflexion of the metatarsals and midtarsal bones in relationship to the rearfoot (B). It may also present with a posterior cavus resulting in a significant supination of the rearfoot and an increase in the calcaneal inclination (C). Most frequently, however, a cavus foot is the combination of both an anterior and posterior cavoid deformity referred to as a global cavus (D).

219

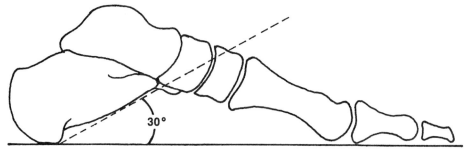

Figure 163

The calcaneal inclination angle is determined by drawing a line along the inferior surface of the calcaneus and another paralleling the weight-bearing surface. Normal values are between 15–30°.

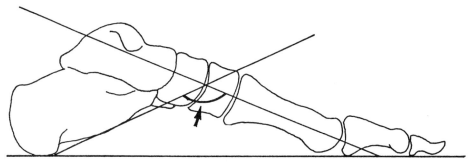

Figure 164

The calcaneal-first metatarsal angle is formed by a line drawn through the first metatarsal and one drawn along the inferior surface of the calcaneus.

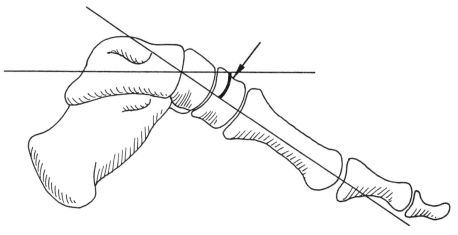

Figure 165

To determine the apex of a cavus foot deformity, draw a line through the middle of the talus and another through the center of the first metatarsal. The point in which they intersect is considered the apex.

foot pathology. Conservatively, an in-shoe orthotic device (Shaeffer plate, pronated orthosis, etc.—see Chapter 13) can be extremely beneficial in helping to redistribute the weight stress and maintain position. This is advantageous in the mild forms of cavus feet with minimal deformity of the toes and limited varusing of the calcaneus. It is also effective in the positional (flexible) type cavus foot. It should be advised that posting an orthotic to a cavus foot deformity may lead to complications. A rearfoot varus post, for example, should not be applied to the degree of varus present in the calcaneus. If applied, it may cause the foot to twist easily in inversion and produce an ankle sprain and/or ankle injuries. It may also cause severe lateral wear of the shoes due to the rigid calcaneal varus condition. A rectus posting (0 degrees) or even a slight valgus post will prevent this tendency toward inversion and yet control the foot adequately. The forefoot should either allow the 1st metatarsal to function freely as in a Root orthosis, or brought to rectus when casting a flexible type. If the first metatarsal or forefoot is in a nonflexible plantarflexed valgus position, then forcing this position can cause degenerative changes in the midtarsal

Plantar release

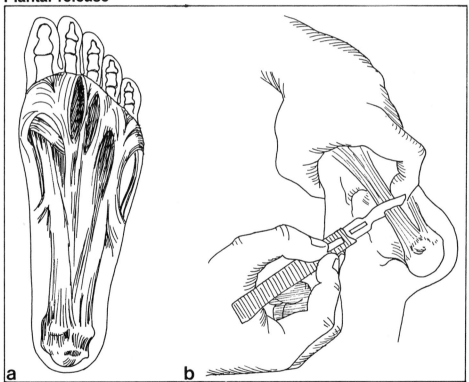

Figure 166

A Steindler stripping is the release of both the plantar fascia and all the plantar muscular attachments to the calcaneus. The procedure is best performed through a medial approach with all the structures incised from medial to lateral. This will include both slips of the plantar fascia as well as the musculature.

joint and tarso–metatarsal joints. Children most often will present with a more flexible type foot and are therefore more capable of being controlled in a rectus attitude.[12,14]

Surgically, several procedures have been offered for correction. A Steindler stripping of the plantar fascia and plantar musculature has been advocated for several years to release the intrinsic tightness (**Figure 166**). This author has found that even when performed in the totally flexible cavus foot, there is not sufficient correction, due to the refibrosing of the structures, to allow the foot to reduce to a more functional attitude. This procedure in combination with the following will produce a reasonably well functioning and comfortable foot (**Figure 167**). An osseous correction of the varus calcaneus (Dwyer calcaneal wedge osteotomy); lengthening of the Achilles tendon when necessary; elevation of the first metatarsal (EHL tendon suspension, dorsiflexory wedge osteotomy of the first metatarsal) and/or elevation of all the metatarsal (Hibb's suspension, midtarsal-ostectomy Japas or Cole Procedure, tarso–metatarsal or metatarsal osteotomy); and correction of claw toes. Occasionally there is a need for a tendon transfer in the mid and rearfoot when a neurological deficit has left one muscular group weakened or paralytic or a triple arthrodesis when indicated (see **Figure 155C**). Postsurgical follow-up in an orthotic device will allow maintenance and functional control as well as adequate weight distribution in the foot.[2–4,6–11,13,15]

When a cavus foot is found in a child with no neuromuscular disorder contributing to its cause, conservative care should be employed initially until

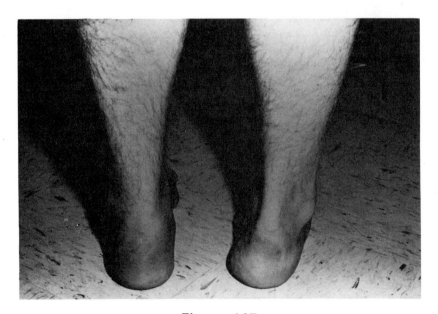

Figure 167

Left, *Postop Dwyer calcaneal osteotomy.*
Right, *Preop Dwyer calcaneal osteotomy.*

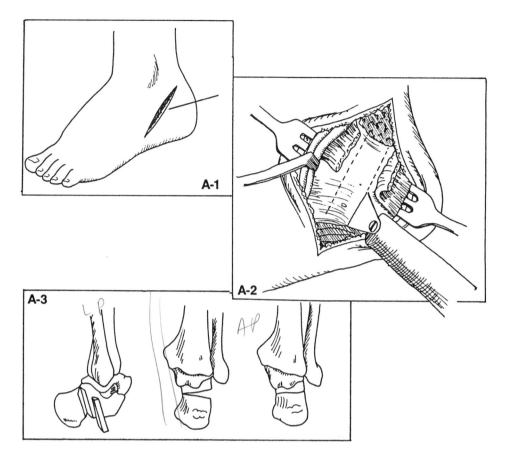

Figure 167(A)

A Dwyer calcaneal osteotomy is performed through a lateral incision (1) with the removal of an appropriate wedge of bone from the calcaneus (2). The base of the wedge is lateral and the apex medial (3). With the removal of the wedge, the calcaneus can be redirected from a varus position to a rectus attitude. Note that the wedge is taken at an oblique angle approximating the angle of the course of the peroneal tendons. This angle allows the posterior segment to move in a tri-plane direction for correction of the varus, inclination and adduction of the calcaneus. (An opening wedge may also be performed from a medial approach using a bone graft to maintain a corrected position).

the child reaches adolescence. Once the foot is full-grown, the degree and position of the deformity can be better evaluated. At this time a surgical procedure may be considered and tailored for proper alignment, if necessary. Performed at too early an age, the surgery may result in a tendency for a reoccurrence with more rigidity secondary to the fibrous changes. Early surgical treatment may also result in an inability to determine all the areas of involvement adequately.

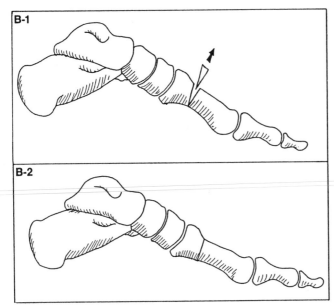

Figure 167(B)

A dorsiflexory wedge osteotomy of the first metatarsal (1)(2) will reduce a local type of cavus foot resulting from a plantarflexed first metatarsal.

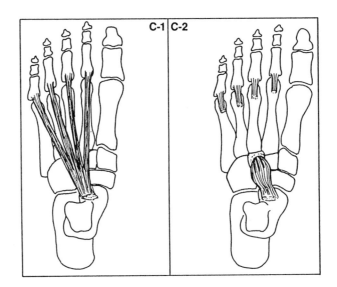

Figure 167(C)

A Hibb's suspension works well in a flexible anterior cavus to bring the forefoot dorsally and concomitantly remove the extensor pull on toes causing a hammertoe deformity. The extensor digitorum longus tendons to all the lesser digits (1) are severed with the distal stump reattached to the extensor brevis tendons. The tendons are then passed through a drill hole in the 3rd cuneiform and suture under tension through the plantar of the foot to reduce the anterior plantarflexion of the forefoot. The foot must be casted for 8–10 weeks to allow adequate tenodesing with vigorous muscle strengthening following the cast removal.

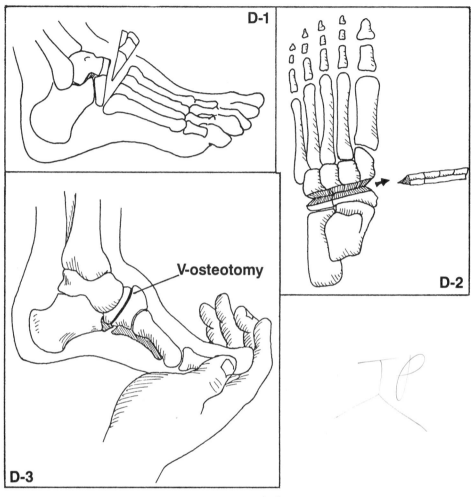

Figure 167(D)

The Cole procedure removes a wedge of bone from the midtarsal area allowing the forefoot to dorsiflex on the rearfoot (1)(2). Similar in effect, the Japas procedure uses a "V" cut through the midtarsal joint area with one arm extending from the first cuneiform to approximately the navicular-3rd cuneiform articulation and the other arm from the navicular-3rd cuneiform articulation to the distal lateral cuboid area. The forefoot can then be dorsiflexed without shortening the foot substantially, as with the Cole procedure (3).

Extensor hallucis longus suspension

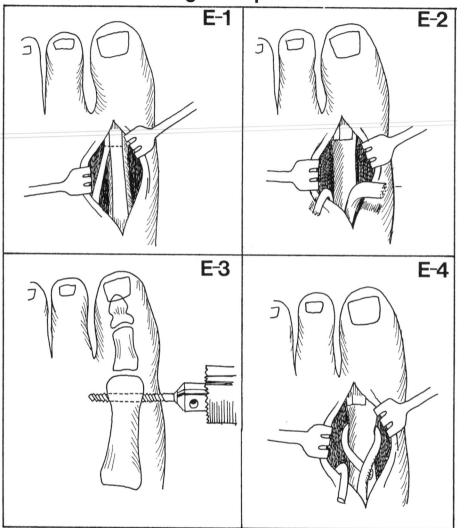

Figure 167(E)

In cases of a flexible plantarflexed first metatarsal, a tendon suspension will reduce the deformity excellently. The extensor hallucis longus and brevis tendons are severed as far distal as possible (1)(2). A drill hole is made transversely through the metatarsal head (3). The extensor hallucis longus tendon is then passed through the hole and sutured to itself under tension to elevate the first metatarsal (4). It is usually necessary to fuse the interphalangeal joint of the hallux to prevent a hallux malleus (cocked hallux).

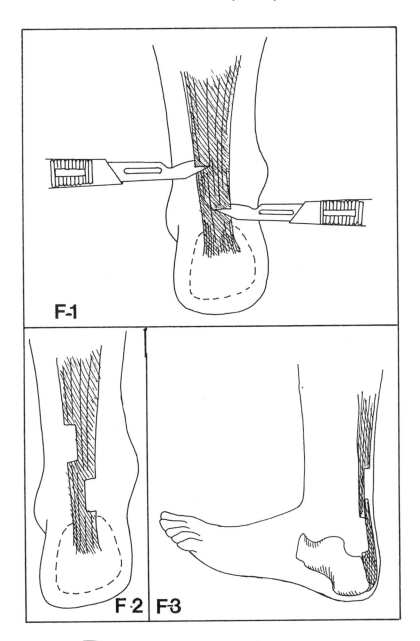

Figure 167(F)

In cases of a flexible plantarflexed first metatarsal, a tendon suspension will reduce the deformity excellently. The extensor hallucis longus and brevis tendons are severed as far distal as possible (1)(2). A drill hole is made transversely through the metatarsal head (3). The extensor hallucis longus tendon is then passed through the hole and sutured to itself under tension to elevate the first metatarsal (4). It is usually necessary to fuse the interphalangeal joint of the hallux to prevent a hallux malleus (cocked hallux).

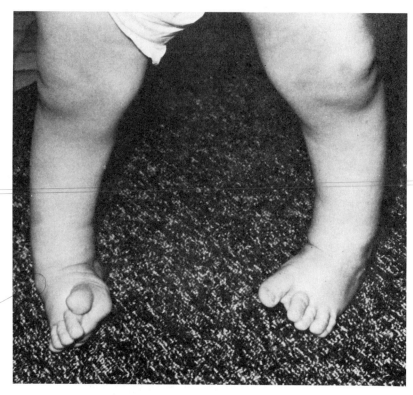

Talar head

Juvenile Clubfoot.

Clubfoot (Talipes Equinovarus)

The first description of talipes equinovarus was offered by Hippocrates in 4 B.C. and since has had an intense history of investigation and treatment regimens. Pathologically, there are primarily three components existing in a clubfoot, i.e., inversion and adduction of the forefoot; inversion (varus) of the heal and hindfoot; and equinus throughout both the ankle and the subtalar joint. Internal tibial torsion has occasionally been described as a fourth component, it is probably not a significant force, but rather a secondary result from the aforementioned deformities.

myofibroblast contractility

Several theories about the etiology of talipes equinovarus have been proposed. One theory suggests that the condition may be caused by the presence of a defect in the germ plasm during the first trimester of pregnancy. A second possible cause is environmental, and a third cause is genetic factors. It is suggested that a great deal of stress is directed toward the developing fetus during the first three months of development, and is especially concentrated at the limb buds where this stress may cause a growth arrestment. This growth arrestment theory appears to be the most sound because clubfeet have been found to exist as early as in a three-month-old fetus. Approximately 15% of the patients with talipes equinovarus have some other major deformity, including: arthrogryphosis multiplex congenita, meningomyelocele, sacral agenesis, dwarfism, and congenital hip dislocation. It is therefore essential that each infant with talipes equinovarus be carefully evaluated for these other anomalies.

Anatomical findings in dissected extremities of clubfeet and normal feet have demonstrated several consistencies: the cross-sectional areas of the legs with talipes equinovarus are comparable to those of normal legs at 6 months' gestation; at term the cross-sectional area of the muscle mass is significantly smaller in the clubfoot leg, as opposed to the normal leg, with the entire muscle mass being diminished totally and not just in selected compartments; the insertion of all tendons were normal with the exception of the Achilles tendon, which inserted more medially; consistently there is seen an abnormal angular relationship of the head–neck of the talus with the body. The talar head is oriented more medially and slightly plantar than is normally found (**Figure 168**); soft-tissue contractures exist at the ligamentous structures between the talo–navicular and calcaneonavicular complex of joints. The posterior tibiotalar and subtalar capsule is also involved. (It was found that with complete detachment of the muscular insertions, correction manually of the clubfoot could not be attained until the ligamentous structures mentioned were sectioned.) The posterior talofibular and calcaneofibular ligaments were also found to be contracted in addition to the deltoid, spring ligaments, talocalcaneal interosseus, and bifurcate (Y) ligaments. Contractures of the plantar fascia are also a consistent finding.[4,8,10,11,14,18,21–24,27,30]

Biomechanically, a normal foot will supinate with plantarflexion and pronate with dorsiflexion. In a clubfoot there is an exaggerated plantarflexion that causes significant movement in the direction of supination, i.e., adduction of the forefoot and varus of the hindfoot.

Clinical Evaluation

Clubfeet have been classified in many ways. Terms such as extrinsic versus intrinsic, primary versus secondary, or flexible versus rigid have been used. There is even a further breakdown including mild–flexible, moderate–less flexible, and severe–rigid. This last classification seems to be most useful to date. A *mild–flexible* clubfoot is one that has peroneal muscle function. This can be tested by tickling the child's foot on the lateral border. The child will normally evert and pull the foot away from this stimulus. The *moderate–less flexible* type exhibits more visible posterior and medial creases of the foot, and the peroneal muscle function is very difficult or impossible to demonstrate. *Severe–rigid* clubfeet present with severe internal rotation of the talus along with medial and plantar angulation of the head and neck. The head of the talus will bulge prominently on the lateral side of the foot, and the navicular

Normal

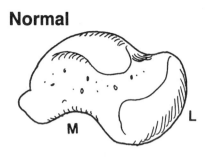

Clubfoot

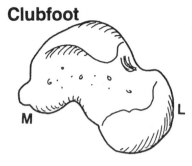

Figure 168

The talar head is directed more medial (M) in a clubfoot than would be found in a normal infant or child of the same age level.

will be articulating principally with the medial malleolus. In corrected clubfeet, the area over the lateral sinus tarsi will show discoloration and creases of the talar bulge. This has been referred to as the "devil's thumbprint."[15,18,19,21,23,24,27]

Radiographic Evaluation

X-ray views that should be exposed for proper evaluation of a clubfoot are: anterio–posterior (AP) of the foot; lateral; stress lateral of foot and ankle; anterioposterior ankle; and axial calcaneal view. The AP view of the foot will show a decrease in the talocalcaneal angle with a talipes equinovarus deformity. An angular value of (+)15–20° is considered normal while in a clubfoot this value is reduced to as much as (−)15–20° (**Figure 169**). On lateral view of the foot, the talocalcaneal angle is normally between (+)30–45° while in a clubfoot deformity this is usually reduced to 0° or even (−)10–15° from the parallel position (**Figure 170**). An index can be arrived at for the values of both the AP and lateral talocalcaneal angle. Examples of normal values are 45° (lateral) and 15° (AP) = 60°. When correcting a clubfoot, a good surgical result would occur if the talocalcaneal index would approach 40°. The axial calcaneal view will reveal the degree of varus positioning of the os calcis and the talocalcaneal positioning.[9,15,23,24]

Treatment

The treatment of a clubfoot may require both conservative and surgical care depending on the classification and degree of deformity. Stretch casting is indicated in all forms of clubfoot to allow a better evaluation of the residual contractures. Some clinicians have suggested that a tendo-Achilles lengthening be performed before any casting is attempted. This is performed to avoid the possibility that overstretching might produce a rocker-bottom foot. This author would concur with this thinking due to the short tendo-Achilles in-

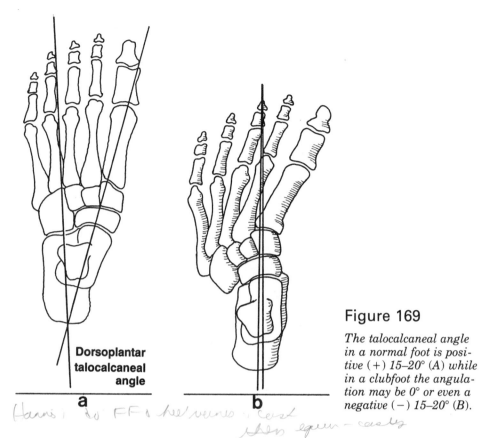

**Dorsoplantar
talocalcaneal
angle**

a   **b**

Figure 169

*The talocalcaneal angle
in a normal foot is posi-
tive (+) 15–20° (A) while
in a clubfoot the angula-
tion may be 0° or even a
negative (−) 15–20° (B).*

advertently causing plantarflexion and supination of the foot. Without release
of this tendon, the attempted correction would invariably deviate or sublux
the other joint segments to achieve a desired alignment. It also becomes next
to impossible to grab the calcaneus properly and to plantarflex the posterior
aspect when casting. The desired procedure for lengthening the Achilles tendon
is through two stab incisions, as shown in **Figure 171**. This method minimizes
wound exposure to facilitate quicker healing and prevents the surgical contractures and scarring often found in the open tendon-lengthening procedures.

Casting

In casting the foot, manipulation should be performed for approximately
10–15 minutes prior to the application of plaster. A double layer of webril is
applied prior to the plaster application. When necessary, tincture of benzoin
should be applied to the skin to control dermatitis conditions, etc. Thicker
layers of webril will lessen the effect of the cast and should be avoided. Padding
over any pressure areas (i.e., malleoli, base 5th metatarsal, etc.) can be increased slightly.

All three components of the clubfoot should be manipulated: abduction of

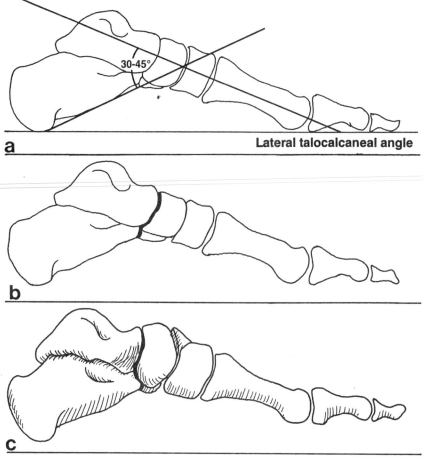

Lateral talocalcaneal angle

Figure 170

The lateral talocalcaneal angle in a normal foot is positive (+) 30–45° (A) while in a clubfoot this may be reduced to negative (−) 10–15°. The lateral cyma line is normally found as in (B); however, in the clubfoot the cyma line will be in a negative position with the talonavicular joint being posterior to the calcaneocuboid joint (C).

the forefoot, eversion of the hindfoot, and dorsiflexion of the ankle should be performed (**Figure 172**). This can be accomplished by placing the first two or three fingers over the medial of the heel and pushing the heel in a valgus position. At the same time with the other hand, force the fore and midfoot into abduction and valgus concomitantly. Elevation of the first metatarsal to a rectus position should be incorporated in the manipulation. Without proper elevation of the first metatarsal, one cannot reduce the forefoot valgus deformity that exists. Simultaneous dorsiflexion of the foot on the ankle to stretch the Achilles and posterior ankle joint capsule should be performed. This is not necessary if an Achilles lengthening was performed.

The casts should be removed by either the parents' soaking them off or

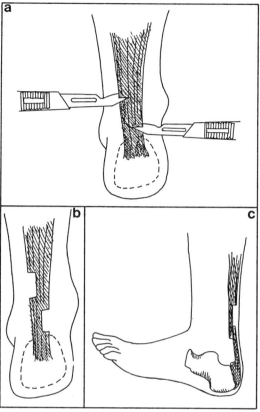

(A) *Using a #15 or #64 blade, a tenotomy of the Achilles tendon can be performed through an initial stab over and lateral to the tendon fibers. Approximately one-half of the tendon is incised. A second incision is then made medially similar to that performed laterally. The two incisions should have approximately 4–8 cm of distance between them to allow adequate lengthening without total separation of the sections. (B) By dorsiflexing the foot, the fibers should glide past one another providing adequate dorsal motion. A void will be noted in the areas where the tendon has separated. (C) This is a side view of the appearance of the tendon after lengthening. The child should be casted for approximately 6–8 weeks in a 90° position with weight-bearing. Vigorous exercise is needed following a cast removal. A calcaneus gait may be noted for several months afterward until sufficient strength is regained. The use of a removal cast may be advantageous in allowing early rehabilitation by passive strengthening with reduction in muscle atrophy.*

Figure 171

by the clinician approximately every 4–7 days with the manipulation procedure repeated. Casting should begin as early as possible in an infant. Cast changes should be every 2–3 days in the nursery and every week after the child is 7–10 days of age. Casts should not be left on longer than one week as the efficiency level is usually lost beyond this amount of time. After correction is achieved, maintenance casts should be employed for a period of 4–8 weeks to ensure adequate positioning. Follow-up to the casting should include the use of out-flared shoes or straight last shoes to continue maintaining correction. Several years of use is necessary for an adequate position to be maintained. It may become necessary to institute additional castings if a regression of the correction occurs. Do not hesitate to reapply castings even as old as 4, 5, or 6 years when necessary.[12,13,15,16,18–21,23–25,28]

Surgical Correction

It has been realized that a reoccurrence of this deformity may frequently occur in the growth and development of a child. Percentages as high as 50–60% have been found to exist between the ages of 10 months and $5\frac{1}{2}$ years

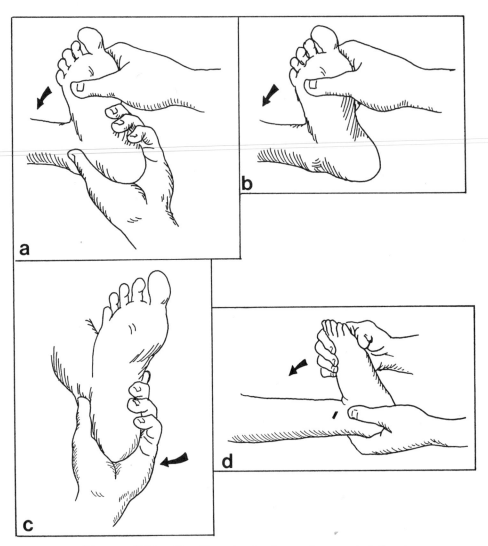

Figure 172   Casting technique for a clubfoot.

Grasp the foot as in (A) by using the first 2–3 fingers to grasp the calcaneus and evert at the subtalar joint to reduce the varus component (C). The other hand should grasp the forefoot and produce abduction and valgus positioning. This will reduce the adduction and varus deformity. The first metatarsal should be dosiflexed while the foot is manipulated into this position (B). Dorsiflexion at the ankle should be performed concomitantly with the other two maneuvers to reduce the equinus deformity (D).

following correction castings with concomitant tendo-Achilles lengthening.[16,19,25] Second reoccurrences (post-first reoccurrence) were found in approximately 18% of the clubfeet and occurring between 15 months and 5 years with 10% having a third reoccurrence between the ages of 3–8 years. It becomes paramount to follow these children until approximately the age of 8–10 years in order to treat any recurrence.

Several surgical procedures have been described for correction of resistant clubfeet. As previously mentioned, a lengthening of the tendo-Achilles becomes critical not only in conservative treatment but also in surgical realignment procedures. Very often a reoccurrence of this deformity post-serial casting requires a surgical release of the foot to accomplish an adequate positional alignment. A review of the procedures most frequently employed follows. Surgical treatment can be categorized into two classifications: soft-tissue procedures and bony procedures.

Soft-tissue procedures commonly utilized are: tendo-Achilles lengthening; posterior capsulotomy; posterior tibial lengthening; medial joint release; Heyman–Herndon–Strong procedure; plantar fasciotomy; posterior tibial tendon transfer; and anterior tibial tendon transfer.

A *tendo-Achilles lengthening* described in **Figure 173** should be performed

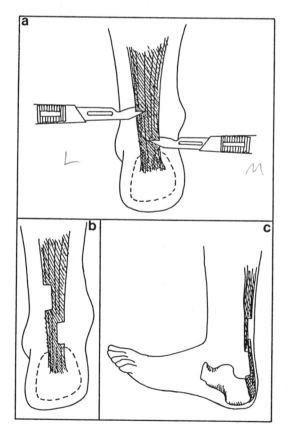

Figure 173

See Figure 171 for a description of a tendo-Achilles lengthening through a two-stab incision.

prior to serial castings in the more resistive type clubfoot and in conjunction with other surgical procedures to be described.

A *posterior capsulotomy* can be frequently employed with a tendo-Achilles lengthening in congenital clubfeet. It is not indicated in cerebral palsy children as it seems to add to the morbidity. In performing this procedure, a release of the posterior ankle and subtalar joint is necessary. This procedure should be performed later than 3 months of age due to the size of the joints and should be performed simultaneously with the Achilles lengthening (**Figure 174**).

A *posterior tibial lengthening* can be performed as an independent procedure but is most commonly combined with a medial joint release. In a more flexible clubfoot, the release of this tendon can allow for better forefoot correction in combination with serial castings. As an independent procedure it can be performed at the lower third of the leg as shown in **Figure 175**.

A *medial joint release* is commonly performed in the following: in cases where a reocurrence has resulted post serial casting; in the older infant (over 7 months of age) with other congenital problems such as arthrogryposis multiplex congenita, sacral agenesis, or meningomyelocele; or in the older child before 11 years of age. The goal of the medial joint release is to allow the foot to be placed back into an anatomic position allowing a proper articulation of the talus with the navicular with the hope that remodeling will occur in this corrected position. Beyond 11 years of age this becomes reasonably impossible. This procedure consists of sectioning the spring ligament, deltoid ligament, talonavicular capsule, navicular joint, cuneiform capsule, talocalcaneal ligament, interosseous talocalcaneal ligament, and lengthening the posterior ti-

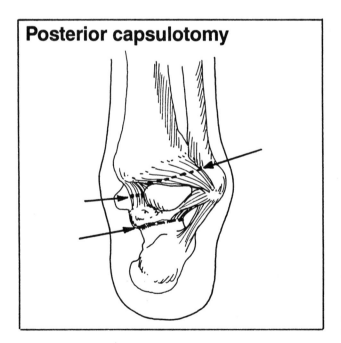

Posterior capsulotomy

Figure 174

A posterior capsulotomy includes the incising of both the posterior ankle joint structures and the posterior subtalar joint.

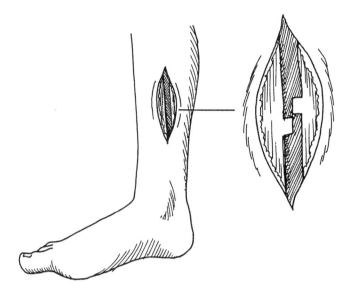

Figure 175

Lengthening of the posterior tibial tendon is best performed at the lower one-third of the leg using a linear medial incision. The tendon is located and a Z-plasty lengthening is performed with the tendon sutured in its lengthened state.

bial, flexor hallicus longus and flexor digitorum longus tendon. Casting should be maintained for 12–16 weeks to achieve a proper position (**Figure 176**).

The *Heyman–Herndon–Strong procedure* releases the ligamentous and capsular attachments at the bases of the five metatarsals (**Figure 177**). Its purpose is to reduce the metatarsus adductus and metatarsus adductovarus commonly found in the clubfoot. This procedure should be performed prior to squaring (**Figure 178**) of the metatarsal bases which occurs at approximately 7–8 years of age.

The *plantar fasciotomy* (Steindler stripping) is not only a release and lengthening of the plantar fascia but also a release of the muscular attachments at the base of the calcaneus. It is advantageous to release the plantar fascia in at least two different areas to reduce the likelihood of contractures after healing. This procedure is commonly performed in combination with the other procedures described, and not as a single independent procedure (**Figure 179**).

Posterior tibial tendon transfer can be performed as a total transfer laterally in the foot to produce eversion, or may be split and one half transferred laterally when there is a need for medial muscle function. This procedure is not performed prior to 18 months of age in order for the surgeon to be able to clearly define what muscles are functioning; to know how well they are functioning; and to know exactly what deforming forces are existing. Additionally, one is unable to have the child cooperate in an examination of this muscle properly below this age level (**Figure 180**).

Anterior tibial tendon transfer, like the posterior tibial transfer, can either be performed in toto or as a split transfer. One must be aware of the functioning of the peroneal muscles in this transfer. If the peroneals are reasonably strong, then a transfer too far laterally of this tendon will cause an eversion (valgus) instead of a correction of the varus deformity. In these cases, it is advised not

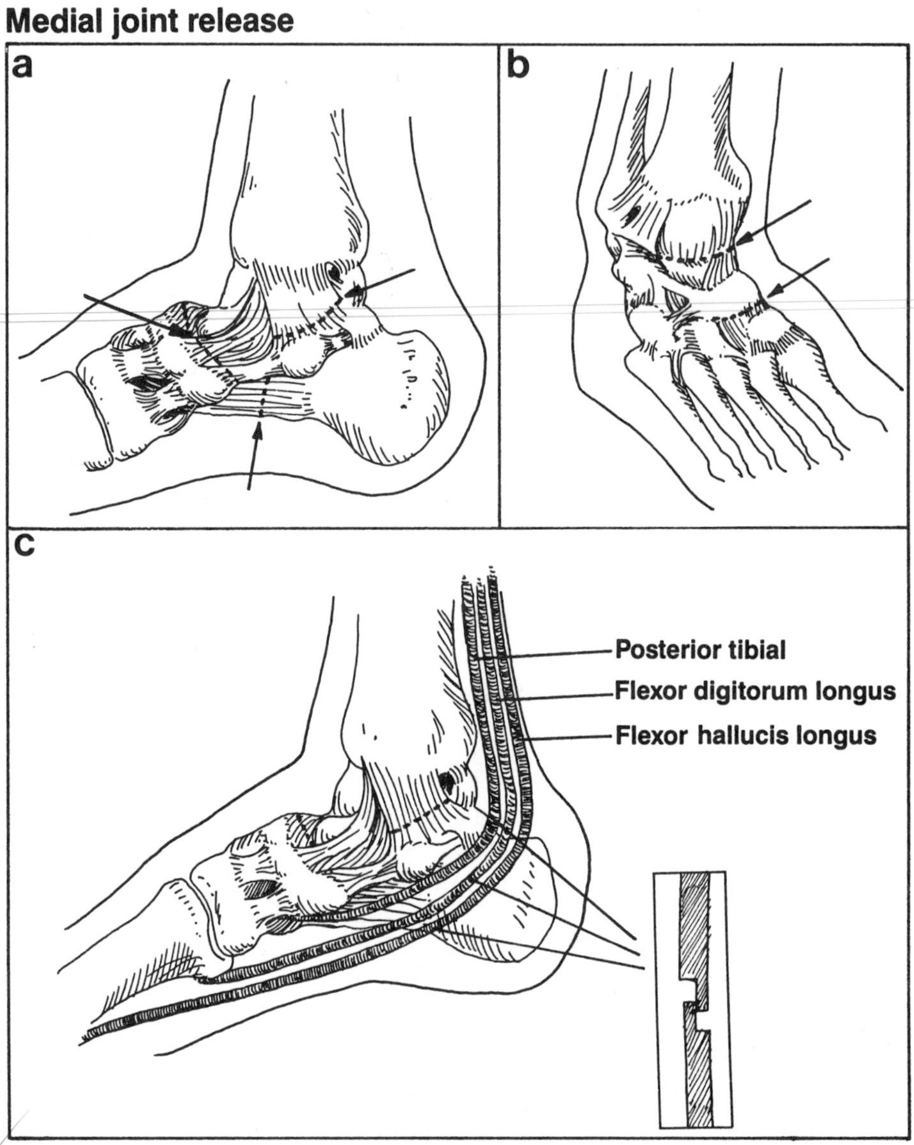

Medial joint release

Figure 176

To perform a medial joint release, the spring ligament, deltoid ligament, talonavicular capsule, navicular joint, cuneiform capsule, talocalcaneal ligament, and interosseous talocalcaneal ligaments are incised (A) (B). A lengthening of the posterior tibial tendon, flexor hallucis longus, and flexor digitorum longus tendons are also necessary to achieve adequate reduction (C).

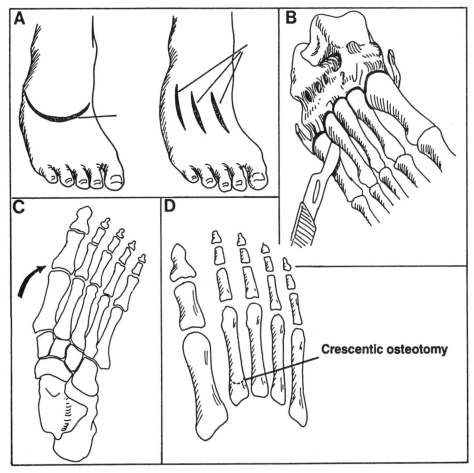

Figure 177

The Heyman–Herndon–Strong procedure can be approached by either a transverse or three linear incisions to expose the bases of the metatarsals (A). The dorsal, medial, lateral, and the medial one-third of the plantar ligament of each metatarsal base is incised (B). The metatarsals are then manipulated laterally (abduction) to reduce the metatarsus adductus or adductovarus deformity (C). The foot is casted for 8–10 weeks in this corrected position. Occasionally it is necessary to perform a crescentic osteotomy of the second metatarsal (D) to allow this metatarsal to shift laterally. The reason for this is that the mortise effect of the 2nd metatarsal may not allow the base to shift laterally after the capsule release.

to transfer any further than the 3rd cuneiform bone. However, if the peroneals are atrophic, it may be advantageous to transfer the tendon as far laterally as the cuboid to correct the varus deformity properly (**Figure 181**).

 Bony procedures frequently employed by surgeons are: cuboid decancellation; cuboid–calcaneal fusion; metatarsal osteotomies; Dwyer calcaneal osteotomy; triple arthrodesis; and talectomy.

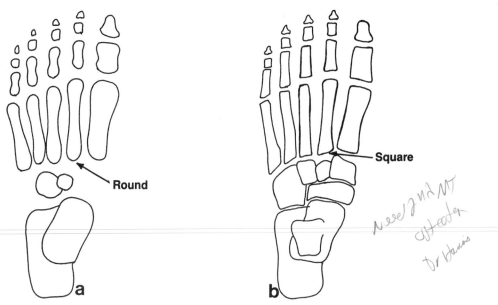

Round

Square

need 2nd MT
osteotomy
Dr Harris

Figure 178

Rounded metatarsal bases (A) will allow reduction with readaptation of the cartilagenous surfaces of the tarso-metatarsal joints. This is usually lost around age 7–8 years with a squaring (ossification) being visualized (B). The squaring indicates loss of cartilagenous tissue at the bases and therefore an inability for correction and readaptation.

Plantar release

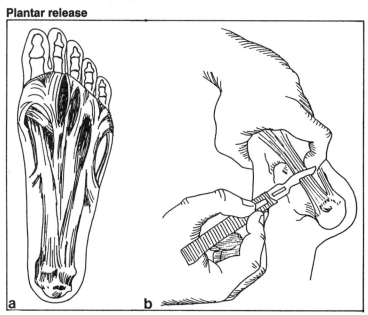

Figure 179

Both the medial and lateral slips of the plantar fascia should be released along with the muscular attachments to the calcaneus. Removing a section of the plantar fascia reduces the likelihood of refibrosing and reshortening.

Posterior tibial tendon transfer

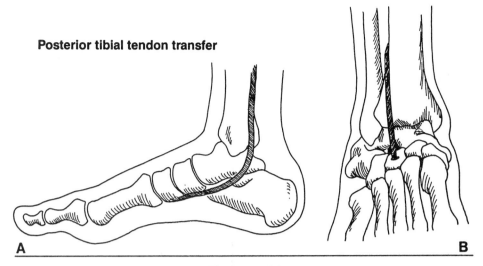

A   **B**

Figure 180

Transferring of the posterior tibial tendon is best performed by a detachment either partially or totally from the medial aspect of the foot (A) and inserting it through a drill hole, trephine plug, screw-washer fixation, etc. at the third cuneiform. The tendon is placed under tension while the foot is held in a corrected position. Casting is performed for 8–10 weeks followed by vigorous physical therapy.

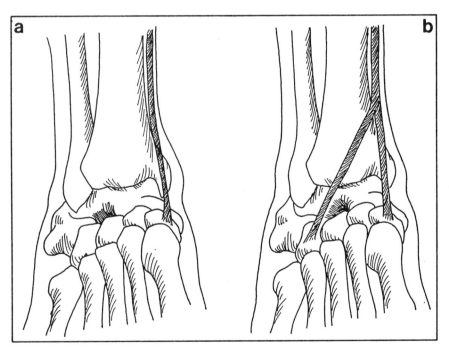

Figure 181

An anterior tibial tendon transfer can be performed either totally or split as in (A) and (B). The tendon should either be transferred to the cuboid if the peroneals are atrophied or to the third cuneiform if there is adequate peroneal function.

241

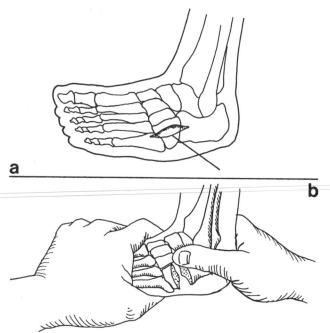

Figure 182

Decancellation of the cuboid is approached by an incision over this bone (A) and removal of the cancellous portion after osteotomizing the bone (B). The foot is then manipulated into an abducted position with the opposing bone surfaces compressing each other. A potential problem with this procedure is the loss of the peroneus longus groove.

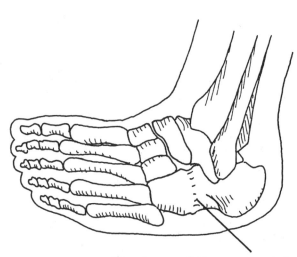

Fusion of the cuboid-calcaneal joint

Figure 183

With removal of an appropriate wedge from the calcaneocuboid joint to correct the adduction deformity in the forefoot, a fusion is performed to maintain this correction. The use of staples, pins, screws, or plates will accomplish this correction well. Casting may be necessary for 10–12 weeks for proper fusion.

Cuboid decancellation—This procedure evacuates the cancelleous bone through an opening at the lateral of the cuboid with compression of the bone followed by abductory manipulation. It will correct a forefoot adduction deformity by shortening the lateral column of the foot. This procedure is not performed prior to 6 years of age. An apparent advantage of this procedure is its ability to maintain intact the articular surfaces (**Figure 182**).

Cuboid–calcaneal fusion—As described by Evans, this procedure removes a lateral wedge from the calcaneo–cuboid joint with fusion of the area. Similar

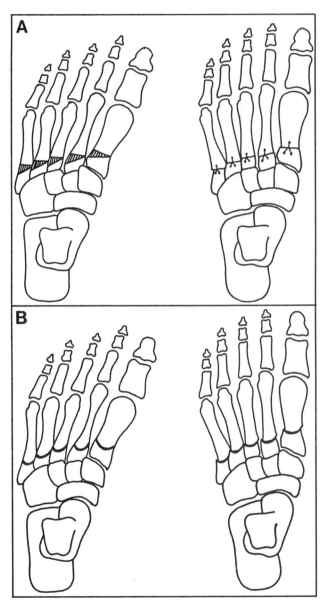

Figure 184

Two types of metatarsal base osteotomies may be performed to correct an adductus deformity. The lateral closing wedge (A) achieves adequate reduction but with a reasonable amount of difficulty. Properly removing equal portions of bone to allow each metatarsal a correct position with the adjacent metatarsals is difficult. The crescentic osteotomy (B) more easily allows movement of all the metatarsals evenly. Pin fixation of the first and possibly the fifth metatarsal may be necessary for stability, but may not be necessary in all cases. A lateral closing wedge of the first metatarsal with crescentic osteotomies of the lesser metatarsals offers the best stability of the two procedures aforementioned. The foot should be casted into correction for 6–8 weeks.

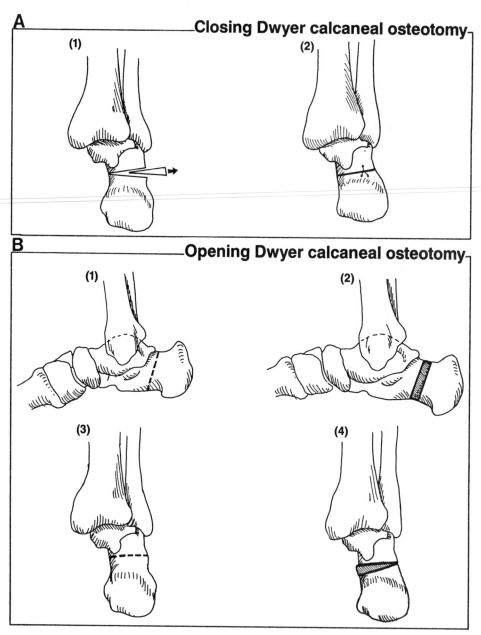

A _____Closing Dwyer calcaneal osteotomy⌐

(1)   (2)

B _____Opening Dwyer calcaneal osteotomy⌐

(1)   (2)

(3)   (4)

Figure 185

Closing wedge osteotomy of the calcaneus (A) is performed laterally for reduction of a varus deformity. An appropriate wedge is removed (A-1) and the osteotomy may be fixated with a staple, pin, or screw. If adequate closure is achieved with dorsiflexion of the foot on the ankle, one may choose not to use fixation. Casting is for 6–8 weeks with weight-bearing as tolerated. The opening calcaneal osteotomy (B) is approached from the medial side of the calcaneus. Care must be taken to avoid the neurovascular bundle in this area. After osteotomizing the calcaneus an appropriate wedge of bone either from a donor site or from a bone bank may be used to maintain the position (1)(2)(3)(4).

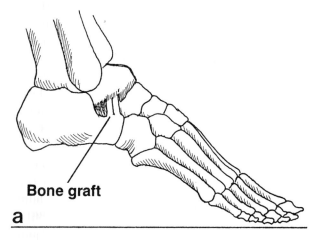

Bone graft

a

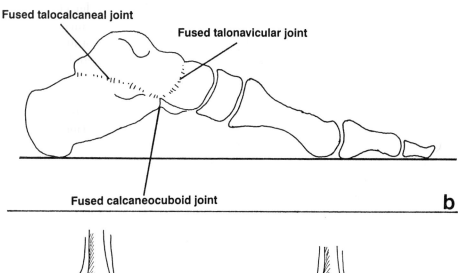

Fused talocalcaneal joint

Fused talonavicular joint

Fused calcaneocuboid joint

b

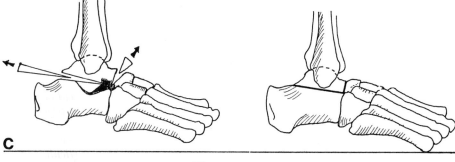

c

Figure 186

Fusion of the talonavicular, subtalar, and calcaneocuboid joints will stabilize the rearfoot in a clubfoot and allow proper correction when adequate and appropriate wedges of bone are removed. The forefoot may need further bone correction procedures when indicated.

to the cuboid decancellation, it allows for correction of the forefoot adduction. This procedure should be left for the older child beyond 6 years of age to properly appreciate the degree of deformity that will persist (**Figure 183**).

Metatarsal osteotomies are also performed to correct a metatarsus adductus in children beyond 7–8 years of age when the bases of the metatarsal are ossified. Wedge osteotomies or crescentic type osteotomies can be performed to correct the adductus deformity followed by an appropriate period of casting (**Figure 184**).

Dwyer calcaneal osteotomy can be performed to correct the varus deformity in the calcaneus. Either an opening medial wedge or a closing lateral wedge will accomplish this result. Again, this is not performed prior to age 6–8 years of age due to the size of the calcaneus, and the exact degree of varus is not known until after this age level (**Figure 185**).

Triple arthrodesis is a fusion of the calcaneo–cuboid, talonavicular, and subtalar joints with appropriate removal of wedges to allow for correction of the deformities. This procedure is usually left as a salvage for the adult clubfoot and should not be used in children or the adolescent (**Figure 186**).

Talectomy is the complete removal of the talus from the ankle joint (**Figure 187**). This procedure becomes the operation of choice in the older child with either the untreated or poor result type of clubfoot. When performed, the foot should be maintained for 12 weeks in a cast to achieve good stability. It is primarily used for the bilateral clubfoot in order to avoid a limb shortage problem which would occur in a unilateral situation. It also becomes an excellent procedure in patients with arthrogryposis multiplex congenita, meningeomyelocele, etc. With this procedure a pseudoarthrosis occurs between the tibia and calcaneus and the navicular articulates with the anterior aspect of the tibia.[1–3,5–7,15–19,21,23,25–27,29]

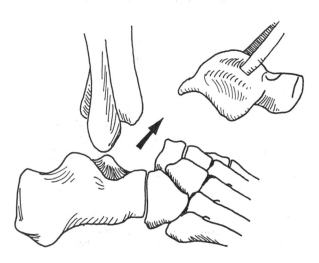

Figure 187

Complete removal of the talus allows the tibia–fibular complex to articulate with the calcaneus and the navicular to articulate with the anterior of the tibia. This procedure is an excellent salvage procedure in the older child or adult clubfoot.

References

Pes Cavus:
1. Barenfeld, P.A., Weseley, M.S., Shea, J.M.: The congenital cavus foot. *Clinical Orthopedics,* Number 79, September 1971.
2. Dwyer, F.C.: The etiology, clinical features, and treatment of calcaneus deformity. *J.A.P.A.,* 71:Number 5, May 1981.
3. Dwyer, F.C.: The present status of the problem of pes cavus. *Clinical Orthopedics,* Number 106, 1975.
4. Fenton, C.F., McGlamry, E.D., Perrone, M.: Severe pes cavus deformity secondary to Charcot-Marie-tooth disease. *J.A.P.A.,* 72:Number 4, April 1982.
5. Garceau, G.J., Brahms, M.A.: A preliminary study of selective plantar muscles denervation for pes cavus. *Journal of Bone and Joint Surgery,* 38-A:1956.
6. Japas, L.M.: Surgical treatment of pes cavus by tarsal V-osteotomy. *Journal of Bone and Joint Surgery,* 50-A:1968.
7. Kaplan, E.G., Kaplan, G.S.: Triple arthrodesis. *The Journal of Foot Surgery,* 15:Number 3, 1976.
8. Kate, A., Keasel, L., Kay, A.: Arthroplasty of the forefoot. *Journal of Bone and Joint Surgery,* 49-B:1967.
9. Mann, R.A.: Tendon transfers and electromyography. *Clinical Orthopedics,* Number 85, 1972.
10. Pandey, S., Shanhar, J.H.A., Pandery, A.K.: Ostectomy of the calcaneus. *Int. Orthop.,* 4:1980.
11. Reinherz, R.P., Pupp, G.R.: Biplane calcaneal osteotomy for severe pes cavovarus deformity. *J.A.P.A.,* 70:Number 1, January 1980.
12. Schoenhaus, H.D., Jay, R.M.: Cavus deformities—Conservative management. *J.A.P.A.,* 70:Number 5, May 1980.
13. Tachdjian, M.O.:*Pediatric Orthopedics.* W.B. Saunders Co., Philadelphia, PA, 1972.
14. Tax, H.R.: *Podopediatrics.* Williams and Wilkins Co., Baltimore, MD, 1980.
15. Weseley, M.S., Barenfeld, P.A.: Mechanism of the Dwyer calcaneal osteotomy. *Clinical Orthopaedics,* Number 70, 1970.

Clubfoot:
1. Adelaar, R.S., Kyles, M.K.: Surgical correction of resistant talipes equinovarius: Observations and analysis—Preliminary report. *Foot & Ankle,* 2:Number 3, 1981.
2. Bose, K.: Place of calcaneal osteotomy in the treatment of varus deformity of resistant clubfoot. *J. West. Pacific Orthop. Assoc.,* 15:1978.
3. Brill, L.R., Lepow, G.M.: The Arnold-Chiari malformation with an associated pes equinovarus deformity. *J.A.P.A.,* 71:Number 9, September 1981.
4. Clark, C.D., Smith, B.W., Harris, E.J.: The intrauterine position and deformities of the lower extremity. *J.A.P.A.,* 71:Number 3, March 1981.
5. DeLangh, R., Mulier, J.C., Fabry, G., Martens, M.: Treatment of clubfoot by posterior capsulectomy. *Clinical Orthop.,* Number 106, 1975.
6. Garceau, G.H.: Anterior tibial tendon transfer for recurrent clubfoot. *Clinical Orthop.,* Number 84, 1972.
7. Hamsa, W.R., Burney, D.W.: Open correction of recurrent talipes equinovarus—A study of end results. *Clinical Orthop.,* 21:1961.
8. Handelsman, J.E., Badalamente, M.A.: Neuromuscular studies in clubfoot. *Journal of Pediatric Orthopedics,* 1:1981.
9. Heywood, A.W.B.: The mechanics of the hindfoot in clubfoot as demonstrated radiographically. *Journal of Bone and Joint Surgery,* 46-B:1964.

10. Irani, R.N., Sherman, M.S.: Pathological anatomy of clubfoot. *Journal of Bone and Joint Surgery,* 45-A:1963.
11. Isaacs, H., Handelsman, J.E., Badenhorst, M., Pickering, A.: The muscles in clubfoot—a histological histochemical and electron microscopic study. *Journal of Bone and Joint Surgery,* 59-B:1977.
12. Kaplan, D.G.: A method of application of a clubfoot cast. *Clinical Orthopedics,* Number 84, 1972.
13. Kite, J.H.: Nonoperative treatment of congenital clubfoot. *Clinical Orthopedics,* Number 84, 1972.
14. Lichtblau, S.: Etiology of clubfoot. *Clinical Orthopedics,* Number 84, 1972.
15. Lovell, W.W., Hancock, C.I.: Treatment of congenital talipes equinovarus. *Clinical Orthopedics,* Number 70, 1970.
16. Ono, K., Hayashi, H.: Residual deformity of treated congenital clubfoot. *Journal of Bone and Joint Surgery,* 56-A:1974.
17. Ono, K., Hiroshim, K., Tada, K., Inocie, A.: Anterior transfer of the toe flexors for equinovarus deformity of the foot. *Int. Orthop.,* 4:1980.
18. Pokrasoa, M.A., Rodgveller, B.: Talipes equinovarus. *J.A.P.A.,* 71:Number 9, September 1981.
19. Ponseti, I.V., Campos, J.: Observations on pathogenesis and treatment of congenital clubfoot. *Clinical Orthopedics,* Number 84, 1972.
20. Shaw, W.E.: The early management of clubfoot. *Clinical Orthopedics,* Number 84, 1972.
21. Siegel, N.R.: Clubfoot. *Arch. of Pod. Med. and Foot Surg.,* 3:Number 2, 1976.
22. Simons, G.W.: External rotational deformities in clubfeet. *Clinical Orthopedics,* 126:1977.
23. Tachdjian, M.O.: *Pediatric Orthopedics.* W.B. Saunders Co., Philadelphia, PA, 1972.
24. Tax, H.R.: *Podopediatrics.* William and Wilkins Co., Baltimore, MD, 1980.
25. Tayton, K., Thompson, P.: Relapsing clubfeet. Late results of delayed operation. *Journal of Bone and Joint Surgery,* 61-B:1979.
26. Tuell, J.I.: Anterior transposition of posterior tibial muscle in equinovarus. *Clinical Orthopedics,* 21:1961.
27. Turek, S.L.: *Orthopedics,* Ed. 2, J.B. Lippincott, Philadelphia, PA, 1977.
28. Vesely, D.G.: A method of application of a clubfoot cast. *Clinical Orthopedics,* Number 84, 1972.
29. Wesley, M.S., Barenfeld, P.A., Barrett, N.: Complications of the treatment of clubfoot. *Clinical Orthopedics,* Number 84, 1972.
30. Wynne-Davies, R.: Genetic and environmental factors in the etiology of talipes equinovarus. *Clinical Orthopedics,* Number 84, 1972.

An osteochondrosis of any type is best described as an avascular necrosis of unknown etiology. The appearance will be either fragmentation and/or increased density with diminishment of its normal size. The avascularity is the primary reason for the more dense appearance taken on by the bone. If the affected bone is allowed to revascularize, it will develop normally and produce a bony structure comparable to that of a nonaffected bone. The density of the bone will also achieve a comparability to the other surrounding osseous structures when revascularized. Several bones may be affected in the foot; therefore, each will be described separately.

Sever's Disease

Sever's disease has been commonly described as an osteochondrosis of the calcaneal apophysis. Some other descriptive terms used for this condition are calcaneal apophysitis and adolescent calcaneodynia. The condition was first described by Sever in the early 1900s when he had noted an increase in the density of the calcaneal apophysis along with fragmentation occurring (**Figure 188**).[9–11] The presenting symptom is pain in the heel area occurring with ambulation and on direct pressure to the calcaneal apophysis.

Since this description by Sever was offered as the cause for this condition, other investigators have viewed this same or similar appearance existing in normal asymptomatic feet. This is confusing to those proponents of Sever's philosophy. Presently, most investigators and clinicians agree that this abnormality is not the result of avascularity of the calcaneal apophysis as was first described. The presence of fragmentation and altered bone density *may* or *may not* accompany the classical complaints of a painful heel in a youngster presenting with this condition.

The painful heel syndrome ascribed to Sever's disease occurs between the ages of 8–15 years with the average around 10–11 years of age. Boys tend to be more affected than girls. With more female participation in strenuous sports

249

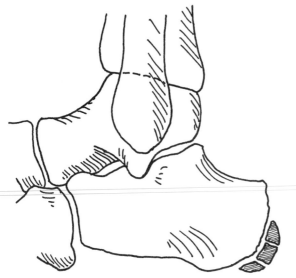

Figure 188

An avascular necrosis of the apophysis of the cal- caneus has been referred to as Sever's disease. This may not be truly the dis- turbance of the apophysis as described in the text. An increased density or fragmentation of the growth center may be the result of a traumatic fracture or a synovitis of the Achilles tendon rather than an avascu- larity.

Calcaneal apophyseal disturbance

coming about the frequency is now equalizing. Traction injury to the apophysis as a result of a tight Achilles tendon may be one possible etiology. A rapid growth spurt in the child or a tenosynovitis at the insertion of the Achilles tendon to the apophysis would cause this form of symptomatology. Another possible cause is a microstress fracture of the apophysis as a result of trauma. This could result secondarily to running and jumping activities commonly participated in by these youngsters.

Clinically, the examiner will elicit pain over the posterior plantar aspect of the calcaneus with compression. Side-to-side pressure over the same area will also produce discomfort. There is a higher incidence of this form of heel pain in the overweight child, suggesting again that increased trauma is the more probable cause.

Historically, this condition has predominated in males. It was theorized that, because of its occurrence at the time of puberty, the apophysitis was secondary to hormonal changes. As mentioned earlier, with the acceptance of females into active sporting activities, the frequency among females has equaled that among males; this implies that puberty, hormonal changes, or the physical makeup of a male, as opposed to a female, do not affect the outcome; rather, trauma and stress appear to be the primary etiology. It is known that the epiphyseal plate of the calcaneus is the weakest during the age period when this apophysitis arises. Combined with athletic activity and resulting trauma, the cause could easily be an apophyseal plate fracture (Salter type 1 fracture), which is not demonstrable radiographically.

A good history will often reveal a form of trauma followed by heel pain. An example would be onset of heel pain shortly after a child begins a sporting program. Improper shoe gear or spikes may be indicated as the cause of the heel trauma.

Treatment is primarily directed to reducing the amount of stress imposed on the heel. With elevation of the heel $\frac{1}{2}$–1 inch, the pull of the Achilles tendon will be reduced at the apophysis. If the cause is a traction injury or a tenosynovitis of the insertion of the Achilles tendon, then this elevation should relieve the symptoms. Heel cups (MF cup, Tuli cups, etc.) also are advantageous in helping to reduce trauma to the apophysis. Their function is to compress the fat pad from side to side, allowing greater shock absorption. Orthotic control may also be indicated when a pathologic condition exists in the foot that may be contributing to calcaneal stress. Occasionally it becomes necessary for adequate healing to rest the heel completely. This can be accomplished either by complete elimination of all strenuous activities causing trauma to the heel or by using a walking cast or crutches when the problem persists. The treatment may last as little as 2–4 weeks or as long as 1–2 years. Since this condition does not occur beyond the age of approximately 14–15 years, protection is only necessary until then.

Several other conditions must be differentially diagnosed when the examiner is confronted with a child complaining of heel pain. This should include a septic heel, hematogenous osteomyelitis, juvenile rheumatoid arthritis, and an apophyseal or calcaneal fracture. Synovitis T A

Köhler's Disease

Köhler's disease is considered an osteonecrosis occurring at the navicular in the foot. This disorder is found relatively infrequently among children. It affects youngsters between the ages of 3–9 years, and affects males and females approximately equally. Subjective symptoms may include complaints of vague pain over the dorsal and medial aspects of the foot accompanied by limping. Objectively, there may or may not be a thickening and/or swelling over the area of the navicular. The history obtained may or may not reflect any acute injury. An acute injury may mask the true condition of the navicular. Children within this age range should be suspected for this disorder, which should be included in the differential diagnosis.

When a child with Köhler's disease is observed during gait, it is common to see a limp with an attempt to place the weight on the lateral aspect of the foot. Any attempt at active inversion will be avoided, with the child guarding the area protectively. Compression of the area surrounding the navicular will often elicit a certain degree of pain or discomfort. With sufficient swelling and joint changes, the foot will assume a greater degree of pronation (collapse in the rear and midfoot). This is likely the loss of ligamentous integrity along the medial joints of the foot allowing them to break down.

The radiographic appearance of a Köhler's disease is one of thinning and/ or narrowing of the navicular ossification center. There is found an increase in the density of the entire bone with fragmentation occurring occasionally (**Figure 189**). Careful interpretation is advised when evaluating this area. The navicular can be developing from multiple growth centers and appear fragmented without exhibiting a true osteonecrosis or Köhler's disease.[3,4,8–11] Radiographs of this disease should be compared with a view of the healthy foot for proper interpretation.

Treatment should be directed toward supporting and resting the affected area. The acute stage may best be treated by having the child avoid weight-

Navicular

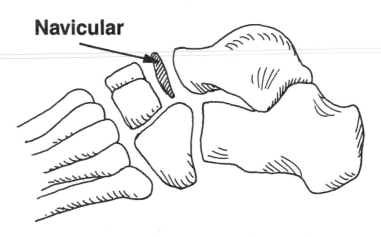

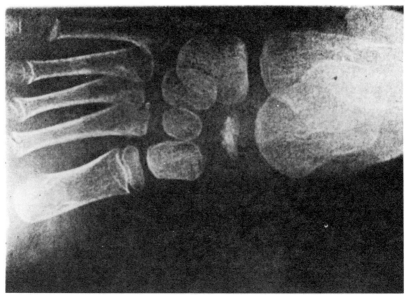

Figure 189

Köhler's disease will radiographically exhibit a narrowing of the navicular with an increase in density. Care is needed not to confuse this with a multiple ossification center or even an osteomyelitic process.

bearing by using crutches and/or a cast, when indicated. Following the non-weight-bearing period, orthotic control is advised in order to maintain a proper structural alignment of the medial joint structures. The orthotic control should be continued until adequate bone revascularization and sufficient growth have resulted. Approximately 1–2 years, sometimes more, are needed for the foot to achieve an adequate resolution of the condition with proper alignment. Shoe padding has been used to relieve the stress along the medial arch area. Unfortunately it cannot adequately control the overall biomechanics of the foot. Therefore, if shoe padding is to be considered, it should be left for the foot with a normal structural attitude presenting with an early stage of Köhler's disease.

Freiberg's Disease (Osteochondrosis of the lesser metatarsals)

Freiberg's disease seems to affect only the lesser metatarsal heads (2nd, 3rd, 4th, and 5th metatarsals), with the second metatarsal being the most frequently afflicted. The metatarsal head will take on an appearance of flattening and collapse with a trumpet appearance (**Figure 190**). The exact etiology is still unknown although several theories have been proposed. Trauma to the second toe or fracture of the epiphysis at the metatarsal head, osteonecrosis secondary to a metabolic disorder, necrosis as a result of lost vascularity to the metatarsal head, and the presence of a short first metatarsal producing an undue amount of stress to the second metatarsal have all been suggested

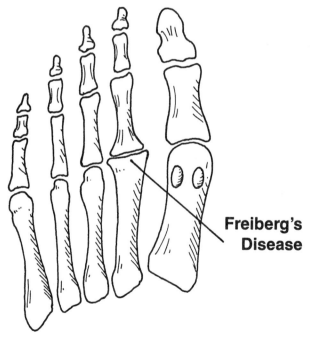

Freiberg's Disease

Figure 190

Freiberg's disease will show radiological evidence of compression and flattening of the metatarsal head with a flaring or "trumpet" appearance. The second metatarsal is the most affected with the third next most and the fourth and fifth metatarsals the least involved.

as possible explanations, but no conclusive etiology has yet been determined.[1,2,4,6,9-11]

This disorder is most frequently encountered in adolescents, occurring between the ages of 13–15 years, and in approximately 3 females for every 1 male. It may occur either unilaterally or bilaterally, and is often symmetrical. There is documentation that two metatarsals may be affected within the same foot. These occurrences lead one to suspect that trauma, either sudden or gradual, is a very likely cause.

The presenting complaint is usually pain over or around the affected metatarsal. Local swelling and thickening of the joint area will be noted. The range of motion at the metatarso-phalangeal joint will be limited or guarded.

The radiologic appearance of the metatarsal head is flattened, irregular, and trumpet-like. The process is usually gradual so that early x-rays may not readily reveal these signs. Serial radiographs are needed to make a proper differential diagnosis of this disorder.

The pathologic findings are similar to those found in other avascular necrotic epiphyses when viewed microscopically. There has been no suggestion that an infection process may be the cause.

Treatment consists initially of reducing any pressure under the affected metatarsal head. This is continued until the pain subsides or further treatment is necessary. The acute phase will last approximately 1–1½ years. This period may persist longer in certain cases. The use of balanced forefoot orthotic devices is advantageous and suggested in the relief of the stress to the affected metatarsal(s).

An adult who presents with an incidental finding of a Freiberg's disease often will relate a period during his adolescence in which he experienced mild to moderate pain in the area. He will frequently relate no apparent discomfort in the area at present and only a short period of pain during the acute phase experienced during adolescence. It therefore behooves the clinician to reduce the pressure to the area by using an accommodative type of orthosis with a cutout for the respective metatarsal. This will allow this active phase to reach a stage of remission without a great degree of destruction.

If a sufficient period of time is allowed for conservative treatment to relieve the discomfort during the acute phase, and the pain persists or intensifies, then further treatment is necessary. This may occur in up to 50% of the cases presenting with this disease. Surgical intervention is necessary but should be postponed, when possible, until the epiphyseal closure of the metatarsal heads.

Many surgical procedures have been devised to alleviate the discomfort from this disorder. A procedure that should be performed selectively is the total metatarsal head resection. This often creates other debilitating conditions. For example, a transference of weight to an adjacent metatarsal causing an intractable plantar keratosis or a dorsal dislocation of the second toe will result secondarily to the loss of joint stability. Therefore, if the surgeon would only remodel the metatarsal head without disturbing a great deal of the plantar condylar surface, the result would be an adequate amount of bone to allow for proper weight-bearing, and less disturbance of the stability of the joint.

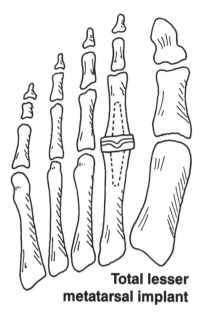

Total lesser metatarsal implant

Figure 191

A total double-stemmed implant is advantageous in treating Freiberg's disease. It will reduce the possibility of toe retraction, maintain alignment of the joint, and allow adequate joint motion of ambulation. This is necessary only in cases where total joint destruction has occurred and adaptation has not resulted.

When complete removal of the metatarsal head is required, then the use of a double-stemmed implant is advised (**Figure 191**). This is used to maintain a joint space and to avoid the retraction of the respective toe. The use of a follow-up orthosis is recommended to maintain a more balanced weight stress across the metatarsal head area.[7]

Ilfeld's or Treve's Disease (Osteochondrosis of the sesmoid)

An osteonecrosis may occur in either the tibial or fibular sesmoid located below the first metatarsal head. The incidence is greater among females with the frequency of occurrence being primarily during adolescence and young adulthood. On examination, tenderness is found with palpation of the affected sesmoid. Significant pain will occur on active or passive dorsiflexion of the hallux. Axial sesmoid and dorsoplantar projections radiographically will reveal fragmentation of the sesmoid without any apparent changes in the metatarsal head or its articular surfaces (**Figure 192**). Do not mistake this condition for a bi or tripartite sesmoid or a fractured sesmoid. A proper history will help in arriving at a correct diagnosis.

When treating an osteochondrosis of a sesmoid, all conservative forms of therapy should first be exhausted. Accommodative padding, steroid injections, physical therapy, etc., should all be tried initially. It has been the experience of this author and others that these forms of therapy have a very poor success rate. Therefore it frequently becomes necessary to surgically remove the affected sesmoid to relieve the persistent symptomatology. Caution is advised to not produce secondary complications. Cases of a hallux varus are documented

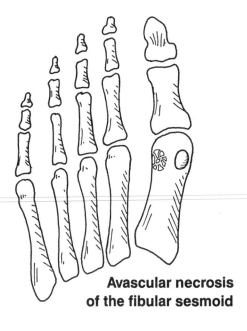

**Avascular necrosis
of the fibular sesmoid**

Figure 192

Avascular necrosis of a sesmoid will appear fragmented radiographically. It can affect either the tibial or fibular sesmoid. Care must be taken to distinguish this from a multipartite sesmoid or a fracture.

by excision of the fibular sesmoid without adequate stabilization, or a hallux valgus from the removal of the tibial sesmoid.

Other less frequent osteochondroses of the foot include:

Diaz or Mouchet's Disease—an osteochondrosis of the talus as a result of trauma.

Buschke's Disease—an osteochondrosis of the three cuneiforms in the foot. This condition is relatively rare in occurrence.

Islin's Disease—an osteochondrosis of the base of the fifth metatarsal as a result of some form of trauma.

All the osteochondroses should be treated by conservative means initially with surgical intervention when lesser treatments do not respond adequately.[1,2,4,9–11]

Osteochondritis Dissecans

Osteochondritis dissecans is a condition in which a portion or fragment of an articular cartilage detaches itself either partially or totally from the subchondral bone. It may then become lodged in the joint, causing avascularity and thus necrosis. The condition occurs equally in children and adults, with males more frequently affected than females. The more commonly affected joints are the knees, ankles, hips, and elbows. Cases have also been reported in which the first metatarso-phalangeal joint, subtalar joint, and other joints in the foot were affected, though more rarely. The etiology may involve heredity, trauma, or ischemia. Trauma probably plays the most significant role in this disorder. Hereditary predisposition is the greatest secondary cause in combination with trauma. Ischemia may be the result of the formation of emboli in the subchondral bone resulting in necrosis and eventual fragmentation with dislodgement.

The presenting symptomatology is intermittent pain within the affected joint upon any form of physical activity. There may be swelling, stiffness, and/ or a popping or clicking sensation within the joint. Occasionally, the joint may lock, usually as a result of the fragment detaching itself and freely floating in the joint space.

With radiographic evaluation, a fragment may be distinguished by its dense appearance and a radiolucent line of demarcation surrounding the fragment (**Figure 193**). Occasionally it may be necessary to employ a laminogram (tomogram) or computerized axial tomography (CAT) scan to demonstrate the presence of a fragment in an early stage of development.

In children, treatment for an osteochondritis dissecans is conservative unless the fragment truly becomes detached. The probability that the fragment will heal is high. However, the joint must be protected from any undue stress during weight-bearing. A walkling cast applied after an initial period of non-weight-bearing is beneficial. There should be a period of partial weight-bearing with crutches prior to complete weight-bearing with the walking cast. The period of nonweight-bearing should be between 2–4 weeks followed by protective weight-bearing for approximately 2–10 months. With the advent of the removable cast, passive exercising of the limb and joints will greatly help to maintain muscle tone and range of motion. It thereby avoids the common cast

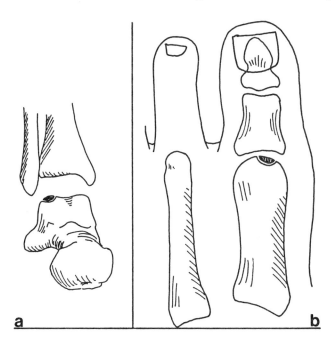

a   b

Figure 193

An osteochondritis dissecans can occur in a variety of joints. In the foot the two areas frequently encountered are the talar dome either medially or laterally (A), and the first metatarsal head (B). The occurrence rate is relatively rare in the foot, however.

disease that follows immobilization. Swimming can also be encouraged as a
form of exercise to maintain muscle tone and m゛゛゛ ゛゛
cast.

Periodic radiographic evaluations ⱥ
of healing or nonhealing that is occurr
diographic evidence of healing is necessa

When an osteochondritis dissecans o
is a lesser likelihood that healing of the f
of the fragment becomes indicated. The
fragment must also be allowed to fill in
This can be accomplished by drilling ho
site of the void, which will result in a fil
producing a smooth surface for joint art
should be properly informed of the inciden
to occur in the joint in the ensuing years
than leaving the fragment alone in the jo

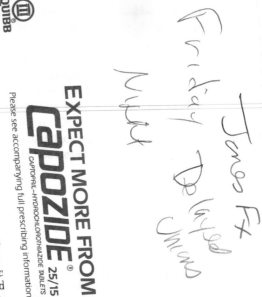

Reference

1. Alrgerter, E., Kirkpatrick, J.A.: *Orthopedic
   Radiology,* Ed. 4. W.B. Saunders Co., Philad
2. Brashear, R.H., Beverly Raney, R.: *Shand's*
   9. C.V. Mosby, St. Louis, MO, 1978.
3. Dobas, D.C., Cachat, P.T.: Köhler's disease. *J..* _____ ᴢ, ʀᴇʙruary 1978.
4. Gamble, F.O., Yale, I.: *Clinical Foot Roentgenology,* Ed. 2. Krieger, New York, 1975.
5. Hill, J., Jimenez, L., Langford, J.H.: Osteochondritis dissecans treated by joint
   replacement. *J.A.P.A.,* 69:Number 9, September 1979.
6. Johnson, H.: Osteochondritis of the second metatarsal head (Freiberg's). *J.A.P.A.,*
   43:1953.
7. Kehr, L.E.: A new surgical technique for the correction of Frieberg's disease. *J.A.P.A.,*
   72:Number 3, March 1982.
8. Sinclair, G.G., Uhlman, R.E., Zeichner, A.M.: Osteochondrosis of the tarsal navicular bone—Köhler's disease. *J.A.P.A.,* 71:Number 2, February 1981.
9. Tachdjian, M.O.: *Pediatric Orthopedics.* W.B. Saunders Co., Philadelphia, PA. 1972.
10. Tax, H.R.: *Podopediatrics.* Williams and Wilkins, Baltimore, MD, 1980.
11. Yale, J.F.: Growth center injuries of the foot. *Arch. of Pod. Med. and Foot Surg.,*
    1:Number 2, October 1973.

Chapter 11

METATARSUS ADDUCTUS, VARUS, ADDUCTOVARUS

*M*uch confusion is evident in the literature regarding the terms and their definitions in respect to forefoot and metatarsal in-toeing abnormalities. It is therefore necessary and appropriate for us to describe and define each term prior to our discussion of the etiology, diagnosis, and treatment.

METATARSUS ADDUCTUS—a transverse plane deformity at the tarso–metatarsal joint in which all five metatarsals are adducted (transverse plane). The first metatarsal will be most adducted with the fifth metatarsal being the least (**Figure 194**).

METATARSUS VARUS—a frontal plane deformity at the tarso–metatarsal joint with all the metatarsals inverted. Minimal or no adduction is present (**Figure 195**).

METATARSUS ADDUCTOVARUS—a combined frontal and transverse plane deformity at the tarso–metatarsal joint (i.e., adduction and inversion occurring simultaneously). This combined deformity is the most frequently encountered abnormality (**Figure 196**).

FOREFOOT ADDUCTUS—this condition can be either a single or combined plane deformity occurring at the midtarsal joint area. The attitude of the metatarsals at the tarso–metatarsal joints exist independently and can assume a normal or adducted position in respect to the midtarsal joints (**Figure 197**).

Subclassifications of these forefoot abnormalities can concurrently be offered for a better description. These subclassifications include the *nonrigid–rigid* type and the *nonfunctional–functional* type. In the nonrigid deformity, a reduction to a normal position can be achieved by manipulation into a corrected attitude. The rigid type may be only partially reducible or may be totally nonreducible. The nonrigid type is the precursor to the rigid type with the age

259

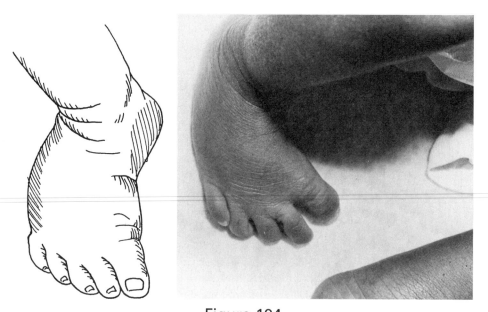

Figure 194

Metatarsus adductus—transverse plane deformity.

of the child and the persistence of the deformity allowing a more fixed attitude to eventually result.

The classification of the *nonfunctional* type is one in which the deformity is existent from birth and will persist throughout the child's development if not treated. The etiology for this type is somewhat obscure although inheritance, fetal positioning, abnormal muscular insertion, and muscular or neuromuscular imbalance have been offered. The *functional type* is the result of a compensatory mechanism from a rearfoot condition. In pronation, the forefoot

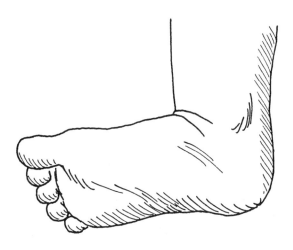

Figure 195

Metatarsus varus—frontal plane deformity.

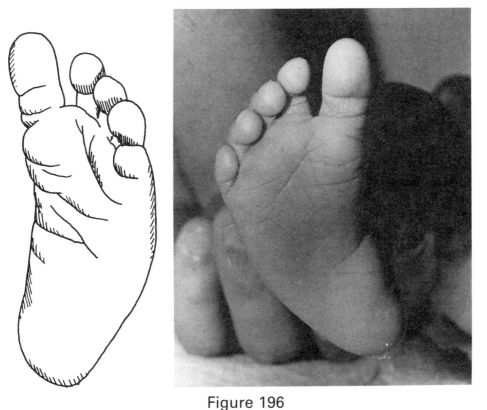

Figure 196

Metatarsus adductovarus—transverse and frontal plane deformity.

= most common

Dr. H says MA
– most common 95%
M ad var = 4%

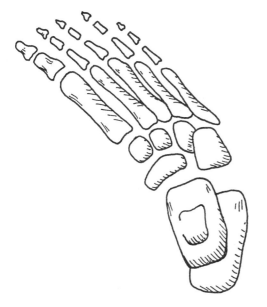

Figure 197

Forefoot adductus—occurs irrespective of the metatarsal attitude.

may be inverted in relationship to the rearfoot as the rearfoot moves into a valgus position. In the cavus foot one will observe an adductus or adductovarus of the metatarsals. This is the result of the rearfoot supination causing the forefoot to assume this position. The reason for this position occurring lies in the mechanical advantage given to the medial muscular attachments (i.e., tibialis anterior, tibialis posterior, abductor hallucis, etc.) to allow greater pull. These positional deformities must not be confused with those found at birth and those resulting in a pronation syndrome as compensation. This can be easily distinguished with a proper history.

One may hear references to metatarsus adductus, varus or adductovarus as a form of clubfoot (talipes equinovarus). It should be apparent to the reader that these two conditions are grossly dissimilar. With the metatarsus deformities, the rearfoot will be in a normal position or even in a valgus position. Dorsiflexion will be sufficient. This is in contradistinction to the clubfoot having a rigid rearfoot varus and limited dorsiflexion. Additionally, the metatarsal deformities (adductus, varus, adductovarus) have their apex at the tarso–metatarsal joints while the clubfoot has concomitant mid and rearfoot articular abnormalities. Therefore, it is grossly inappropriate to attempt to equate the two conditions as similar.

Another frequent statement made with adduction and varus deformities of the metatarsals is the presence of an associated internal tibial torsion. It is this author's opinion that this concomitant finding of internal tibial torsion with a metatarsus deformity is the result of an overpowering or imbalance in the musculature affecting the medial aspect of the leg–foot. It is not felt that there exists a true torsional abnormality in the tibia but rather a positional change as was described in the section on *internal genicular position*. The overpowering and imbalance occurs medially resulting in limited external rotation of the leg at the knee and an internal leg position. The overpowering will also occur in the medial foot musculature resulting in an adductus, varus, or adductovarus condition. It is known that neuromuscular development occurs from *cephalad* to *caudad*. The level in the spinal cord for control of the internal rotator muscles is below that of the external rotators. It can therefore be postulated that any subtle derangement or delay in development would cause aberrant impulse to occur to the internal rotator muscles more persistently than the external rotator muscles.

Another common finding with the metatarsus deformities (i.e., adductus, varus, adductovarus) is the increase in arch attitude in children prior to ambulation. This can be ascribed to the results of overactivity of the tibialis anterior and tibialis posterior muscles. Functionally, the tibialis posterior muscle is primarily a stance phase muscle while the tibialis anterior is a swing phase muscle. Recent electromyographic studies have shown that both of these muscles are overactive at birth in children with these forefoot deformities.[2,12,18]

The current literature has also shown a correlation among metatarsus adductus, varus or adductovarus, and hip dysplasias and dislocations. Anywhere between 3–10% of incidence has been reported. It behooves the examiner to further evaluate these children and infants with these metatarsus deformities to rule out any hip abnormalities. There have also been concomitant findings of this deformity with spina bifida, arthrogryposis multiplex congenita, and Fredrick's ataxia.[4,10,12,14,16,17]

Clinical Examination

The clinical features of the various metatarsus deformities will vary with the type and classification. With metatarsus adductus and adductovarus, the foot will assume a "C" or "comma" shaped appearance (**Figure 198**). The lateral border of the foot will be convex and the medial border concave. The styloid process of the fifth metatarsal base will frequently be prominent. The interval between the hallux and the second toe will often be increased. The rearfoot in these metatarsus deformities is usually in a normal or even valgus position. The arch of the foot may be raised, as was discussed previously in this section.

True metatarsus varus, as defined in this text, will not exhibit the "C" or "comma" shaped appearance. Its appearance is one of complete inversion of the metatarsals and occasionally the entire foot. The rearfoot more often is in a normal attitude with a possible slight varus position that is easily reducible. Adequate dorsiflexion at the ankle is present as well as plantarflexion. Of caution is to not categorize this foot with talipes equinovarus (clubfoot), though its resting appearance may be similar. A clubfoot has limitation of dorsiflexion with a rigid forefoot and rearfoot deformity. This has been completely outlined in Chapter 9.

When examining the foot, it is important to determine the degree of re-

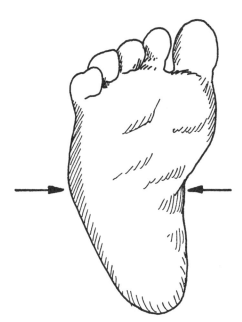

Figure 198

Metatarsus adductus or adductovarus will show a "comma" or "C" shaped appearance laterally. The medial aspect of the foot will be concave due to an increased arch position.

ducibility of the deformity. The examiner should grasp the rearfoot with one hand and place it in a neutral position. This is found by locating the maximum degree of pronation and supination and determining the midpoint between these two. The opposite hand should then grasp the metatarsals on the transverse plane and carefully, but forcibly, attempt reduction (**Figure 199**). The thenar aspect of the hand holding the rearfoot should be sufficiently proximal to be behind the base of the fifth metatarsal. The hand holding the metatarsals should be firmly placed in its position to avoid bunching or "stairstepping" the metatarsals when reducing the deformity (**Figure 200**).

The examiner will then be able to view the plantar aspect of the foot and determine the degree of reducibility as the foot is being forced into correction. Of note is that this same positioning will be used to manipulate and cast the foot and should therefore be learned with proficiency and accuracy.

Muscular function and action must also be evaluated in the clinical examination of these metatarsus deformities. Determination of tautness, abnormal insertion, and/or spasm in the abductor hallucis, tibialis anterior, and tibialis posterior is critical. An example may be an adduction of the hallux (hallux varus) occurring intermittently in a child's gait and during rest periods. Although not fixed in position, it will occur with regular frequency with an in-toeing deformity. Basmajian and Kerr revealed in their studies that a 19% frequency of a medial insertion of the abductor hallucis muscle occurs. This would cause it to function as a true abductor of the hallux. The other 81% of those examined presented with a plantar–medial or plantar insertion of the abductor hallucis. In these cases the muscle functioned not as a pure abductor

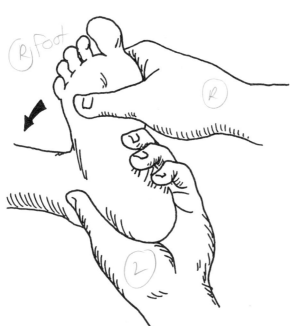

Figure 199

To determine reducibility, place one hand across the metatarsals and the other around the calcaneus. Care is necessary to place the subtalar joint into neutral position and maintain it throughout this maneuver. The hand on the metatarsals should attempt to force the metartarsal bones laterally without "stairstepping."

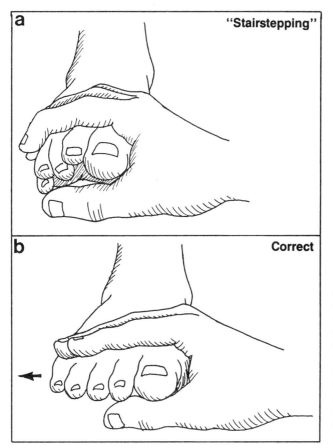

Figure 200

Bunching of the metatarsals is incorrect and will lead to an inaccurate conclusion (A). This error will not allow adequate reduction of the deformity when casting as well. The correct method is to keep all the metatarsals on the same plane with the lateral force being applied evenly (B).

of the hallux, as in the 19% group, but rather as a plantarflexor of the hallux. Therefore in those cases of hallux adductus (hallux varus) accompanied by metatarsus primus adductus, the abductor hallucis muscle will usually insert solely in the medial aspect of the first metatarso–phalangeal joint and function as a true abductor. The result is an adduction deformity when the abductor hallucis muscle contracts. Because anatomically the five metatarsals are joined by the transverse metatarsal ligament, all the metatarsals will be affected if the position of the first metatarsal is altered. With adduction of the first metatarsal and hallux, the respective metatarsals will follow the direction of the first.

This explains the minimal adduction of the fifth metatarsal and maximum adduction of the first metatarsal in metatarsus adductus or adductovarus.

Overactivity of the tibialis anterior will result in a varus (inversion) of the forefoot. The tibialis posterior will produce an adduction position of the forefoot with some varusing in cases of overactivity. All three of these muscles (abductor hallucis, tibialis anterior, tibialis posterior) should be tested for abnormal tightness or spasm.

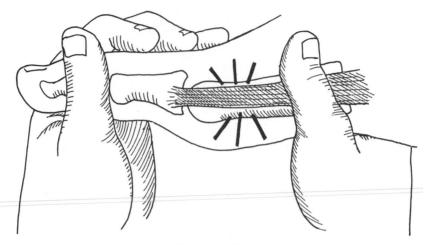

Figure 201

Testing the abductor hallucis muscle is necessary to determine its involvement in a metatarsus deformity. Abducting the hallux toward the second toe will produce tautness along the medial aspect of the foot in a medially inserted tendon. This is easily palpated and/or visualized.

The abductor hallucis muscle is best examined by abducting the hallux while the rest of the foot is stabilized (**Figure 201**). In the presence of abnormal tautness, the tendon of the abductor hallucis will appear markedly bowstrung. The use of a muscle stimulator is another common method of determining the type of action being exerted by this muscle at its insertion. These two testing methods can also be used to examine the tibialis anterior and tibialis posterior muscles. With forcible eversion and plantarflexion of the forefoot, the tibialis anterior can be examined for any abnormal tightness. The presence of bowstringing and significant resistance with this manipulation would indicate an abnormal functioning condition.

Abduction of the forefoot while the rearfoot is kept in neutral position will allow any abnormal degree of contracture in the tibialis posterior muscle to be determined. Muscle stimulation will also help to determine the amount of contractibility remaining in the muscle group.

Radiographic Evaluation

The relationship of the metatarsals and forefoot position should be determined in order to evaluate the extent of the deformity and the progression of treatment.

The infant or young child is limited in the amount of ossified bone structure for referencing. It therefore becomes necessary to alter the points of reference as to those used in the adult. The first line of reference necessary for proper

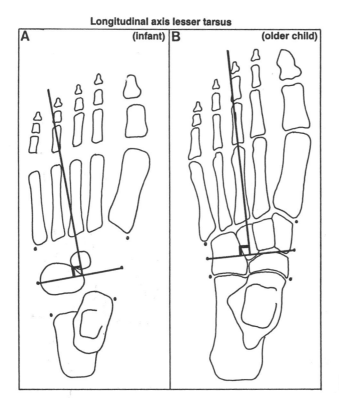

Longitudinal axis lesser tarsus

A (infant) | B (older child)

Figure 202

evaluation is the longitudinal axis of the lesser tarsus (**Figure 202**). This is best constructed in the infant by placing a point at the base of the first metatarsal and another point at the head of the talus. The distance between the two points should be measured and a midpoint marked. On the lateral side, a point should be marked at the base of the fifth metatarsal and another at the distal lateral aspect of the calcaneus. Again measure and locate a midpoint and mark. Connect the two midpoints and draw a perpendicular line from this connecting line at approximately the base of the second metatarsal (**Figure 202A**). With older children or adults, one should use the base of the first metatarsal and the posterior medial aspect of the navicular on the medial side and the distal and proximal articular surfaces of the cuboid on the lateral side. The same procedure is followed to construct the midpoint and perpendicular lines (**Figure 202B**).

To determine the degree of adduction in the metatarsals, construct a bisection line through the second metatarsal intersecting the perpendicular line axis of the lesser tarsus (**Figure 203**). The angle formed is the angle of metatarsus adductus. Normal values for this angle are 5–19°. Values in the range of 20–30° are considered a mild to moderate deformity, while angular values above 35° are considered reasonably severe.[4,15,17]

Metatarsus adductus angle

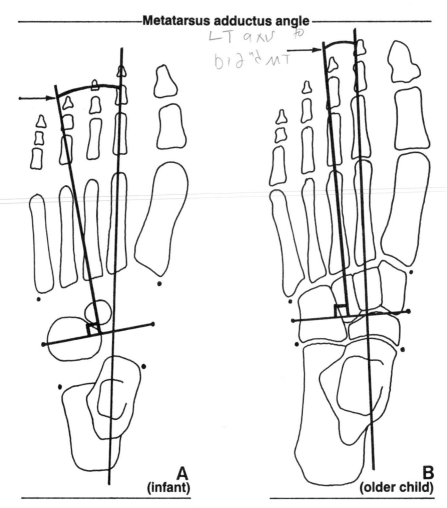

LT axv to
b12nd MT

A
(infant)

B
(older child)

Figure 203

5-19° = Norm
>35° = severe

The amount of adduction present in the lesser tarsus can also be determined by constructing another line representing the axis of the rearfoot. This line is drawn from the anterior–dorso–medial edge of the calcaneus and extended proximally through the center of the calcaneus (**Figure 204**). Once the line is placed properly, it should be extended anteriorly to the toes. The angle created by this axis line of the rearfoot with that of the perpendicular axis line of the lesser tarsus is referred to as the angle of lesser tarsus adductus. Values in excess of 5–15° are considered significant. Greater values of lesser tarsus adduction are most frequently encountered in feet with noted rearfoot supination.

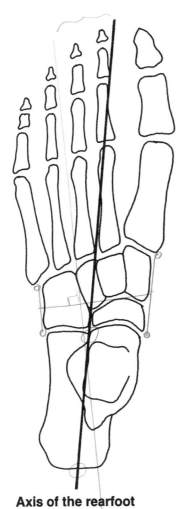

Angle of L-T adductv

Axis of the rearfoot   Figure 204

Normally the lesser tarsus has either minimal or no adduction or even a slight degree of abduction present.

A third angular measurement of value in the radiographic evaluation of metatarsus deformities is the angle of metatarsus primus adductus. This is determined by constructing a bisection line through the first metatarsal and measuring the angular value between it and the bisection of the second metatarsal (**Figure 205**). Values most normally encountered are between 5–10°. Values beyond 10° would be indicative of a metatarsus primus adductus. The adduction may appear as a singular deformity as in hallux adductus (hallux varus) or it may be the true cause of an inwardly adducted appearance of the forefoot. It may also be a concomitant factor in the accentuation and increased severity of metatarsus adductus or adductovarus deformity.

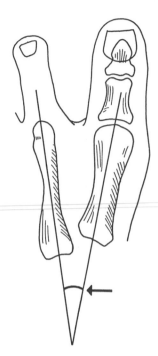

Angle of MT primus adductus

Bi F-MT
B5 2MT

Figure 205

Treatment

When treating the metatarsus deformities (i.e., metatarsus adductus, metatarsus varus, metatarsus adductovarus), one must have a philosophic

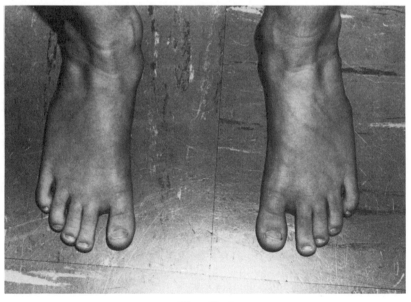

Skew Foot.

understanding of the purpose of treatment and the final results anticipated. Several valid arguments have been made in defense of aggressive treatment of these deformities. When a child exhibits an in-toeing gait abnormality secondary to a metatarsus deformity, his ability to ambulate properly and safely becomes impaired. The tripping and clumsily ambulating child is very likely to lead to harm. For this reason alone, some form of correction is justified. There are, however, equally important consequences to the metatarsus deformities as compensatory changes occur in the foot and leg.

The foot mechanics will alter themselves, allowing the rearfoot and midfoot to collapse architecturally. This occurs to allow abduction of the forefoot for better placement of the center of stress (gravity) in the foot. In biomechanics it has been learned that with pronation of the rearfoot, there will result an abduction of the forefoot, adduction and plantarflexion of the talus, and eversion of the calcaneus. Since our bodies will always attempt to place the center of stress (gravity) over the center of the foot, when possible, the changes that occur are predictable. The adducted attitude of the forefoot in the metatarsus deformities places the center of stress (gravity) laterally in the foot. This will result in an unstable gait pattern. To better adapt to this abnormal center of stress, the foot will pronate and secondarily collapse in structure to allow the gravitational center to move from the lateral position to a more medial position in the foot. This allows for a more stable gait with reduced awkwardness.[14–17,19]

Concomitant with pronation in the foot is the natural internal rotation of the lower leg (tibia and fibula) relative to the calcaneus and forefoot. This internal rotation is the result of adduction of the talus, which is locked in the ankle mortise. The inward rotation of the leg will additionally move the center of stress medial. The leg rotation will have an effect at the knee joint causing rotational stress factors to the cartilage as well as affect the ligamentous and musculotendinous structures. *Note: Forefoot adduction occurs in the cavus foot condition as a secondary result from rearfoot supination. It therefore is not being compensated for as in the metatarsus deformities. It actually is the resulting position from another structural abnormality.*

The structural changes that result in the foot and superstructures eventually provide deleterious effects to the joints and the periarticular structures. Arthritic changes, as a result of deviation or subluxation of the joints affected, will only be recognized once the person is much older and has allowed adequate time for the wearing of these joints. For this reason, treatment should be instituted early to help avoid these anticipated changes. Oftentimes we hear it said that a child will grow out of these metatarsus deformities. In reality the child is actually compensating for the deformity by altering the foot–leg structure rather than "spontaneously correcting" as is often thought. This compensation is not a desired outcome if more correctable means are available and possible. There are other equally important considerations when treating the metatarsus deformities, including shoe fit. The presence of a high degree of metatarsus adductus or adductovarus in excess of 30° and rigid will cause considerable difficulty in shoe sizing and fit. Conversely a flexible type will be easily compensated by pronation in the foot to accommodate the shoe pressures. An early bunion deformity may also easily result from the metatarsus deformities. The presence of a high degree of hallux abductus and hallux interphalangeus in the presence of a low intermetatarsal angle is commonplace. This becomes a difficult deformity to treat because of the minimal intermetatarsal space.

Another secondary change to the metatarsus deformities is the lateral deviation of the extensor tendons in the foot. This positioning leads to contractures of the digits, secondary displacement of the metatarsals with resulting plantar hyperkeratotic lesions, rotation of the metatarsals causing abnormal stress points, etc.

It becomes clear that early treatment of these conditions affords the best possible prognosis with the least amount of secondary changes in the overall foot structure. The "golden age" for treatment is between birth and 1½–2 years of age. The earlier one employs treatment, the shorter the term needed for correction.

Early treatment is comprised of corrective manipulation with serial stretch castings or tape splinting. With very mild metatarsus deformities in a very young infant, manipulation and tape splinting are usually sufficient to reduce the abnormal position (**Figure 207**). The treatment should be continued until adequate overcorrection is achieved.

The method for manipulation that has been described uses one hand to maintain the rearfoot in neutral position while the other hand mobilizes the metatarsals laterally on the transverse plane (**Figure 206**). Avoidance of

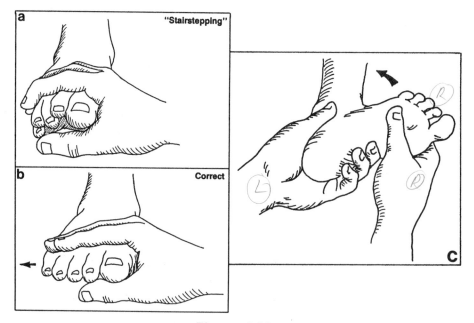

Figure 206

"stairstepping" is paramount. The manipulated foot is held in correction for a period of 15–20 seconds and released. This should be continued for approximately 10–15 minutes when possible. Upon completion of the manipulation, a below or above-the-knee cast or tape splint is applied. The tape splint should be applied as shown in **Figure 207**. It is sometimes possible to allow the parents to apply the tape splint along with manipulation of the foot. It should be at the discretion of the clinician as to their competency and reliability for this to be allowed. Otherwise the clinician should perform both maneuvers every 4–7 days.

The cast application is best performed by:

- Applying tincture of benzoin to the skin for protection and adherence of the padding when necessary.
- Applying a two-layer thickness of padding material of choice. Additional layers should be applied over areas of pressure (i.e., malleoli, heel, upper edge of cast).
- Applying the plaster from beyond the distal aspects of the toes to proximally either below or above the knee.
- Manipulating the foot into its corrected position by using the same hand positioning method described previously until the casting material is set (**Figure 206**).

It becomes important to use a reasonable amount of force to manipulate the cast in order to accomplish an effective position. The child will usually cry or complain if you have overstretched the foot. Therefore, if the child is content while you are manipulating with force, you have not injured or hurt the youngster. This is a usual fear in young inexperienced clinicians. Care should be exerted to avoid pronating the rearfoot when manipulating the cast. For this to be accomplished adequately, the heel should be held in slight varus to supinate the rearfoot while still allowing the forefoot to be manipulated into abduction.

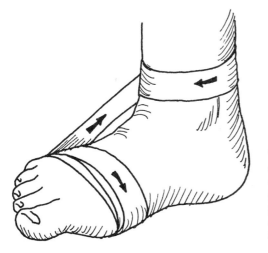

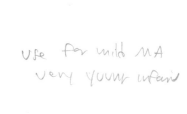

Figure 207

Tape splinting should be applied after adequate manipulation of a metatarsus deformity. The taping can extend to the hallux in a hallux varus deformity or proximal in a forefoot adductus condition. Proper stabilization is necessary to produce a reduction.

When the treatment is for metatarsus adductus or adductovarus, a below-the-knee cast is usually adequate for maintenance. A true metatarsus varus with a rearfoot varus should be treated with an above-the-knee cast to provide adequate stretching of the musculature with avoidance of the cast to be kicked off by the infant. When employing an above-the-knee cast, it is best to first apply the lower leg–foot portion (a below-the-knee cast) and manipulate the foot into correction until the casting material is set. The application of the upper portion is then added and the knee flexed to approximately 35–45° for cast stability. It is the feeling of some clinicians that a small infant needs an above-the-knee cast for any type of casting to prevent the child from kicking the cast off. This author has not found this necessary nor a problem when the cast is applied with the foot–ankle maintained at right angles.

The time frame for cast changes is between 4 and 7 days. Remanipulation is mandatory prior to each cast application to reduce the length of treatment. It has been consistently found that manipulation prior to casting will reduce treatment time to almost one-half. It behooves the practitioner to incorporate manipulation into the casting program without reservation.

For the cast changes, the clinician can remove the cast with the use of a cast cutter or the parents can be instructed on its removal at home. If the parents are cooperative and reliable, then allow them to remove the casts by soaking in a tub of warm water with approximately 1–2 cups of vinegar added. It may take a minimum of 30–60 minutes of soaking to adequately remove the casting material. Caution the parents on the use of scissors or knives in removing the cast so as to avoid any potential harm to the child. Frequently it is sufficient to use only one roll of plaster casting material in the small nonweight-bearing child for a strong below-the-knee cast. When this is possible, the clinician can leave the end of the roll bunched after application, to give the parents a starting point for the removal.

Once a correct attitude has been achieved in overcorrection, a holding cast should be employed for approximately 2–3 weeks to ensure adequate maintenance of the position. A child between the ages of 1–3 months will require approximately 4–6 weeks of casting as an average. Children 3–6 months old will average 6–8 weeks while those children above 6 months of age may require lengthy casting periods to adequately reduce the deformity.

To properly determine the adequacy of correction achieved following the manipulation and stretch castings, a radiograph should be exposed and compared to those taken prior to casting. If an inadequate reduction is found in the positioning, even though clinically it may appear straight, then a continuation of the treatment is necessary to properly ensure an adequate position of the foot. Without strict adherence to the criteria outlined, reccurrence of the deformity may be likely within a short period of time after ending the treatment program.

When a child is in the age period for casting and is found to be resistant to correction after several weeks of manipulation and stretch castings, it may become necessary to release the abductor hallucis tendon to achieve sufficient correction. If contracture of the muscle exists to any substantial degree, stretching by casting may not be capable of adequately reducing the deformity. Determination of its presence has been described under the section *Clinical Evaluation*. To correct this condition, a pericutaneous sectioning of the tendon proximal to the first metatarsophalangeal joint will release the tautness and allow for a better mobilization of the forefoot (**Figure 208**).[8,9,18]

The condition of the metatarsus deformities changes when a child is between 3–8 years of age. There usually exists a semirigid or rigid attitude as a result of the period of time the deformity has been present. At this age level it becomes almost impossible to attempt any correction with serial castings. It therefore requires surgical consideration if a sufficient degree of deformity is existing.

Radiologically, certain conditions must be present for one to consider early surgical procedures. The bases of the respective metatarsals should be cartilagenous, which can be determined by viewing their configuration on anteroposterior x-rays. The appearance of a rounded rather than squared metatarsal bases is indicative of cartilagenous bases (**Figure 209**). When considering a surgical release of the metatarsal bases, there must be sufficient cartilage to allow for readaptation. A moderately severe or severe metatarsus deformity will usually require the surgical release in children at this age level. Metatarsus adductus angles of 30–35° and above should be treated with metatarsal releasing.

The procedure employs the releasing of the dorsal, medial, lateral, and two-thirds of the medial plantar ligamentous–capsular structure which surrounds each metatarsal base. The lateral one-third of the plantar capsule is left intact to reduce the possibility of dorsal migration of the metatarsals. The surgical approach can be either by three linear incisions or one transverse incision (**Figure 210**). The releasing of the first, third, fourth, and fifth metatarsal bases is usually performed without difficulty. The second metatarsal

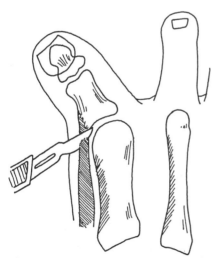

Pericutaneous abductor hallucis tendon release

Figure 208

An abductor hallucis tendon release is performed by a pericutaneous stab incision over the medial aspect of the first metatarsophalangeal joint or just proximal to this joint. The joint should only be incised in cases where the release of the abductor tendon will not sufficiently reduce a hallux varus deformity.

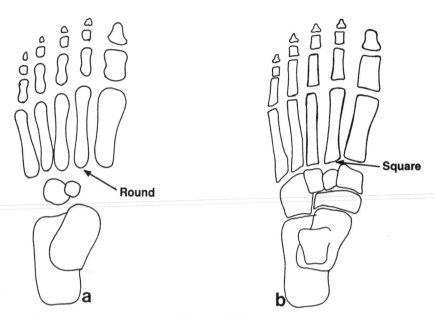

Figure 209

Re: surgery tmt

*Rounded metatarsal bases indicate that adequate cartilage is available for
redirection of the joint surfaces (A). When a squaring appears, then ossification
has advanced to a point that will not allow readaption (B).* *? see anshaul
10-V years later*

base is more difficult due to the mortise in which it is located. To avoid significantly damaging the cartilagenous base and still properly releasing the
base, this author advises osteotomizing the base with a crescentic cut to allow
proper mobilization. The crescentic cut is made through the cartilagenous base
leaving the capsular and ligamentous structures intact (**Figure 211**). Very
often it is advantageous to lengthen or release the abductor hallucis tendon
through the same medial incision to reduce its effect on the deformity. After

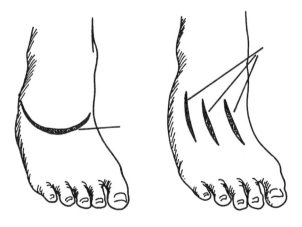

Figure 210

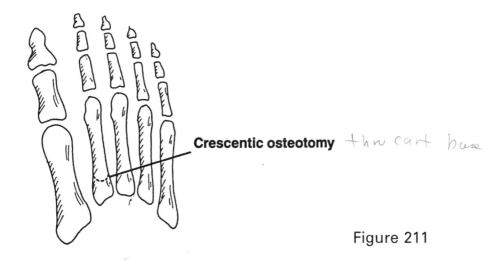

Crescentic osteotomy *thru cart base*

Figure 211

complete release of the metatarsal bases, a well-molded cast should be applied with the foot manipulated into correction. Since the advent of fiberglass casts the use of plaster has been reduced significantly. This author feels that one cannot adequately place the foot in a proper position with the use of the more stiff fiberglass materials. Therefore it is still advisable to use plaster for proper maintenance of the corrected position.[3,5,6,7,11,16]

Cast changes should occur every two weeks with the foot remanipulated prior to each application. Approximately 8–10 weeks of casting is required to achieve a stable and adequate correction. Casting for any time less than this period may allow a reoccurrence. One potential complication of this procedure is the possibility of arthritic changes occurring at the tarso–metatarsal joints 10–15 years later. This will only occur if the procedure is attempted at a later age than suggested or if the metatarsal bases are squared and ossified rather than cartilagenous.

An alternative form of treatment within this age period is the performance of chondrotomies of the lesser metatarsals[2–5] and an osteotomy of the first metatarsal distal to the epiphysis. A chondrotomy is performed by the use of a crescentic blade through the cartilagenous bases of the lesser metatarsals (**Figure 212**). At the first metatarsal base one can either release the dorsal, medial, lateral and plantar two-thirds of the capsule along with the abductor hallucis tendon or perform a crescentic or wedge osteotomy of the metatarsal shaft distal to the epiphysis. This should be then casted for a period of 8 weeks in the corrected position. Occasionally it is necessary to pin fixate the first metatarsal and less frequently the fifth metatarsal to ensure stability. One significant advantage of this procedure is its avoidance of alterations at the tarso–metatarsal joints. The anticipation of cartilage remodeling is not assumed as is the case in the releasing of the metatarsal bases.[7]

Children beyond the ages of 7–8 years with ossified and squared metatarsal bases must be treated according to different criteria. At this age level,

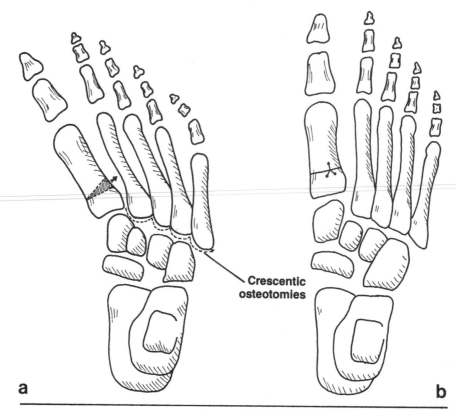

Crescentic
osteotomies

a   b

Figure 212

Chondrotomies through the bases of the 2–5 metatarsals are accomplished by a crescentic osteotomy. The first metatarsal can be reduced by either a closing wedge (A) or crescentic osteotomy. The osteotomy must be performed distal to epiphysis of the first metatarsal. Correction is accomplished by casting the foot into abduction with the achievement of a proper rearfoot–forefoot relationship (B).

the deformity is reasonably fixed and rigid with the articular surfaces fully developed and established. It becomes necessary to consider realignment of the metatarsal shafts by an osseous form of correction. In these cases, a metatarsus adductus angle of 30–35° or greater requires surgical realignment of the deformity. Several methods have been proposed to accomplish an adequate reduction of the osseous condition. Included are: closing base wedge osteotomies of the metatarsals; opening base wedge osteotomies of the metatarsals; and crescentic osteotomies of the metatarsal bases. The most accepted current procedure is the crescentic base osteotomies of the four lesser metatarsal bases with either a crescentic or closing base wedge osteotomy of the first metatarsal distal to the epiphysis, if still open (**Figure 213**). This procedure can be performed through either a transverse incision or three linear incisions. The three

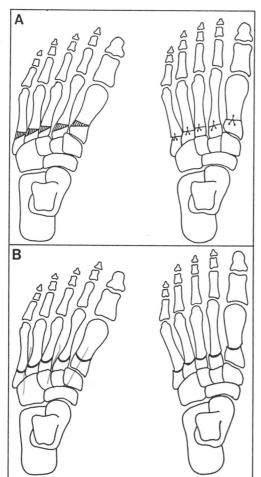

Figure 213

Either a closing wedge osteotomy of each metatarsal (A) or a crescentic osteotomy (B) will allow reduction of a metatarsus adductus deformity. The combination of a crescentic osteotomy of metatarsals 2–5 and a closing wedge osteotomy of the first metatarsal offers excellent stability and reduction of the deformity.

linear incisions are placed one over the first metatarsal base, second between the 2nd and 3rd metatarsal bases, and third between the 4th and 5th metatarsal bases (**Figure 210**). To be remembered is the angulation of the metatarsals as a result of the deformity. Careful tracing of each metatarsal back to its base is necessary to ensure proper placement of your incisions. Pin fixation of the first metatarsal and, when necessary, the fifth metatarsal is advantageous in maintaining proper alignment. There are some surgeons who do not employ any form of fixation and are achieving satisfactory results. The use or nonuse of fixation should then rest with the surgeon and his ability and preference.[1,5,11,12,16]

After the osteotomies are performed, a well-molded paster walking cast should be applied with the foot manipulated well into a corrected position. A period of 6–8 weeks of casting is required for adequate reduction. Casts should be changed every 2–3 weeks with proper alignment of the foot. A fiberglass cast can be used after the first cast, if desired. When using wire fixation, adequate bony healing is needed prior to removal of the pins, which is usually between 3–5 weeks. Radiographic evaluation will best ensure its presence.

After surgery, all patients should be followed with orthotic control to maintain positioning of the rearfoot while supporting and controlling the mid and forefoot structures. The orthosis should be tailored to control the surrounding structural conditions in addition to accounting for the activity and age of the individual. Heel-stabilizing orthoses are advantageous for the young child with a hypermobile foot. The older child will function better with a less confining orthosis (i.e., Whitman–Roberts' plate or functional type) due to the lesser degree of mobility present in the foot. The discretion of the practitioner is needed to determine the most suitable type for his patients and their activities.[13,17,19] *Note:* Following serial casting a child may still assume an improper sleeping or sitting position (**Figure 214**). This will obviously affect the long-term results of your treatment program. It therefore becomes necessary for the clinician to find a means of discouraging this attitutde. The use of night splints (i.e., Fillauer, Denis–Browne, Brachman, Ganley) are extremely effective in discouraging improper sleeping habits. This is accomplished by not allowing the feet and legs to rotate inwardly while the splint is attached to the shoes. When a child grows out of the shoes being attached to the splint, then cutting the toe area out of the shoe will allow for longer use without injury to the foot. The type of shoe used should be with a rigid sole to allow for the attachment of the splint. A word of note, night splints do not offer any

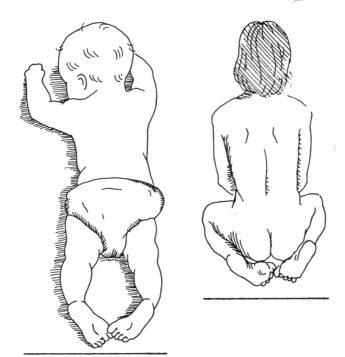

Figure 214

Improper sleeping habits

direct form of treatment to the metatarsus deformities other than to discourage poor sleeping positions.

Sitting positions can be discouraged by having the parents encourage the child to sit on a stool or chair while playing or watching television. This will reduce the excessive forces that will easily reverse the corrections achieved through treatment (**Figure 215**).

Oftentimes shoe therapy has been prescribed for treatment or after treatment to castings. Lateral sole wedges with Thomas heels and medial heel wedge, or the outflare type shoes all have deleterious effects on the overall foot structure. This type of therapy will often cause excessive midtarsal and rearfoot pronation in place of actual correction or maintenance of the metatarsus deformity. This pronatory movement actually allows the forefoot to abduct by the sacrificed stability of subtalar joint and rearfoot. Certainly it is not the intent of a practitioner to allow one deformity to improve at the expense of creating another deformity. Therefore, shoe therapy should be avoided by keeping these consequences in mind. The only exception to this is the usage of straight last shoes. Properly fitted straight last shoes are beneficial in maintaining the alignment of the foot after serial castings for the metatarsus deformities. The use of an orthosis in combination with the straight last shoes

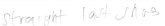

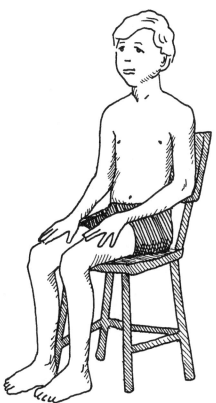

Figure 215

achieves two very important results: proper alignment of the rearfoot is maintained without the compensatory pronation that otherwise results; and an abductory force is being maintained at the metatarsals to ensure stability of the corrected position. The shoes, with the orthoses inserted, can be utilized during the sleeping periods with a night splint as well as during the active daily periods. They should be replaced reasonably frequently to avoid loosening from stretching of the leather and the outgrowing of them by the developing young foot. The shoe is normally fitted with a certain degree of snugness to allow proper maintenance of the correction.[13,17,19]

References

1. Albin, R.L.: The surgical management of metatarsus adductus. Northlake Surgical Seminar Compendium, 1974.
2. Basmajian, J.V., Stecko, G.: The role of muscles in arch support of the foot. *Journal of Bone and Joint Surgery,* 45-A:1963.
3. Brown, J.H., Purvis, C.G., Kaplan, E.G., Mann, I.: Berman-Gartland operation for correction of resistant adduction of the forepart of the foot. *J.A.P.A.,* 67:Number 12, December 1977.
4. D'Amico, J.C.: Congenital metatarsus adductus: An overview. *Archives Podiatric Medicine and Foot Surgery,* 3:Number 4, 1976.
5. Haber, J.: Surgical treatment of metatarsus adductus. *Archives of Podiatric Medicine and Foot Surgery,* 3:Number 4, 1976.
6. Heyman, C.H., Herndon, C.H., Strong, J.M.: Mobilization of the tarsometatarsal and intermetatarsal joints for the correction of resistant adduction of the forepart of the foot in congenital clubfoot or congenital metatarsus varus. *Journal of Bone and Joint Surgery,* 40-A:1958.
7. Johnson, J.B.: A preliminary report on chondrotomies. *J.A.P.A.,* 68:Number 12, December 1978.
8. Jones, R.A., McCrea, J.: Tenotomy of the abductor hallucis for correction of resistant metatarsus adductus. *J.A.P.A.,* 60:Number 1, January 1980.
9. Lichtblau, S.: Section of the abductor hallucis tendon for correction of metatarsus varus deformity. *Clinical Orthopedics,* Number 110, July–August 1975.
10. McDonough, M.W.: Fetal positioning as a cause of right and left-sided foot and leg disorders. *J.A.P.A.,* 71:Number 2, February 1981.
11. Ponseti, I.V., Becker, J.R.: Congenital metatarsus adductus: The results of treatment. *Journal of Bone and Joint Surgery* 48-A:1966.
12. Reimann, I., Werner, H.H.: Congenital metatarsus varus. *Clinical Orthopedics,* Number 110, July–August 1975.
13. Rossi, W.A.: The controversy of corrective shoes. *J.A.P.A.,* 71:Number 4, April 1981.
14. Sharp, J.T.: Assessment of normal motor development in the child. *J.A.P.A.,* 71:Number 2, February 1981.
15. Sgarlato, T.E.: A compendium of podiatric biomechanics. *California College of Podiatric Medicine,* 1971.
16. Tachdjian, M.O.: *Pediatric Orthopedics.* W.B. Saunders Co., Philadelphia, PA, 1972.
17. Tax, H.R.: *Podopediatrics.* Williams and Wilkins, Baltimore, MD, 1980.
18. Thompason, S.A.: Hallux varus and metatarsus varus—A five year study (1954–1958). *Clinical Orthopedics,* 16:1960.
19. Volta, J.J., Weber, R.B.: A nonsurgical treatment regimen for metatarsus adductus utilizing orthosis. *J.A.P.A.,* 71:Number 2, February 1981.

Chapter 12

JUVENILE HALLUX VALGUS AND DIGITAL DEFORMITIES

Juvenile Hallux Valgus

*J*uvenile hallux valgus (hallux–abducto–valgus) presents the practitioner with a challenging problem in both prognosis and treatability. Through the study of biomechanics of the foot, we are aware that a hallux valgus deformity is characterized by the hallux being abducted and axially rotated in eversion as it relates to the first metatarsal. Concomitantly the first metatarsal is medially positioned in relation to the second metatarsal. When viewing a juvenile hallux–abducto–valgus deformity, the characteristics and conditions often differ markedly from those found in the adult-onset type. The juvenile type most frequently has good joint cartilage over its entire first metatarsal head and proximal phalangeal base. The cartilage is adaptable and healthy in contradistinction to that found in the adult type, which usually exhibits degenerative changes.

The foot in a juvenile type presents with a significant degree of abnormality in the first ray mechanics to allow the formation of the metatarsus primus adductus at this early age level. Realizing all these conditions, a method of correction must be tailored to adequately stabilize the components of the deformity for a lifetime of activity without destroying any of the existing congruity or joint architecture.

Biomechanical Considerations

When viewing the first metatarsophalangeal joint, it may be more appropriate to consider it the first metatarso–sesmoidal–phalangeal joint. The reasoning for this consideration is the anatomical makeup of the joint. The intrinsic musculature composed of the abductor hallucis, flexor hallucis brevis, and the adductor hallucis all insert into the sesmoidal apparatus rather than the base of the proximal phalanx of the hallux. These insertions allow the sesmoid to act as a fulcrum with any muscular action of the intrinsics. Any alteration of this function will result in a direct effect upon the stability of the joints that can occur in a surgical intervention or a pathological condition.

283

Biomechanically, the first ray functions around an axis which passes from posterior, medial, and superior to anterior, lateral, and inferior (**Figure 216**). The axis extends through the base of the third metatarsal to the tuberosity of the navicular. The motion that will result from this axis can be considered in two ways. The motion of the first ray above the transverse plane is one of dorsiflexion, inversion, and slight adduction. The range of motion occurring below the transverse plane is one of plantarflexion, eversion, and slight abduction.

Etiologically, a hallux–abducto–valgus deformity is the result of excessive first ray mobility, termed "hypermobility," during stages of gait when limited mobility should be occurring. To have hypermobility, pronation at the subtalar joint or compensatory inversion at the midtarsal joint must exist concurrently. Pronation of the subtalar joint results in an unlocking mechanism of the midtarsal joints. This unlocking allows supination (inversion) of the midtarsal joint. This supination results from the unlocked midtarsal joints along with the hypermobility and instability of the first ray from weight-bearing. The instability not only affects the first ray mechanics but the entire medial column of the foot during the midstance phase of gait.

Biomechanical causes for pronation can include: equinus, compensated nonrigid forefoot valgus, compensated nonrigid forefoot varus, ligamentous laxity, etc. These all allow for first ray hypermobility resulting in a propensity toward the formation of a hallux–abducto–valgus deformity. Other factors that have been ascribed to the predisposition of a hallux–abducto–valgus condition

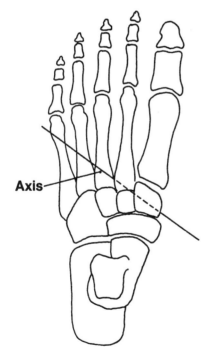

Axis

Figure 216

The axis of motion for the first ray lies obliquely, allowing motion in three planes. Dorsiflexion of the ray will cause inversion and adduction while plantarflexion results in eversion and abduction.

are: hereditary influences, type and shape of the first metatarsal head, length of the first metatarsal and of the phalanges of the hallux, forefoot and metatarsus adductus deformities, first metatarsocuneiform angle, and shoe gear.[2,4,6,7,9–16,19,21,23,24,26]

Radiographic Evaluation

Several considerations are incorporated in the evaluation of a hallux–abducto–valgus deformity. Radiographically, these include the following: proximal articular set angle; distal articular set angle; hallux abductus angle; shape of the first metatarsal head; joint positioning of the first metatarsophalangeal joint; metatarsus primus adductus angle; tibial sesmoid position; first metatarsocuneiform angle.

Proximal articular set angle (PASA) indicates the amount of lateral tilt of the cartilage at the head of the first metatarsal in its relationship to the long axis of its shaft. The normal angular values are 5–8° from the perpendicular (**Figure 217**).

Distal articular set angle (DASA) represents the relationship of the articular surface of the proximal phalanx of the hallux with the long axis of the phalangeal shaft. Five to 8° are the normal accepted angular value (**Figure 218**).

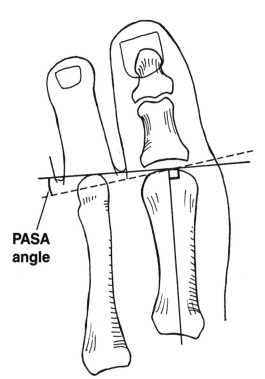

PASA angle

Figure 217

The proximal articular set angle (PASA) is determined by drawing a line bisecting the first metatarsal and a line at right angles to this bisection (solid lines). A line is then drawn along the functioning articular cartilage of the head of the first metatarsal (dotted line). An angle will form at its intersection that normally is between 5–8°. Angles greater indicate lateral deviation of the functional cartilage.

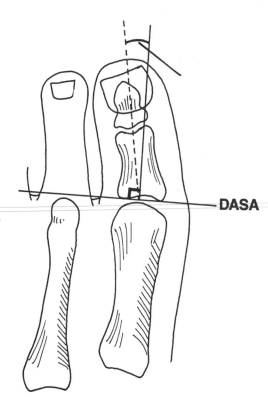

Figure 218

The distal articular set angle (DASA) is determined by drawing a line parallel to the proximal articular cartilage of the proximal phalanx of the hallux. A second line is drawn at right angles to the cartilage (solid lines). A bisection line is then drawn through the proximal phalanx (dotted line) and intersected with the perpendicular line to the articular surface. The angle formed should be approximately 5–8°. Values greater than 5–8° indicate an interphalangeal twist in the bone. Occasionally there may exist a lateral deviation of growth in the distal phalanx with the proximal phalanx remaining straight. This will produce an abnormal lateral position of the distal hallux and place the extensor and flexor tendon in a position to pull the tow into an abduction deformity with a secondary hallux abducto valgus deformity.

Hallux abductus angle demonstrates the amount of abduction of the hallux on the first metatarsal. An angle is formed from the intersecting lines of the long axis of the proximal phalanx and the long axis of the first metatarsal. This angle actually represents the sum total of the proximal articular set angle, the distal articular set angle, and the joint angle. The hallux abductus angle in the nonpathologic foot is normally 10–20° (**Figure 219**).

Shape of the first metatarsal head plays a significant role in the contribution of a hallux–abducto–valgus deformity. There are three types to be considered: the *round, square,* and *square type with a center ridge* (**Figure 220**). In the presence of a deforming force, the round head is the least stable of the three, and is the most likely to become deviated and ultimately subluxed (see joint position of the first metatarsophalangeal joint). The square type is less likely to become deviated and the square type with a center ridge is the least likely to become deviated.

There are three types of positioning of the first metatarso-phalangeal joint: congruous, deviated, or *subluxed* (**Figure 221**). The congruous joint is one in which lines representing the articular surface of the head of the first metatarsal and the base of the proximal phalanx are parallel. In a deviate joint the lines will converge outside of the joint, while in the subluxed joint the lines will converge within the joint space.

Metatarsus primus adductus angle is measured from the intersection of

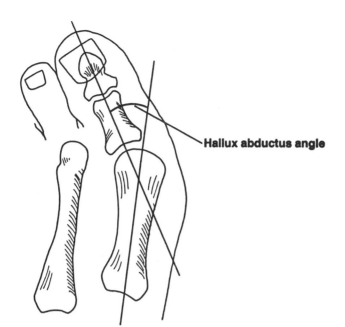

Hallux abductus angle

Figure 219

The hallux abductus angle is formed by a bisection line through the first metatarsal and one through the proximal phalanx. The angle formed is normally between 10–20°. Values greater than 20° are considered pathologic.

the long axis of the first and second metatarsal (**Figure 222**). The normal values are between 5–10°. One must consider the degree of forefoot or metatarsus adductus when totally evaluating this position of the first metatarsal. With greater degrees of adductus, a higher metatarsus primus adductus will exist *without* the concomitant greater angular relationships between the first and second metatarsals (**Figure 223**).

Tibial sesmoid position is determined by examining a dorso–plantar radiograph taken in the normal angle and base of gait. The tibial sesmoid is observed in its relationship to the long axis of the first metatarsal. If the entire tibial sesmoid lies well medial to the long axis of the first metatarsal, the tibial sesmoid position is 1. If it lies central on the long axis of the first metatarsal it is position 4, and if it lies entirely lateral to the long axis it is position 7. This will represent the degree of erosion of the sesmoidal grooves as the number increases in value (**Figure 224**).

First metatarsocuneiform angle is formed by the angular relation of the first metatarsocuneiform joint with the second metatarsal. The degree of angulation will directly affect the position of the first metatarsal along with its degree of stability throughout the first ray mechanics. Angular values greater than 90–105° are considered significant (**Figure 223B**).[6,7,10,12,16,19,21,23,26]

Treatment

Hallux–abducto–valgus begins as a positional deformity that eventually becomes subluxed and structural. Functional bone adaptation will take place

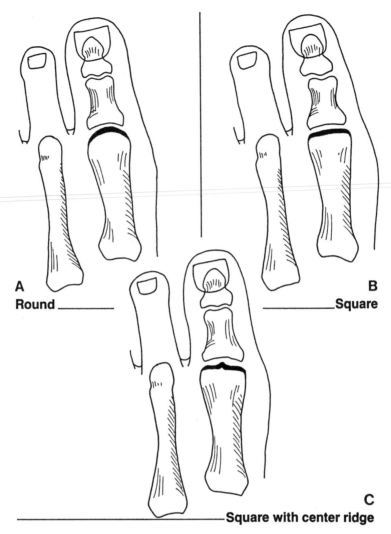

Figure 220

The most unstable metatarsal head is round (A) with the square (B) being more stable and the square with a ridge (C) the most stable.

and the deformity becomes structural as the hallux now functions with its articular cartilage in its new lateral attitude. Due to the motion of the first ray existing above the transverse plane, i.e., dorsiflexion, inversion, and slight adduction, the hallux goes through a triplane deformity and functions oppositely in a laterally inferior and everted relation to the long axis of the first metatarsal. Treatment should be directed to correcting the functional and structural positional deformities in addition to controlling the factors that led to the production of this abnormality. To accomplish this, one should first

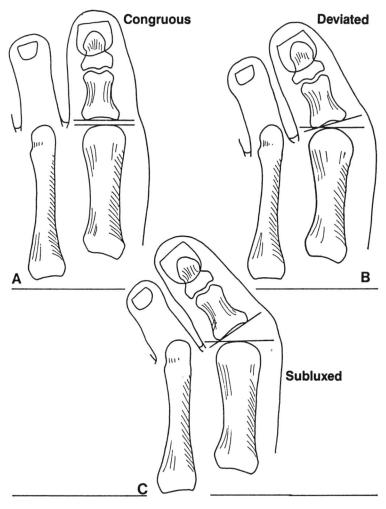

Figure 221

Joint surfaces are normally parallel or congruous (A). With the development of hallux-abducto-valgus, the joints will begin to deviate (B) and eventually sublux (C) in the more severe deformities.

institute mechanical (orthotic) control of the foot pathomechanics and achieve a functionally neutral foot to reduce the first ray hypermobility. Surgical correction should be contemplated when the deformity is significant enough to cause destructive jamming and erosion in the first metatarso–phalangeal joint. The goals of surgery are to: create a low intermetatarsal angle; create a low hallux abductus angle; and produce a reasonably congruous joint. The procedure(s) necessary to overcome this pathologic state must achieve the three goals as well as avoid any injury to the physeal areas. Operative procedures for correcting this abnormality are numerous and may include the structural

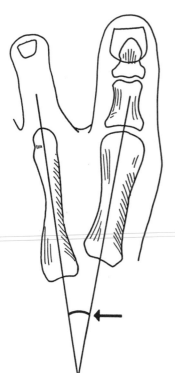

Figure 222

The metatarsus primus adductus angle is formed by a bisecting line through the first metatarsal and one through the second metatarsal shafts. The angle at the intersection of these two lines should be between 5–10° normally. Higher values are an indication of a metatarsus primus adductus deformity.

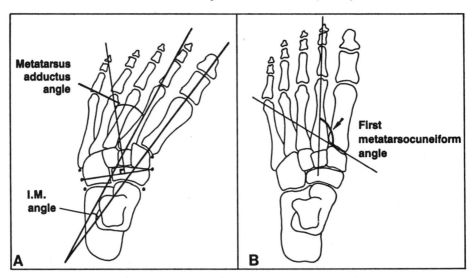

Figure 223

Feet presenting with a high degree of metatarsus adductus will have a reduced inter-metatarsal angle yet have a high degree of metatarsus primus adductus in relationship to the rearfoot (A). The metatarsocuneiform angle also plays a role in the degree of metatarsus primus adductus. This angle is formed by a line paralleling the articular cartilages of the first metatarsocuneiform joint and a line bisecting the second metatarsal shaft (B). Angles greater than 90–105° are considered significant in the contribution to a metatarsus primus adductus deformity.

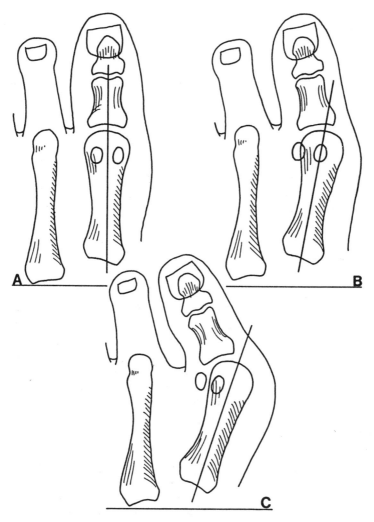

Figure 224

The tibial sesmoid position *helps in evaluating the amount of erosion of the sesmoidal grooves and the degree of medial deviation of the first metatarsal. Tibial sesmoid position lies medial to the bisection of the first metatarsal (A) while position 4 lies on the bisection line (B) and position 7 is in the fibular sesmoid area and lateral to the bisection. The higher the number the greater the metatarsus primus adductus and greater destruction of the sesmoidal grooves.*

corrective procedures of: a closing or opening base wedge or crescentic osteotomy of the first metatarsal to reduce the intermetatarsal angle (**Figure 225**); wedge osteotomy of the proximal phalanx to correct an abnormal distal articular set angle (**Figure 226**); and a medial closing wedge osteotomy of the first metatarsal head to correct the proximal articular set angle (**Figure 227**). Positional correction requires soft-tissue rebalancing and may include the McBride bunionectomy or modified McBride bunionectomy.

In children and adolescents there is little or no erosion or destruction of the articular cartilage. Additionally, the deformity is most often a tri-plane abnormality which therefore requires a tri-plane form of correction. The procedure most acceptable to accomplish this correction is a tri-plane osteotomy of the first metatarsal head (**Figure 228**). Various modifications may be necessary in the adolescent or early adult including ones to correct the proximal articular set angle utilizing a wedge removal (**Figure 227**), wedge osteotomy of the proximal phalanx to correct for an abnormal distal articular set angle as in **Figure 226**, and a shortening osteotomy of the first metatarsal to reduce the metatarsal protrusion (**Figure 229**). The tri-plane osteotomy in children will meet several desirable criteria including: increasing the dorsiflexion of the metatarso–phalangeal joint through plantarflexion of the metatarsal head along with the secondary shortening of the ray; decreasing the metatarsal adduction (intermetatarsal angle) by laterally shifting and displacing the head of the first metatarsal; and reversing the hallux abduction by removing a wedge of bone from the head. The beauty of this procedure is that it does not violate the physis of the metatarsal or the sesmoidal mechanism. Secondarily, it does not invade the first metatarso–phalangeal joint, which will avoid any loss of range of motion as well as avoiding any surgical damage to the cartilagenous surfaces. An adductor hallucis tendon release may be employed when indicated and an additional osteotomy of the proximal phalanx may be incorporated for any phalangeal abductus. The procedure is advantageous in young age groups due to abundant vascular supply and a thickened periosteum, which maximizes the healing potential.

In cases where a reasonably high degree of metatarsus primus adductus is existing, an alternate or adjunctive procedure may be considered. An epiphysidesis of the lateral aspect of the first metatarsal physis can reduce the degree of adductus (**Figure 230**). This must be performed at an appropriate age to achieve a proper correction. A reduction of approximately 4–6° may result if fusion of the lateral epiphysis is performed around 10–12 years in girls and 13–15 years in boys. This may vary with respect to the individual's development and family history. Several methods may be employed for the epiphysidesis including: stapling, a rotating trephine plug, and bone grafting. Stapling offers a possible advantage in that it may be removed if overcorrection occurs. This hopefully will allow the lateral epiphysis to catch up in growth before complete closure has occurred. The reader is referred to the article by Ellis, "A Method of Correcting Mertatarsus Primus Varus: Preliminary Report" for further discussion and information.[8] Other less desirable procedures have been considered; however, serious evaluation is warranted in timing the per-

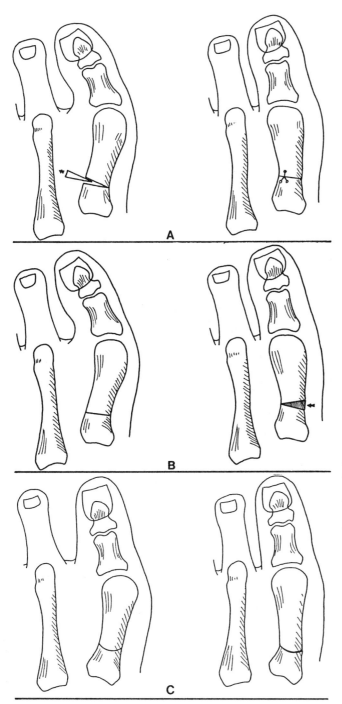

Figure 225

(*A*) *A* closing base wedge osteotomy *should be performed approximately 1 cm distal to the proximal articular surface unless the epiphysis is still open; then it must be distal to the epiphysis.* (*B*) Opening base wedge osteotomy *of the first metatarsal is also placed 1 cm distal to the articular surface. Bone used for the wedge can either come from a bone bank, calcaneus, tibia, or the least desirable, from the medial of the first metatarsal head.* (*C*) *The* crescentic osteotomy *is the least stable of the base osteotomies; however, it is advantageous in correcting any dorsal hypermobility when it is correctly fixated into a plantarflexed position.*

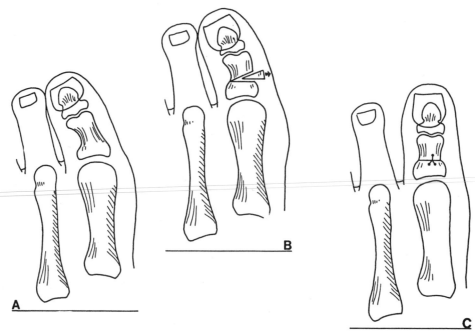

Figure 226

If a high distal articular set angle is present in the proximal phalanx of the hallux (A), a wedge osteotomy is necessary to correct this deformity (B)(C). This will align the flexor and extensor tendons properly over the first metatarsophalangeal joint.

formance of these procedure(s) and one must also consider their long-term results.

As an adjunct to these surgical corrections, the foot must be properly controlled after any corrective procedure is performed. This is to allow the proper maintenance of the correction and to avoid any secondary structural changes from first ray pathomechanics. Orthotic control is the best and only means of maintaining the desirable architectural position needed.[1,3,5,8,9,14,15,17,18,20,22,25,27]

Digital Deformities and Anomalies

Several aberrant forms of digital anatomy can be commonly found in children. Family history will often reveal similar anomalies. The persistence of these conditions or their spontaneous correction is best determined through the family history. It will also afford the examiner a better prognostic result as well as the decision for treatment.

Toe deformities may result from abnormal conditions elsewhere in the foot. An example of this would be the dislocated metatarso–phalangeal joint causing a hammer toe syndrome or an abnormal insertion(s) of the extensor or flexor tendons affecting the configuration of a toe. To properly assess these

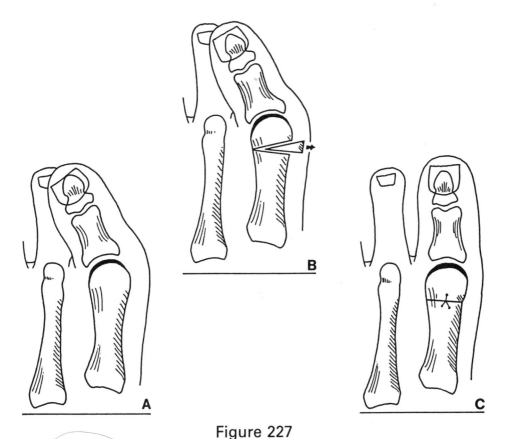

Figure 227

If a high proximal articular set angle exists (A), then a correction can be achieved by removing a medial wedge to align the articular cartilage (B)(C). The osteotomy must be proximal to the sesmoids to avoid degenerative changes to the sesmoid-metatarsal articulation.

conditions, a careful evaluation of the etiological factors with appropriate tailoring of the treatment to the causes is mandatory. Often a congenital toe deformity at birth may spontaneously correct when a child reaches the age of 4–6 years. If a family history relates similar anomalies with spontaneous correction, then nonaggressive treatment should be considered initially.

In the following sections, the more common toe deformities are reviewed, along with discussion of their etiology and appropriate course of treatment.

Clinodactyly (Congenital curly toes)

This condition is one of the most frequently experienced toe deformities in children. It usually affects the four lateral toes, especially the third, fourth, and fifth (**Figure 231**). In clinodactyly, the toe takes on an adducted (transverse

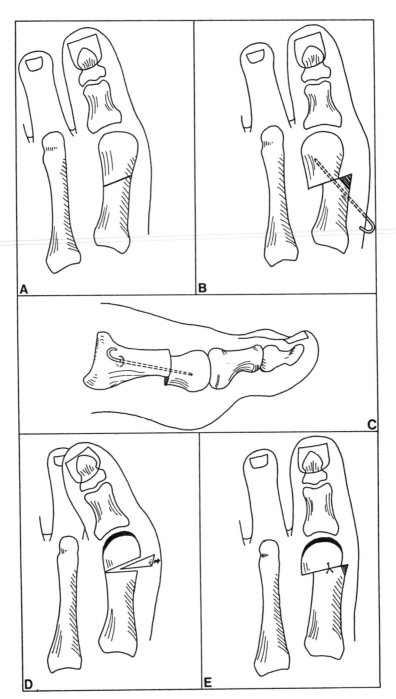

Figure 228

A tri-plane osteotomy of the first metatarsal will allow reduction in the intermetatarsal angle, dorsal hypermobility, and hallux abductus angle. An oblique cut offers the most surface area (A). In a shorter metatarsal, a transverse cut or an oblique cut in the opposite direction to (A) will reduce the degree of shortening. With this cut the head can be transpositionalized laterally as well as rotated and plantarflexed

296

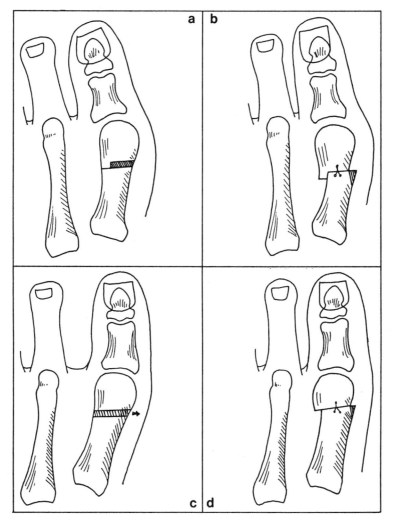

Figure 229

A shortening osteotomy of the first metatarsal with transpositional-ization can be accomplished by a step-down osteotomy (A)(B) using a lateral plug to stabilize the distal fragment. A complete removal of a section with a tri-plane correction (C)(D) may also be employed.

Figure 228 (Continued). (B)(C). Pin fixation is necessary to maintain the position properly. The prominent medial corner of the shaft of the metatarsal should be planed smooth and flush with the surface. This procedure can be performed totally extra-articular avoiding involvement of the joint. This should only be performed in cases where normal cartilage over the head of the first metatarsal exists and a congruous joint surface is present. If the articular surface is laterally deviated, then a wedge may be removed along with transpositionalizing, rotating, and plantarflexing the first metatarsal head (D)(E) to correct for the high proximal articular set angle.

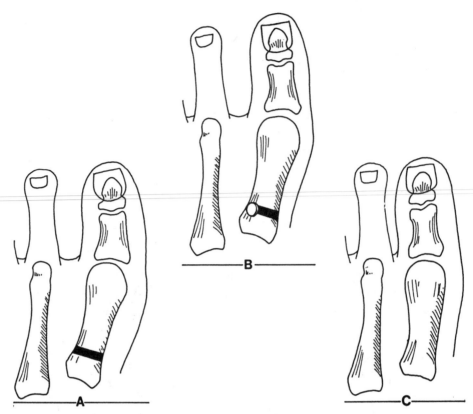

Figure 230

An epiphysidesis of the first metatarsal can be accomplished by either laterally stapling or fusing the epiphysis. The removal of a bone plug from the lateral epiphysis and rotating the trephined plug 90° or inserting a bone graft from the calcaneus or tibial will fuse this portion (A)(B)(C). The medial epiphysis will continue to grow allowing for closure of the intermetatarsal angle and reduction of the metatarsus primus adductus.

plane) and flexed (sagittal plane) attitude. Concomitant with the medial flexed rotation of the third toe may be the dorsal positioning of the second toe with contractures at the metatarso–phalangeal joint. This occurs secondary to the encroachment by the third toe on the space occupied by the second toe. When a child with a dorsally positioned second toe is brought by concerned parents, the examiner must look at the third, fourth, and fifth toes to determine their relative position and determine the probable cause for the second toe deformity.

Concerning the etiology of this condition, we know that the flexor tendon(s) is most often involved in the production of this curly toe syndrome. When rotation and flexion appear to exist only at the proximal interphalangeal joint, the long flexor tendon is either abnormally contracted or contracted and medially inserted. If the apex of the deformity appears to be at the distal interphalangeal joint, then the short flexor is the primary contributor to the

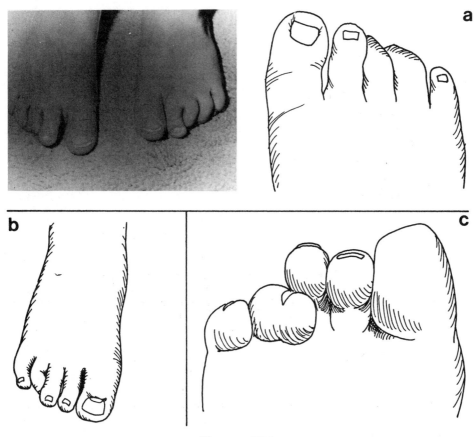

Figure 231

A congenital curly toe deformity may affect the third, fourth, and fifth toes (A). It may also only affect one of the lateral three toes as in (B)(C). The second toe will frequently be elevated secondary to the third toe crowding it out (A). Rarely is the second toe curled as found in the lateral three toes.

deformity. The second toe is usually not rotated but rather appears to be partially dislocated dorsally at the metatarso–phalangeal joint.

TREATMENT

Since spontaneous correction occurs in a vast majority of these conditions, any aggressive treatment should be left for the older child. The use of tape splinting may be moderately beneficial in the infant and very young child (**Figure 232**). When the deformity does not spontaneously correct when the child reaches 4–5 years of age, then a surgical correction should be contemplated. This author has found that by releasing the flexor tendons (long and short flexors) at the apex of the deformity along with a capsulotomy of the

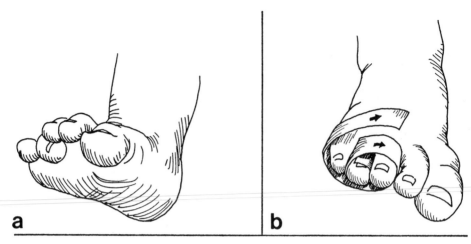

a   b

Figure 232

The use of a ¼" or ⅛" tape splint is beneficial in attempting to stretch the tightness found in a curly toe deformity. The tape splinting should be applied 24 hours a day until correction is achieved or further treatment indicated. Occasionally nonallergenic tape is necessary in children who react to the adhesive.

contracted joint, there will be a correction of the condition very nicely (**Figure 233**). This can be performed as an in-office procedure by anesthetizing the involved toes and possibly employing a mild form of sedation with the less cooperative child. Using either a no. 15 blade or no. 64 Beaver blade, a plantar or medial–lateral (or lateral–medial) approach is made using a stab incision. By manipulating the toe with the blade inserted, one is able to tenotomize the flexor tendons and release the plantar medial and lateral capsule. The dorsal capsule is left intact. Care must be taken to avoid damaging the neurovascular structure. Closure may be either one simple suture or a steri strip. The toes are held in a corrected position by a bandage splint for one week. At this time the skin is usually adequately healed to remove any sutures, when present, and the toes can be allowed into water. The parents are instructed to tape splint (**Figure 232**) for a period of 3–4 weeks. The soft-tissue release works very well in the flexible toe, which can be brought into a corrected position. If in the older child or adolescent the toe is very rigid, then an arthroplastic procedure is required for correction.[7,14,15]

Syndactyly (Web toes)

Frequently the practitioner will see varying degrees of webbing between the toes of young patients. The most common is between the second and third toes, and the next most common between the third and fourth toes (**Figure 234**). This condition is often familial and usually does not present with any adverse problem in function. Though soft-tissue webbing is most often expe-

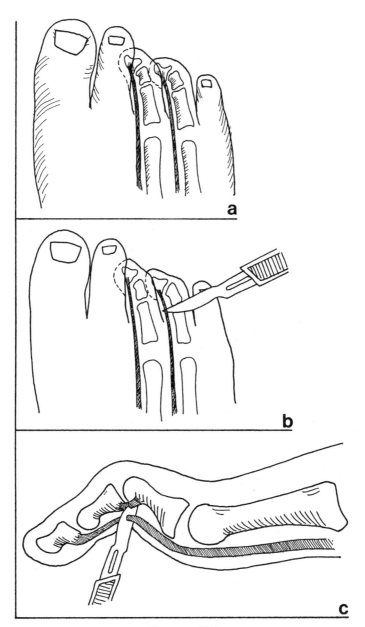

Figure 233

Surgical correction for flexible curly toes requires the release of the flexor tendons (long and short) and release of the capsule at the joint affected. A medial or medial-plantar approach offers the best position to release the dorsomedial, medial, and plantar capsule and the flexor tendons (A)(B)(C).

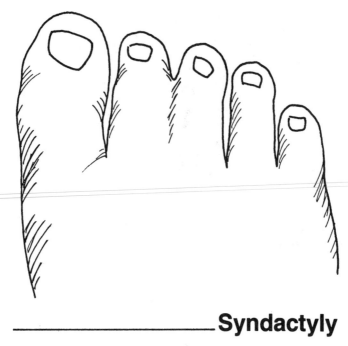

Syndactyly

Figure 234

rienced, an osseous bridging may present as well. Neither condition warrants any form of correction unless it begins to cause a problem or the patient wants it resolved for cosmetic and aesthetic reasons. *Treatment* is by desyndactylization using a variety of methods depending on the particular condition (**Figure 235**).[8]

Polydactyly (Supernumerary Toes)

Extra toes are not at all uncommon in children. The most frequent areas in which an extra toe may be found is at the medial aspect of the hallux and the lateral aspect of the fifth toe (**Figure 236**). Rarely is an accessory digit present among the middle three toes.

TREATMENT

Resolution of the problem is often necessary to allow adequate shoe fit and foot function. To remove a supernumerary toe, one must plan an approach surgically to allow the toe with the best position, function, and articulation with the metatarsal head to remain. It may be found that the extra toe is composed of only phalanges or that it may coexist with a partial or total metatarsal. It becomes extremely advantageous for the surgeon to wait until adequate growth in the bones has occurred to determine their position and

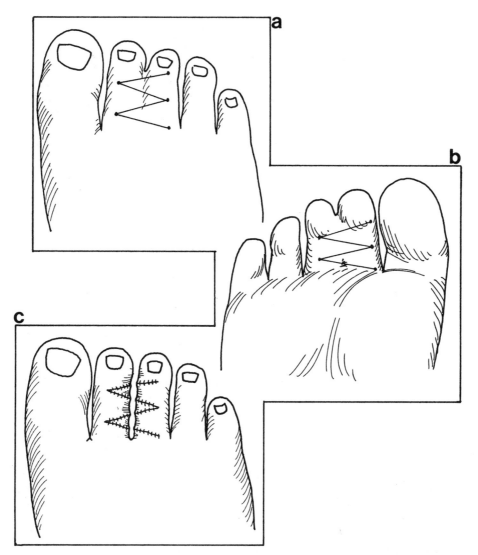

Figure 235

*Desyndactylization of web toes can be accomplished by using the W-flap approach
with the dorsal and plantar flaps opposite each other (A)(B). With the toes separated,
the flaps can be sewn in place covering the space created. There will be some exposed
area left which must epithelialize by second and third intention.*

availability for correction. After removal of an accessory toe that has extended
from a metatarsal head area (**Figure 237**), an awareness by the surgeon of
the potential for overgrowth of bone occurring later in the development of the
child or adolescent is necessary. This will usually arise from the epiphyseal
area and may require further surgical reduction. This possible complication

Polydactyly

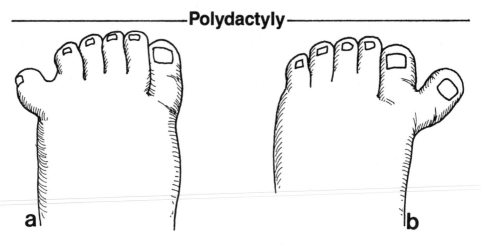

Figure 236

should be discussed with the parents at the time of surgical removal of the toe to avoid future problems.[3,10,11,14-16]

Congenital Overlapping 5th Toe (Digiti Minimi Varus)

A common condition found in infants and children as well as in adults, this familial deformity has the components of a dorsally displaced fifth toe with contracture at the metatarso–phalangeal and interphalangeal joints (**Figure 238**). The fifth metatarso–phalangeal joint is partially dislocated dorsally with contractures being noted at the extensor tendon, dorsal capsule, and dorsal

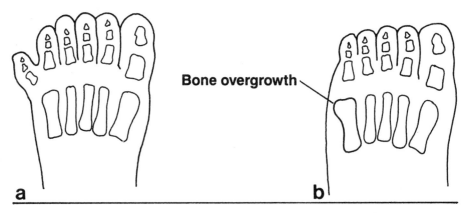

Bone overgrowth

Figure 237

Removal of an accessory toe that may be arising from or near an epiphysis may result in an overgrowth of bone at the site later in the development of the child (A)(B). This must be anticipated and prepared for by the surgeon, patient, and parents.

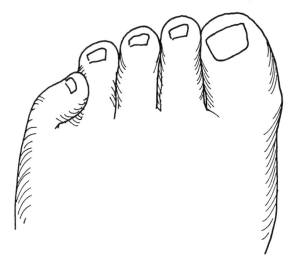

Congenital overlapping 5th toe   Figure 238

skin. Secondarily, the flexor tendons are producing flexure of the interphalangeal toe joints as a result of their mechanical advantage. Concomitant with this dorsal positioning may be a rotation in the fifth toe toward the fourth toe. This is a result of the medial pull of the flexor tendons on the toe.

Treatment is directed toward relocating the toe by: surgically releasing the skin by using a V–Y skin plasty; a lengthening tenotomy of the extensor digitorum longus tendon; a capsulotomy of the dorsal, medial, and lateral capsule of the fifth metatarsophalangeal joint; and either performing a flexor release and capsulotomy of the interphalangeal joints in a flexible toe or an arthroplastic procedure of the interphalangeal joint in the more rigid toe to allow for proper alignment (**Figure 239**).[1,7,15,17]

Hammer Toes, Mallet Toes, Claw Toes

These three toe deformities will be discussed together although each has its own characteristic abnormality. A *hammer toe* is characterized by a plantar flexion contracture of the proximal interphalangeal joint and dorsiflexion contracture at the metatarso–phalangeal joint (**Figure 240A**). A *mallet toe* has a plantar flexion contracture of the distal interphalangeal joint (**Figure 240B**), while a *claw toe* has plantar flexion contractures at both the proximal and distal interphalangeal joints, with dorsiflexion at the metatarsophalangeal joint (**Figure 240C**).

Etiologically, there may be an imbalance in the intrinsic musculature of the toes causing an abnormal movement with a resulting malposition of the toe. Not to be discounted is the long toe syndrome, which is affected by shoe pressure. Wearing short or tight shoes and/or tight stockings will produce a

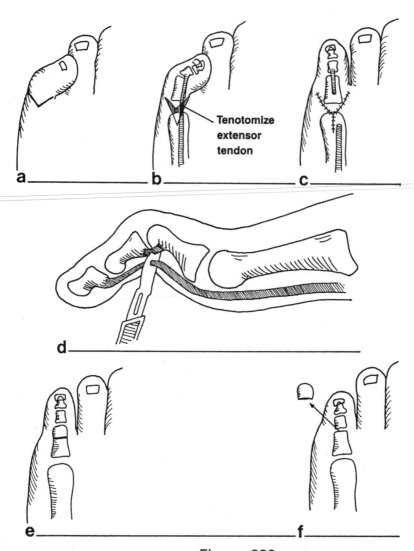

Figure 239

A congenitally overlapping fifth toe needs to be corrected by a V–Y skin-plasty performed at the fifth metatarsophalangeal joint (A), tenotomy of the extensor digitorum longus tendon with complete capsulotomy of the metatarsophalangeal joint (B), and suturing the toe in a corrected position with the skin lengthened (C). A flexor release of the interphalangeal joint is also performed to achieve a straight alignment of the toe (D). An arthroplastic procedure may be necessary in the rigid toe deformity. This requires a removal of a portion of the proximal phalangeal head (E)(F). The V–Y skin-plasty and metatarsophalangeal joint release are still necessary with the arthroplastic procedure to achieve a proper position of the toe.

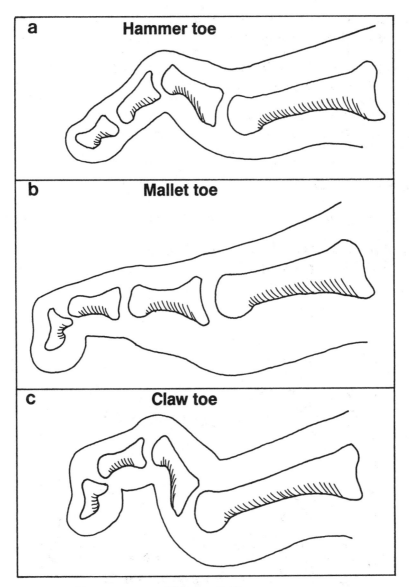

Figure 240

retrograde force on the toes, leading to a deformity. High arched (cavus) feet very often will have the coexistence of claw toes secondary to the metatarsal declination. This allows an imbalance to occur in the extensor and flexor pull resulting in the toe deformation.

Treatment should be directed toward rebalancing any imbalance in the musculature. Discouraging the use of short shoes or socks is also important. When correcting any muscular imbalance conditions, a careful look at the total foot structure is necessary. The determination of the presence of a cavus foot or flatfoot deformity will help to evaluate the causes and the areas for correction. These foot conditions must be appropriately treated simultaneously with the toe correction if treatment is to be maintained adequately. Surgical correction of a flexible toe deformity may be easily performed by releasing the flexor and/or extensor contractures (**Figure 241**). The more rigid toe deformity will require an arthroplastic procedure with fusion of the interphalangeal joints, when indicated, to allow proper balance of the flexor and extensor tendon function.[7,12,14,15]

Hallux Interphalangeus

The section *Juvenile Hallux Valgus* described a condition in which the distal articular set angle was affected by the amount of curvature in the proximal phalanx of the hallux (**Figure 242A**). Not only can this exist in the proximal phalanx but may also occur in the distal phalanx of the hallux

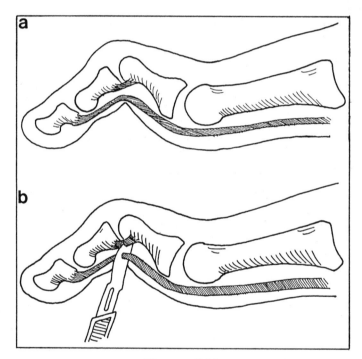

Figure 241

A flexor release of the long and short flexor tendons along with the plantar interphalangeal capsule (A)(B) is useful in correcting the flexible hammer toe in a young person. It may be necessary to release the extensor tendons to the toe at the metatarsophalangeal joint for proper correction.

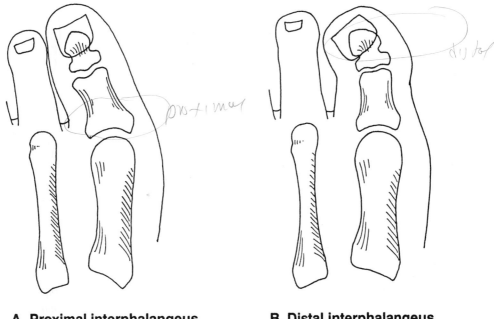

A. Proximal interphalangeus   **B. Distal interphalangeus**

Figure 242

(**Figure 242B**). When an abnormal degree of lateral curvature occurs it is referred to as *hallux interphalangeus*. The etiology for this lateral growth, with an abduction deformity in the hallux, is the result of an abnormal amount of shoe pressure in the presence of a reasonably stable first metatarso–phalangeal joint. With excessive medial pressure being exerted on the epiphysis of the distal and to a lesser degree the proximal phalanx, a stimulation in growth as a response to the tension will occur. This commonly follows the principles of Wolf's law. The increase in medial growth will result in a disproportionate configuration in the bone structure causing the medial surface to be longer than the lateral surface. The examiner is cautioned to carefully evaluate for this condition in a child presenting with an apparent hallux valgus problem. The first metatarso–phalangeal joint in this condition will be very normal in architecture while the interphalangeus of the hallux is the actual cause for the abducted hallux appearance. There may also exist a combination of both conditions, (i.e., hallux interphalangeus and hallux valgus). *Treatment* should only be considered when the condition is abducted sufficiently to cause pressure on the second toe or may be causing a problem with daily comfort. In the absence of any first metatarso–phalangeal joint deformity, an adductory wedge osteotomy of the proximal phalanx may be performed to correct the condition (**Figure 243**).

    This procedure should only be performed after complete epiphyseal closure to ensure proper correction along with the avoidance of any damage to the

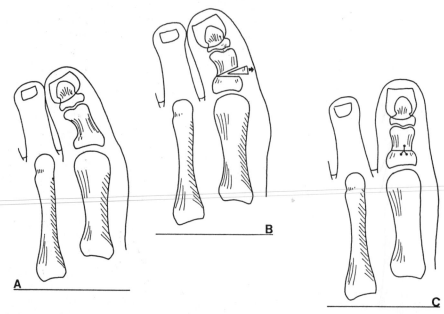

Figure 243

If a high distal articular set angle is present in the proximal phalanx of the hallux
(A), a wedge osteotomy is necessary to correct this deformity (B)(C). This will align
the flexor and extensor tendons properly over the first metatarsophalangeal joint.

epiphyseal growth of the proximal phalanx. A medial epiphyseal arrest may
be performed at an appropriate age to allow for correction when possible.[2,15]

Hallux Varus (hallux adductus)

This adduction deformity found in a hallux is often the result of an aberrant insertion of the abductor hallucis muscle tendon located primarily at the
medial aspect of the hallux (**Figure 244**). Approximately 20% of the population
will present with a functioning abductor hallucis muscle truly acting as an
abductor. The remaining 80% of the populace functions with the abductor
hallucis muscle as a plantarflexor with a slight degree of abduction at the
hallux (**Figure 245**). When the insertion occurs more medially, an adductus
(varus) deformity may occur as the muscle fibers contract. Small infants and
young children may exhibit a hallux adductus condition prior to their beginning ambulation. The clinical appearance observed by the examiner can be
easily mistaken for a metatarsus adductus deformity. Although there may
exist concomitantly a hallux varus and a metatarsus adductus condition, the
two should be separately distinguished by the use of both clinical and radiographic evaluation. Previously mentioned under the section on *Metatarsus
Adductus,* the abductor hallucis muscle may insert at the medial aspect of the

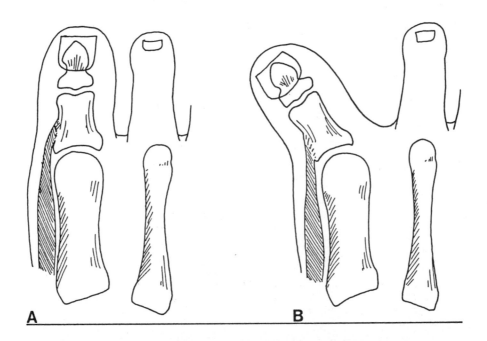

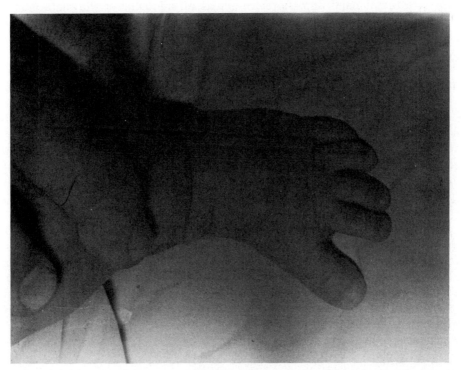

Figure 244

The abductor hallucis muscle is often the cause for a hallux varus deformity due to a medial insertion rather than a medial-plantar insertion (A)(B). This occurs in approximately 20% of the population, causing an adduction deformity.

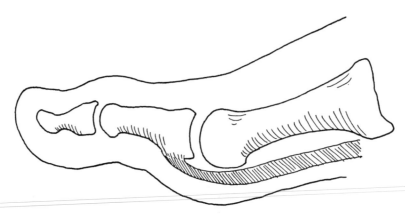

Figure 245

The majority of the population (80%) has a medial-plantar or plantar insertion of the abductor hallucis tendon causing primarily plantarflexion rather than adduction of the hallux.

first metatarsal head and therefore act as an adductor of the metatarsals. However, if the insertion occurs more distal into the base of the proximal phalanx, then a hallux adductus (varus) deformity may arise. A weakening of the adductor hallucis muscle may also provide a mechanical advantage for this condition. It is this author's feelings that the abnormal contractions of this muscle, which eventually results in a contracture, is the end product of a mild form of muscular spasticity. The cause may be a pre, peri, or postnatal injury, or an abnormal innervation of the muscle. Clinical examination will frequently allow one to distinguish the tautness in the abductor muscle by abducting the hallux and palpating along the muscular course. A bulge present along the medial aspect of the foot with palpable medial tendon fibers along its course and its insertion, is a reasonable indication of a contracture. Muscle stimulation, using an electrical stimulator, will also help to distinguish this abnormality.

Treatment is primarily directed toward stretching the muscle and any of the secondary contractures which may have resulted from the continued presence of the adduction deformity. Manipulating the hallux into abduction for approximately 10 minutes, followed by a below-the-knee or foot–ankle cast is effective in correcting this deformity. Tape splinting can be used if the parents and the child are cooperative (**Figure 246**). The casts should be changed weekly with remanipulation prior to reapplication. Once a corrected attitude is reached, which is dependent on the age of the child, a straight last shoe should be fitted for maintenance of the correction. Make certain that the shoe fits tightly enough across the width to hold the hallux in a rectus attitude. The shoes should be worn for approximately 6 months to 1½ years with reevaluation every 4–6 months to determine the progress. In milder cases, straight last shoes may be the only necessary treatment. This method does not produce an effective result in the smaller infant due to the limitation in size and fit of the shoes.

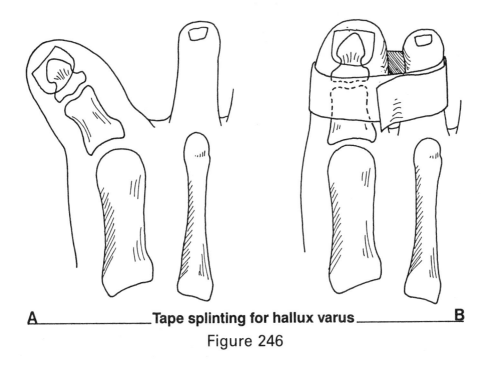

A _____ **Tape splinting for hallux varus** _____ **B**

Figure 246

Therefore, children prior to walking will correct faster and more effectively if treated by stretch castings or tape splinting.

Certainly there will be cases in which correction cannot be maintained. Reoccurrences may present several months after an appropriate correction has been achieved. These instances may require a release of the fibers of the abductor hallucis tendon to avoid continued involvement. This is accomplished by a pericutaneous release performed at the first metatarso–phalangeal joint (**Figure 247**). A stab incision using a small blade such as no. 15 or no. 64 Beaver blade is inserted at the dorsal medal aspect of the first metatarso–phalangeal joint. Subcutaneously, the blade is passed plantarward and the fibers of the abductor tendon incised. If the correction is adequate, no further releasing is necessary. Occasionally however, there may be needed additional releasing at the medial capsule of the first metatarso–phalangeal joint to achieve a more normal rectus position. Once the releasing is completed, a closure with steri strips or one simple suture is all that is required. The hallux is then bandaged in an abducted position. When necessary, a cast is applied to protect the correction. The maintenance of this position is required for approximately 3–5 weeks. The cast and/or dressings are only necessary for maintenance of position for a period of two weeks. This should then be followed by a tape splint for the remaining period (**Figure 246**). Once the cast and/or dressings are removed, the child is allowed to bathe as long as the toe is properly positioned with a splint during any activities. Straight last shoes are recommended for follow-up. To be avoided are the abductory type shoes which will

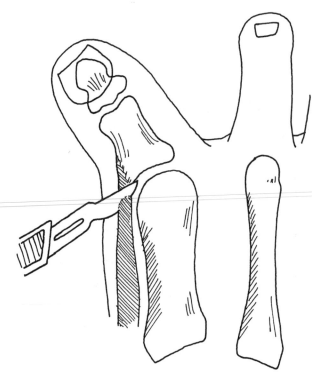

Pericutaneous abductor hallucis tendon release
Figure 247

exert a considerable degree of stress toward the rear and midfoot. The potential result from this type of shoe may be a pes planus deformity and/or a hallux–abducto–valgus abnormality.[4,6,9,14,15]

References

Hallux Valgus:
1. Auerbach, A.M.: Review of distal metatarsal osteotomies for hallux valgus in the young. *Clinical Orthopedics,* Number 70, May–June 1970.
2. Cralley, J.C., McGonagle, W., Fitch, K.: The role of adduction hallucis in bunion deformity. *J.A.P.A.,* 68:Number 7, July 1978.
3. Curda, G.A., Sorto, L.A.: The McBride bunionectomy with closing abductory wedge osteotomy. *J.A.P.A.,* 71:Number 7, July 1981.
4. D'Amico, J.C., Schuster, R.O.: Motion of the first ray. *J.A.P.A.,* 69:Number 1, January 1978.
5. Dintcho, A.: Procedures to correct hallux abducto valgus and metatarsus primus adductus. *Journal of Foot Surgery,* 15:Number 1, 1976.
6. Duke, H., Newman, L.M., Bruskoff, B.L., Daniels, R.: Hallux abductus interphal-

angeus and its relationship to hallux abducto valgus. *J.A.P.A.,* 72:Number 1, January 1982.

7. Duke, H., Newman, L.M., Bruskoff, B.L., Daniels, R.: Relative metatarsal length patterns in hallux abducto valgus. *J.A.P.A.,* 72:Number 1, January 1982.
8. Ellis, V.H.: A method of correcting metatarsus primus varus: Preliminary report. *Journal of Bone and Joint Surgery,* 33-B:1951.
9. Fenton, C.F., McGlamry, E.D.: Reverse buckling to reduce metatarsus primus varus. *J.A.P.A.,* 72:Number 7, July 1982.
10. Greenberg, G.S.: Relationship of hallux abductus angle and first metatarsal angle to severity of pronation. *J.A.P.A.,* 69:Number 1, January 1979.
11. Grode, S.E., McCarthy, D.J.: The anatomical implications of hallux abducto valgus. *J.A.P.A.,* 70:Number 11, November 1980.
12. Hardy, R.H., Clapman, J.C.R.: Observations of hallux valgus. *Journal of Bone and Joint Surgery,* 33-B:1951.
13. Helal, B.: Surgery for adolescent hallux valgus. *Clinical Orthopedics,* Number 157, 1981.
14. Holstein, A.: Hallux valgus: An acquired deformity of the foot in cerebral palsy. *Foot and Ankle,* 1:1980.
15. Houghton, G.R., Dickson, R.A.: Hallux valgus in the younger patient: The structural abnormality. *Journal of Bone and Joint Surgery,* 61-B:1979.
16. Johnson, K.A.: Chevron osteotomy of the first metatarsal: Patient selection and technique. *Contemporary Orthopedics,* 3:1981.
17. McBride, E.D.: Hallux valgus, bunion deformity: Its treatment in mild, moderate and severe stages. *J. Int. Col. Surg.,* 21:1954.
18. McCrea, J.D., Lichty, T.K.: The first metatarsocuneiform articulation and its relationship to metatarsus primus adductus. *J.A.P.A.,* 69:Number 12, December 1979.
19. McGlamey, E.D.: Reverdin modification of the McBride technique for correction of hallux valgus. *Journal of Foot Surgery,* 14:Number 1, 1975.
20. McNeiney, J.E., Johnston, B.: Generalized ligamentous laxity, hallux abducto valgus, and the first metatarsocuneiform joint. *J.A.P.A.,* 69:Number 1, January 1979.
21. Mitchell, C.L., Fleming, J.L., Allen, R., Glenney, C., Sanford, G.A.: Osteotomy–bunionectomy for hallux valgus. *Journal of Bone and Joint Surgery,* 40-A:January 1958.
22. Piggott, H.: The natural history of hallux valgus in adolescence and early adult life. *Journal of Bone and Joint Surgery,* 42-B:1960.
23. Schuberth, J.M., Cralley, J.C., Wingfield, E.J.: Extensor hallucis tendons of normal and hallux abducto valgus feet. *J.A.P.A.,* 72:Number 3, March 1982.
24. Silberman, F.S.: Proximal phalangeal osteotomy for the correction of hallux valgus. *Clinical Orthopedics,* Number 85, June 1972.
25. Simmonds, F.A., Menelaus, M.B.: Hallux valgus in adolescents. *Journal of Bone and Joint Surgery,* 42-B:1960.
26. Winston, L., Wilson, R.C.: A modification of the Hohmann procedure for surgical correction of hallux abducto valgus. *J.A.P.A.,* 72:Number 1, January 1982.

Digital Deformities and Anomalies:

1. Cockin, J.: Butler's operation for an over-riding fifth toe. *Journal of Bone and Joint Surgery,* 50-B:February 1968.
2. Duke, H., Newman, L.M., Bruskoff, B.L., Daniels, R.: Hallux abductus interphalangeus and its relationship to hallux abductus valgus. *J.A.P.A.,* 72:Number 12, December 1982.
3. Gastwirth, B., Mauro, G., Karrat, I.O.: Congenital polydactyly with polymetatarsia in a ten-month old child. *J.A.P.A.,* 70:Number 10, October 1980.
4. Hawkins, F.B.: Acquired hallux varus: Cause, prevention and correction. *Clinical Orthopedics,* Number 76, May 1971.

5. Jamecki, C.J., Wildle, A.H.: Results of phalangectomy of the fifth toe for hammertoe. *Journal of Bone and Joint Surgery,* 58-A:October 1976.
6. Jones, R.A., McCrea, J.: Tenotomy of the abductior hallucis for correction of resistant metatarsus adductus. *J.A.P.A.,* 70:Number 1, January 1980.
7. Jordan, R.P., Caselli, M.A.: Overlapping deformity of the digits in the pediatric patient. *J.A.P.A.,* 68:Number 7, July 1978.
8. Ketai, N.H., Ketai, R.S., Tilles, S.J., Sherman, A.M.: A simple, complete, single syndactyly: A case report. *Journal of Foot Surgery,* 15:Number 1, 1976.
9. Miller, J.W.: Acquired hallux varus: A preventable and correctable disorder. *Journal of Bone and Joint Surgery,* 57-A:March 1975.
10. Ogden, J.A.: An unusual case of polydactylisn. *Clinical Orthopedics,* Number 84, May 1972.
11. Perdicie, R.L., Mason, W.H., Bernard, T.N.:Macrodactyly: A rare malformation. *J.A.P.A.,* 69:Number 11, November 1979.
12. Sgarlato, T.E.: A compendium of podiatric biomechanics. *California College of Podiatric Medicine,* San Francisco, CA, 1971.
13. Shaw, A.H.: Pseudohypoparathyroidism. A review of the syndrome with particular reference to pedal symptomatology. *Archives of Pod. Med. and Foot Surgery,* 1:Number 2, October 1973.
14. Tachdjian, M.O.: *Pediatric Orthopedics.* W.B. Saunders Co., Philadelphia, PA, 1972.
15. Tax, H.R.: *Podopediatrics.* Williams and Wilkins, Baltimore, MD, 1980.
16. Tozzi, M.A., Penny, H.L.: Post axial polydactyly with polymetatarsia. *J.A.P.A.,* 71:Number 7, July 1981.
17. Wilson, J.N.: V–Y correction for varus deformity of the fifth toe. *British Journal of Surgery,* 41:1953.

Chapter 13

ORTHOTIC CONTROL IN CHILDREN

*T*hroughout the preceding chapters, the reader was informed of many structural and functional disorders that may affect a child. Whether the disorder existed in the hip, femur, knee, tibia–fibula, ankle, or foot, often some form of control is required in the foot biomechanics. It was realized throughout the discussions of these various lower extremity disorders that the foot was either directly or indirectly affected, therefore necessitating some form of control.

A child with an in-toeing or out-toeing condition, as an example, will often compensate for these deformities by pronating his feet. Equally frequent is the flatfoot condition secondary to muscular or ligamentous abnormalities. Whatever the particular etiology, the outcome is still the need for some form of control of the foot structure.

The feet of children are very malleable and moldable to their environment. Conditions that forcibly cause the foot to assume a position other than that of a normal "neutral" position will eventually produce adaptations and eventual complications. The goal of the foot specialist is not only to attempt to alleviate any structural disorders that will lead to abnormal compensations in the foot, but also to protect the foot during the period of time in which other forms of treatment are being instituted. In those cases where the deformity is within the structural confines of the foot–ankle, corrective orthotic control is certainly necessary and mandatory. It behooves the practitioner to be cognizant of not only the flatfoot or high arched foot conditions which are commonly controlled by an orthosis but also the rotational, muscular, and functional abnormalities of the superstructures from which the foot must be protected.

Modern orthotic therapy involves many types and forms of devices. The materials in which these are being fabricated vary from the rigid (fiberglass and rohadur) to the very flexible (plastizote, rubber, sponge). In between are materials that have greater flexibility than fiberglass and rohadur but more rigidity than plastizote and rubber (i.e., polypropylenes and cork and leather). The types of orthoses being commonly used for children include: Whitman plate; Roberts' plate; Whitman–Roberts' plate; Shaffer plate; heel stabilizers types A,B,C,D, and E; out-toeing gait plate (Reverse Roberts' plate); and functional posted orthoses.[3,4,5,9,10,12]

317

The function and effect of each of these types of orthoses will be discussed; we must first realize that a child's foot does not function like an adult's foot (see Chapter 5). Biomechanically, the foot is changing rapidly with growth and development. It becomes difficult to apply static adult biomechanics to a dynamically changing foot. The child additionally has greater soft-tissue mass (i.e., fat, cartilage) in the foot than an adult and greater motion in the joint structures. Equally important is the fact that children need to be controlled and protected until they reach full bone maturity. At this point it may be possible to discontinue orthotic treatment temporarily if normal structural integrity is assumed. This will allow one to observe if the foot will maintain itself structurally and function comfortably. Using careful follow-up with x-ray evaluation and biomechanical determinations, the examiner will be able to decide whether a need for reinstitution of orthotic therapy is necessary.[2,4,5,9,12]

The adaptable foot of a child should be allowed to develop into a normal position whenever possible. The foot specialist must always be aware of any abnormalities lending itself to the production of compensation in the foot. Care in maintainence of a normal foot architecture is mandatory. Different than a child's, an adult foot has achieved a matured attitude and position. Adaptation and changes may still occur with time in the adult, but there is no chance for stimulation of the structures to reassume a normal neutral position. This can only be anticipated in a developing foot of a child.

Furthermore, if superstructural problems or abnormal foot structural conditions persist into adulthood, then it will be necessary to continue orthotic control to prevent any secondary changes in the foot. Do not allow a patient to undermine or alter the practitioner's intentions and convictions for the course of treatment just for cosmetic reasons or through their noncompliance. This will only lead to them losing confidence in the effect of the therapy and in the abilities of the practitioner.

Whitman Plate

The Whitman plate was developed by Royal Whitman, an orthopedic physician, in the early 1900s. The principle on which this device works is to consciously remind the wearer, through painful pressure on the medial aspect of the foot, to supinate the foot (**Figure 248C**). The intended net result would be strengthening of the medial musculature of the foot, thus stabilizing the joint structures. In theory the principle was somewhat sound but in practice it was difficult to implement. The wearer constantly felt such a considerable degree of pain that the medial flange of the device was eventually modified to a more Shaffer plate type so that less pressure was being exerted on the medial arch structure. The small lateral flange is not to allow the heel to slip laterally, thus keeping the calcaneus vertical to the ground.

The use of this type of orthosis, with its present modification for a pronated or compensatorily pronated foot, is advantageous in the child older than 8–10

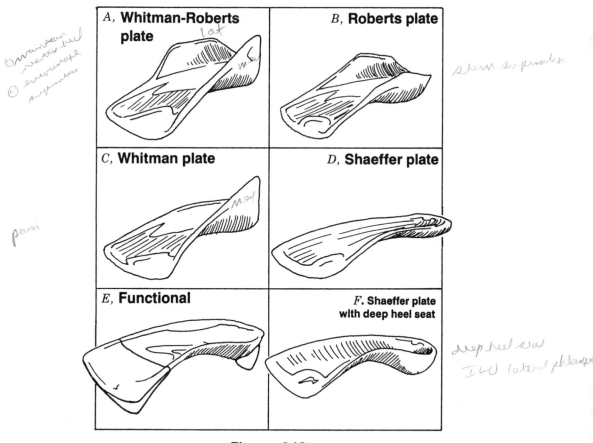

Figure 248

years of age. The younger child exhibits too much flexibility and soft-tissue mass to be adequately controlled with this form of an orthosis.

Roberts' Plate

The Roberts' plate, developed by Dr. Percy Roberts, is based on a different principle of control from the Whitman plate. The theory behind this device is that the calcaneus can be controlled by maintaining it in a vertical or varus position with the ground, and parallel with the lower leg (**Figure 248B**). It does not support the arch area of the foot as well, nor does it control any forefoot position. The eventual outcome from its use is to again strengthen the medial musculature of the foot by encouraging supination. With the biomechanical understanding we have today of the foot, this device does not prove to be useful in most instances since not only does the musculature play a role in the attitude of the foot but so does the amount of ligamentous looseness and bony structural position.

Whitman–Roberts' Plate

This type of orthosis was eventually developed to employ both principles of control, i.e., to maintain a rectus heel and to stimulate supination with adequate support in the arch area. This device employs a reasonably high medial flange to limit medial motion of the talus as well as a lateral flange to limit lateral movement of the heel. When taking an impression of a child's foot for this type of device, a neutral rectus position should be employed. This positioning places the rearfoot in neutral position (talus neither maximally supinated nor pronated) and the midtarsal joints loaded to maximum pronation. If there exists any varusing or valgusing of the metatarsals, it should be corrected in the casting to achieve a parallel rearfoot to forefoot relationship (see casting technique). If this method is followed carefully, the resulting orthosis will be able to maintain the rearfoot in neutral position and allow the forefoot to achieve a balanced rectus position.

The Whitman–Roberts' plate is useful in the child above the age of 8 or 9 years. It may become too confining in the adolescent patient who is very active in sports. Its use is effective to control pronation problems secondary to superstructural conditions or abnormalities primarily inherent in the foot (**Figure 248A**).

Shaffer Plate

This type of plate is commonly referred to as an "arch support." Though it does contribute to the support of the arch, it will also maintain the heel position when a heel post is incorporated into the device. It is possible to maintain the forefoot alignment if the impression casting of the foot is placed into rectus (**Figure 248D**). The device has a medial flange that supports the foot well without causing pain, as is found in the true Whitman plate. It does not, however, have a lateral flange to maintain lateral heel slippage. A deep heel seat will help to avoid this slippage in the milder forms of pronation (**Figure 248F**).

The Shaffer plate should be employed in the older child or adolescent who exhibits a mild degree of structural collapse in the foot. If a reasonable degree of eversion of the calcaneus and pronation in the foot exist, then a more confining orthotic device is recommended such as the Whitman–Roberts' plate or an appropriate heel stabilizer.

The impression casting can be taken either in semiweight-bearing or nonweight-bearing depending on what the forefoot structure exhibits. If a reasonable degree of forefoot varus or valgus exists, then a rectus nonweight-bearing impression is better utilized. If a rectus forefoot is present, then a semiweight-bearing impression is acceptable along with a neutral rearfoot position.

Heel Stabilizers

Five types of heel stabilizers are currently in use: types A,B,C,D, and E (**Figure 249**). The construction is either of fiberglass or rohadur. This author has found that fiberglass is more acceptable due to less bulk in the shoe. Children as well as adults may benefit by these types of orthoses, depending on their activities and age. Children will usually tolerate heel stabilizers until approximately 8–10 years of age. At this point their weight, structural development, shoe types, and activities will have changed. The child who is very active in sports may be uncomfortable using the confining heel stabilizer. It therefore becomes necessary to change to an orthosis, which will control as well as afford the availability of greater ranges of motion in these children.

Adults may also benefit by heel stabilizers if their feet have adequate flexibility to allow for rigid control. Unfortunately, the medial and lateral aspects of these devices extend to just below the malleoli and therefore limit the type of shoe that will contain them. They also are reasonably hard on socks due to the talus attempting pronation while being limited by the medial flange. The result is a wearing of the stocking material at the impact point of the talar head and the orthosis. One will also note a callus formation over the medial head of the talus due to the restrictive control. With the exception of these shortcomings, the heel stabilizer actually controls the foot better than any other form of orthotic device.

Type A Heel Stabilizer

A type A heel stabilizer primarily functions as a control of the calcaneal position. The construction of the device limits inversion or eversion of the calcaneus by confining the heel rigidly (**Figure 249A**). It has minimal support in the arch area of the foot and no control over the forefoot positioning. Its use is limited to a narrow spectrum of patients exhibiting only calcaneal eversion with little or no midtarsal or forefoot alterations or changes. Realizing that this type of patient is reasonably rare, the use of this type of stabilizer will be infrequent.

Type B Heel Stabilizer

This stabilizer employs two forms of control: maintenance of proper heel position and support and control of the mid and forefoot (**Figure 249B**). It extends distally to just behind the metatarsal heads to establish a balanced forefoot. Medially the supporting flange extends past the talo-navicular joint

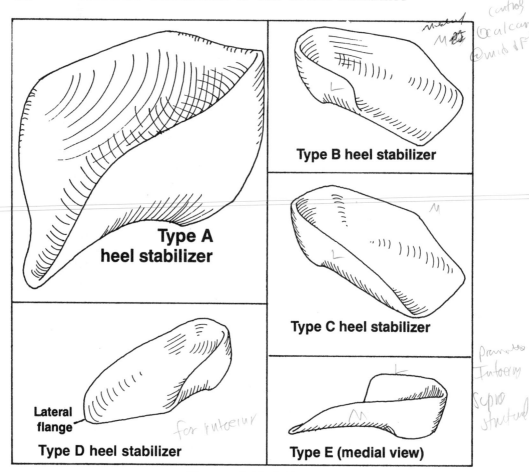

Figure 249 A-E

limiting subtalar pronation while the lateral flange is reducing lateral movement of the calcaneus.

The use of a type B heel stabilizer in the mild to moderately pronated foot or as a maintenance therapy for superstructural abnormalities is beneficial. It should not be used in the moderately severe or severe flatfoot condition or in certain rotational abnormalities (i.e., overpowering tibialis anterior and tibialis posterior, internal genicular position, etc.) This type will also work reasonably well in the adult foot. Compliance must be assured to the practitioner before dispensing this type of orthosis to an adult patient. The foot should be casted in a neutral rectus position to establish the best and most desirable attitude. This can only be accomplished by a nonweight-bearing impression technique. It is also mandatory to place the plaster sufficiently high on the sides of the foot to capture the complete impression of the calcaneus and the talonavicular joint.

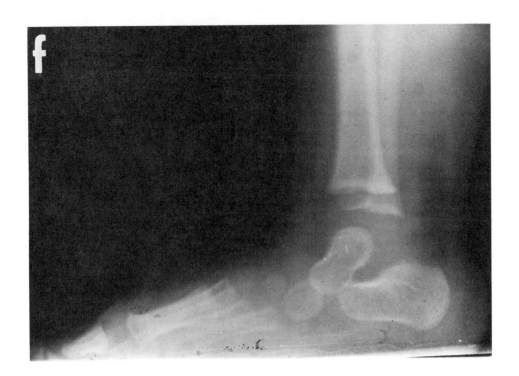

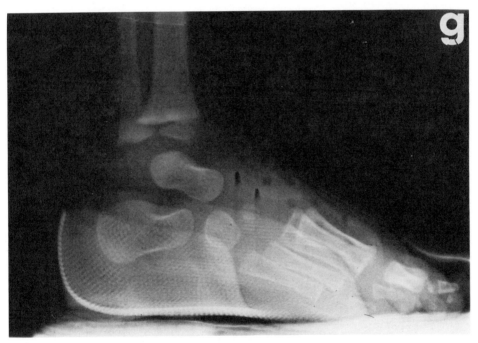

Figure 249 F–G

F) Juvenile flatfoot
G) Same child as F with foot aligned in an orthotic in a shoe

323

Type C Heel Stabilizer

Feet which exhibit a reasonable degree of laxity and splaying benefit greatly by the type C heel stabilizer (**Figure 249C**). The construction of this device is different than the type B in that the medial flange area extends along the entire medial surface of the foot up to the first metatarso–phalangeal joint. The lateral flange extends to just behind the fifth metatarsophalangeal joint as well. The confinement of this type heel stabilizer allows: rigid control of the rearfoot; proper support of the entire midfoot; limitation of medial–lateral splaying of the metatarsals; and proper forefoot positioning in relationship to the rear and midfoot. Its use is for the ligamentous lax foot which most frequently is the type of flatfoot encountered in children. This author would encourage its use initially in early childhood where a need for some form of orthotic treatment is necessary regardless of the degree of laxity. The reason for this advice is that the developing foot can use good support to encourage proper architectural development. It will be beneficial in these children until they have reached an age when a lesser confining orthosis is required. The impression casting for this type of orthosis is in a nonweight-bearing neutral rectus position.

Type D Heel Stabilizer

Children who present with various forms of in-toeing may benefit from this type of an orthosis. Its function is to stimulate an out-toeing gait pattern by altering the mechanics of the foot. *Note:* It does not correct any of the many causes for in-toeing; however, the D type stabilizer will help to change and stretch the mechanical pull of the tibialis anterior and posterior.

This heel stabilizer is constructed with a lateral plantar flange that extends beyond the fourth and fifth metatarsophalangeal joints (**Figure 249D**). The medial area of the forefoot is left without any form of support. The rearfoot is controlled by a medial and lateral flange that confines the heel and also supports the talonavicular joint. The medial flange does not extend beyond the talo-navicular joint as is found in a type B or C stabilizer.

The principle on which this device works is that a rigid lever arm will cause changes in propulsion of the foot. Better explained, the lateral plantar flange has to extend beyond the fourth and fifth metatarso–phalangeal joints to limit the dorsiflexion of the joints in gait. We know that in gait the weight stress passes along the lateral aspect of the foot, across the metatarsals, and out through the hallux (**Figure 250**). With the presence of a rigid lever arm under the fourth and fifth metatarso–phalangeal joints, the foot is unable to propulse over these joints. The foot therefore must roll medially to allow dorsiflexion to occur at the first three metatarsophalangeal joints. The result of this medial rolling is that the forefoot is forced to abduct. The more pronation that is allowed at the mid and rearfoot, the more abduction will be allowed to occur in the forefoot. Cosmetically, this will produce an abducting gait, which may be aesthetically desirable but has a negligible effect on function and

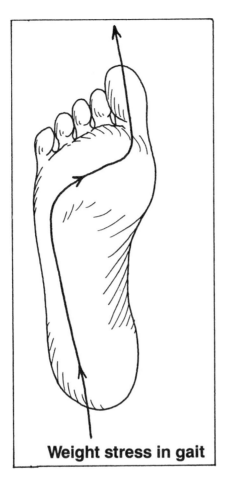

Weight stress in gait

Figure 250

correction. The fact that a certain degree of pronation in the rearfoot is needed to allow abduction of the forefoot is disadvantageous. The pronation, however, can be controlled and therefore can be considered a reasonable adjunctive therapy for the various in-toeing deformities.

The practitioner must periodically evaluate the function of this type of device due to normal foot growth. If the lateral flange is proximal to the fourth and fifth metatarsophalangeal joints, then its function is lost and replacement should be considered.

Since a type D heel stabilizer does not correct any of the etiologies for in-toeing, it should be used primarily for control of secondary (compensatory) pronation. The practitioner, as well as the parents, must be aware that with the use of a device of this nature the foot may continue to in-toe. As an example, if any degree of compensatory pronation has existed in the foot, then resupination of the foot will actually accentuate the in-toeing appearance. By employing a type D heel stabilizer, one is resupinating the foot while at the same time attempting to stimulate an out-toeing gait pattern. The stimulated out-toeing gait pattern may only negate the increased in-toeing that resulted from the supination of the rearfoot. Therefore, it may not necessarily improve the general gait appearance of the child. The parents should be informed of this factor and comforted by the fact that the foot is not being allowed to continue to compensate as a result of the in-toeing deformity.

The type D heel stabilizer can be used in children up to complete maturity. Some cases may warrant changing to an out-toeing gait plate (reverse Roberts' plate) to allow for greater mobility in the foot. For fabrication, the foot is placed in a neutral rectus position to achieve a proper impression casting.

Type E Heel Stabilizers

Children who need orthotic therapy to promote an in-toeing gait benefit well by this type of heel stabilizer. Opposite from the type D stabilizer, this device has a long medial flange extending distal to the medial three metatarso–phalangeal joints (**Figure 249E**). As was the case in the type D stabilizer, the flange acts as a rigid lever arm limiting motion at the metatarso–phalangeal joints. With limitation of dorsiflexion at the medial three metatarso–phalangeal joints, the foot must roll laterally in propulsion. This lateral positioning will naturally supinate the foot as well as promote adduction.

The use of this type of orthosis is beneficial in out-toeing gait problems from superstructural conditions (i.e., retroversion, retrotorsion, external tibial torsion, etc.) or from intrinsic pronation conditions of the foot. It should not be used in the severely ligamentous lax foot due to its limited medial–lateral stability in the forefoot. It will, however, work well in the less severe pronation conditions. Casting is performed in a neutral rectus position nonweight-bearing. Care should be taken periodically to examine these children for growth beyond the end of the orthosis so as not to lose its effectiveness.

Reverse Roberts' Plate (Out-Toeing Gait Plate)

This device is similar in function to the type D heel stabilizer. It only differs in the respect that it does not confine the rear and midfoot to the same

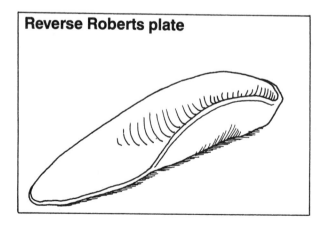

Reverse Roberts plate

Figure 251

degree that the heel stabilizer does (**Figure 251**). Most frequently it is employed in children older than 8–10 years who are exhibiting an in-toeing deformity. The impression casting is the same as in the type D heel stabilizer.

Functional Type Orthosis

This form of orthotic control should be left for the older child or adolescent. As previously mentioned, this type of device does not confine the young foot adequately to reduce medial–lateral instability resulting from joint laxity (**Figure 241E**). Additionally, there is usually minimal rearfoot and forefoot bony abnormality to warrant any form of posting. As discussed under the section on *Pes Planus,* the forefoot only assumes a position (varus or valgus) after it has been forced to function there for a period of time. A child has not had sufficient time to force the structural positioning to become rigid. Therefore it does not warrant any type of posting. It may even be detrimental to the child to attempt to force a foot into a posted position if a more rectus position could be achieved by maintaining a rectus attitude of the foot throughout development.[5,6,9,11]

Therefore, only consider using this type of orthotic control in the older child or adolescent who has achieved complete bone maturity and development.

Casting Techniques

Most children do not present with any significant form of rigidity in their foot structure to consider modification of any of the impression castings. In all of the types of orthoses mentioned, with the exception of the functional orthotic, a neutral rectus impression is the most desirable. This is accomplished by placing the subtalar joint in neutral position (the talar head is neither maximally supinated or pronated) and the midtarsal joint maximally pronated while the forefoot is held in a parallel (rectus) position with the calcaneus (**Figure 252**). Maximum pronation of the midtarsal joint is established by forcing the fourth and fifth metatarsal heads dorsally to maximum resistance. Care must be taken to avoid pronating the subtalar joint. This can be avoided by just forcing the forefoot in a dorsiflexing movement (with the rearfoot in neutral position) without abducting or adducting the midtarsal joints. Using the same hand that is maximally pronating the midtarsal joints (use your thumb to press on the fourth and fifth metatarsals), place your index and adjacent finger over the dorsum of the medial side of the foot to press down any apparent varus positioning to a rectus attitude (**Figure 253**). If a valgus forefoot position exists, then use the opposite hand to elevate the medial aspect of the forefoot to a rectus position while ensuring a neutral rearfoot (**Figure 254**).

The neutral rectus impression casting can only be accomplished by utilizing a nonweight-bearing prone position (**Figure 255**). Some attempts have been made to position the foot into neutral rectus using a semiweight-bearing

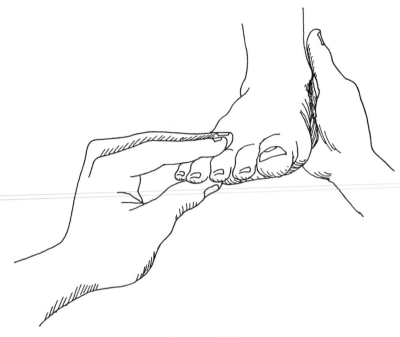

Figure 252

impression. This becomes difficult due to the inability by the practitioner to control the forefoot. When difficulty presents in casting an uncooperative youngster, it may become necessary to employ a semiweight-bearing impression or alternatively to take a neutral nonweight-bearing impression and manipulate the cast on a flat surface to place the fore and rearfoot rectus.

In casting for a functional orthosis, one need only to establish a neutral position. The forefoot is not manipulated into rectus. Posting can then be applied to balance any rear and forefoot positioning.

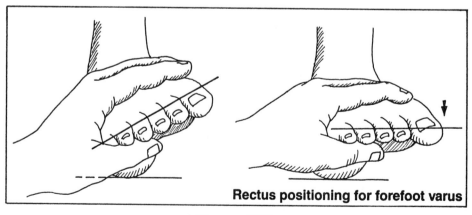

Rectus positioning for forefoot varus

Figure 253

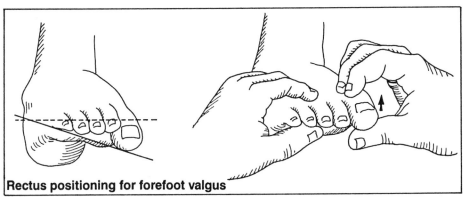

Rectus positioning for forefoot valgus

Figure 254

Various materials have been suggested for impression casting including plaster splints, containers of plaster in which the foot is placed semiweight-bearing, vacuum casting, semiweight-bearing foam, etc. This author still feels that employing plaster splints to capture the foot in a corrected position is the most effective and reproducible method. Each practitioner, however, must choose the method most suited to his abilities and needs.

Bars, Night Splints, Twister Cables, Etc.

Many devices have been developed in the course of the past several decades for the treatment of rotational deformities, positional problems, poor sleeping

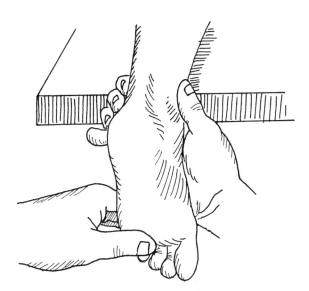

Prone position casting in neutral position   Figure 255

habits, etc. The use of bars, splints, and twister cables have been offered as a treatment mode for these deformities or disorders. A review of some of the more common types along with their advantages and disadvantages will be discussed.

Bars and Night Splints

Fillauer bars, Denis–Browne bars, Brackman skates, counter splints, and Ganley splints (**Figure 256A–D**) have all been used to correct various types of rotational or positional deformities. These splints will primarily provide: help in avoiding a sleeping position that will promote a positional or soft-tissue contracture; a varus or valgus position to the foot–ankle with the bending of the bar when necessary; a stretch to the soft-tissue structures around the hip with full extension of the limbs; a stretch to the soft-tissue structures around the knees when the knees are maintained in a flexed position. The bars and

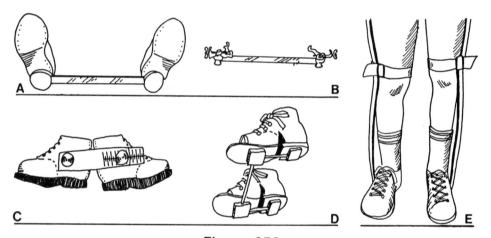

Figure 256

(A) Brackman Skate. *Dynamic splint that can be used both during ambulation and sleep. Somewhat cumbersome for a normal active child.* (B) Fillauer Bar. *There are several types, but the ones with clamps offer the best convenience. This can be removed from the shoes during activities and reattached when the child naps. Probably the most diverse splint and the most widely used.* (C) Counter Splint. *This attaches to the shoe and has several disadvantages: it cannot be removed; it can only correct for internal contractures by turning the feet outward; it cannot independently stretch one side without affecting the other.* (D) Ganley Splint. *Offers an excellent ability to splint independent abnormalities in the foot and maintain good leg position as well. Can only be used during nonambulation and is fixed to the shoes. It does not offer the same degree of independent control of the legs and hips as a Fillauer bar.* (E) Twister cables *are strapped onto the legs with an attachment to the shoes. The amount of tension placed on the cables will affect the degree of external rotational force applied. The torque force is being applied primarily at the distal end (shoe) in dynamic function.*

splints will not affect any bony structural abnormality as has been described thoroughly in the past several chapters.

When using a bar or splint to discourage an improper sleeping position, place a bend in the center of the bar (splint) to provide a slight varus position to the foot attached. This will help avoid any excessive valgus force on the feet, causing stretching and weakness to the medial joint structures. An opposite bend should only be used to maintain a correction for a varus deformity in the foot–ankle.

If a splint or bar is to be used for stretching of hip soft-tissue contractures, then a rotation of the foot on bar should be gradually increased. Do not rotate excessively in either direction. An injury to the soft tissue as well as bony structures may ensue.

The length of the bar should be no longer than 1–2 inches wider than the width across the anterior superior iliac spines of the pelvis. Greater widths will force the limbs and hips into excessive abduction and produce forces on the medial ankle–foot, medial knee, and hip joints that may alter the stability.

Removable bars offer the best versatility and avoid the need for reattachment to new shoes. These can be applied during napping and sleeping times to a stiff sole pair of shoes. When the child is active the bar can be removed and the shoes may continue to be worn. If the child outgrows the shoes before the cessation of bar therapy, then a new pair can be purchased and applied to the same bar.

Parents must be encouraged to tolerate the complaints of a child with the initiation of bar–splint therapy. Usually within a couple of days the presence of the bar (splint) will not disturb the child's sleep. Encouragement to the parents to apply the splint routinely is mandatory for proper result. The institution of bar–splint therapy is commonplace after stretch-casting and should be maintained for 6–12 months following this treatment. Children older than $2-2\frac{1}{2}$ years will not cooperate or tolerate bar–splint therapy. They are knowledgeable enough at this age to remove the splint or shoe to avoid its presence. At this age the child is usually not sleeping in one position and therefore one need not be as discouraged as with the younger infant or child.

Twister Cables

Twister cables have been used to correct many rotational deformities (**Figure 256E**). Torsional or versional abnormalities of the hip, torsional problem in the leg, and soft-tissue deformities in the foot–ankle have all been treated by this device. This author would discourage anyone from using this method of treatment for any rotational problem that may present. Several cases have been observed in which a partial rupture or tear of the tibialis posterior and/ or tibialis anterior tendon attachment in the foot have occurred. This is the result of the valgus external force being placed on the foot by the cable to rotate the limb outward. Not only will this brace produce a significant valgus force on the medial ankle–foot but will produce a similar stress to the medial knee structures. These reasons alone would be sufficient to avoid its usage along with the psychological effects on the child with such an awkward brace. Since no real benefit is gained by weighing all of the detrimental effects, this form of therapy should never be considered in the treatment of children's rotational abnormalities.

References

1. Ciacchiolo, A.: Office practice: Footwear and orthotic therapy. *Foot and Ankle,* 2:Number 4, 1982.
2. Di Geovanni, J.E., Smith, S.D.: Normal biomechanics of the adult rearfoot. *Journal of the American Podiatry Association,* 66:1976.
3. Polokoff, M.M.: An approach to children's foot orthopedics. *Journal of the American Podiatry Association,* 66:Number 6, June 1976.
4. Root, M.L., Orien, W.P., Weed, J.H.: *Biomechanical Examination of the Foot,* Vol. 1, Clinical Biomechanics Corp., Los Angeles, CA, 1971.
5. Root, M.L., Orien, W.P., Weed, J.H.: *Clinical Biomechanics,* Vol. 2, *Normal and Abnormal Function of the Foot.* Clinical Biomechanics Corp., Los Angeles, CA, 1977.
6. Ross, A.S., Gurnick, K.L.: Elevator selection in rearfoot posted orthosis. *Journal of the American Podiatry Association,* 72:Number 12, December 1982.
7. Rossi, W.A.: Children's shoes. *Journal of the American Podiatry Association,* 71:Number 10, October 1981.
8. Rossi, W.A.: The controversy of corrective shoes. *Journal of the American Podiatry Association,* 71:Number 4, April 1981.
9. Sgarlato, T.E.: A compendium of podiatric biomechanics. *California College of Podiatric Medicine,* San Francisco, CA, 1971.
10. Tax, H.R.: *Podopediatrics.* William and Wilkins, Baltimore, MD, 1980.
11. Weed, J.H., Ratliff, F.D., Ross, S.A.: A biplaner grind for rear posts on functional orthoses. *Journal of the American Podiatry Association,* 69:Number 1, January 1978.
12. Wickstrom, J., Williams, R.N.: Shoe correction and orthopaedic foot supports. *Clinical Orthopedics,* Number 70, May–June 1970.

Chapter 14

GAIT ANALYSIS

*T*his chapter will discuss the differences found in the mechanics of the limb function in a child and an adult, the various neuromuscular gait abnormalities and their characteristics, and finally what is exactly being viewed in gait with the common structural abnormalities that are often experienced.

Biomechanics of Gait

We will assume first that the reader has a basic working knowledge of the mechanics of gait. If you feel that you are deficient in this area, then a review of the article by Inman et al. on "The Major Determinants of Gait in Normal and Pathological Gait" and "The Mechanics of Walking" by Perry is suggested.[6,8] To capsulize these articles, there are six determinants that affect the pathway of movement: rotation of the pelvis, tilting of the pelvis, lateral movement of the pelvis during weight shifts from one limb to the other, flexion of the knee during heel strike and push off, motion around the foot and ankle during stance, and reduction in ankle motion by knee flexion during push off and heel strike. These determinants must be understood to appreciate what is occurring during gait. Also, the weight stress that is transmitted through the foot normally occurs at the lateral posterior aspect of the heel at heel strike; extends along the lateral aspect of the foot through early midstance; passes across the metatarsal head through the period of late midstance and early push off, and exits out the hallux in the final stage of push off. The various phases of gait including heel strike, mid-stance, push off, and swing phase must all be clearly appreciated. Recent studies have found that children up to the ages of 3–4 years will exhibit a markedly different mechanism of gait than that found normally in the older child or adult (Chapter 5). A child under 4 years of age will ambulate with a knee flexed position through both swing phase and most of stance phase, which are different than that found in an adult gait pattern. The knee joint never fully extends in position at heel strike but rather is partially flexed throughout this first phase of weight acceptance. As a result of this, the foot does not meet the weight-bearing surface in the typical heel-to-toe pattern. Instead, the foot will contact the ground with a foot-flat attitude at the initiation of weight-bearing. From heel strike (foot-flat) to midstance, the knee will extend from its flexed position. This extension does not approach the fully extended position found in the older child or adult.

During the propulsive phase of gait, the knees of these young children will again begin to flex and will continue throughout the swing phase to and including the next heel strike (**Figure 257**). This difference in gait accounts for the apropulsive attitude in ambulation and the awkward (toddling) function. A child therefore does not achieve a characteristic heel-to-toe gait with sufficient lateral stability until around 3–4 years of age, and in some cases much later. These factors and characteristics must be understood and taken into account when evaluating the gait of a youngster.

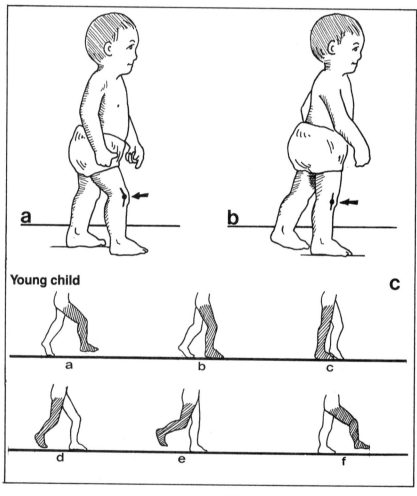

Figure 257

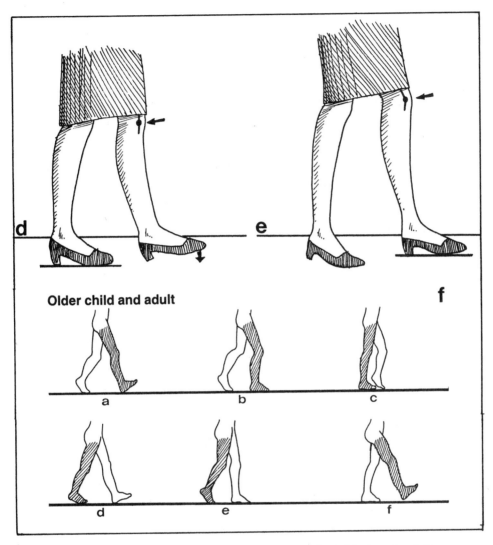

A child ambulates with a knee flexed position at the initiation of weight acceptance (A) and extends the knee through midstance (B). He will flex again at propulsion and maintain this position until initiating weight acceptance again (C). An adult has a knee extended attitude at true heel strike (D) and flexes the knee at midstance. The knee will again extend at propulsion and flex through swing phase (F).

Neuromuscular Gait Abnormalities

Spastic Gait

Hypertonicity with a muscular imbalance is the characteristic finding of this abnormal gait. The child may ambulate with a flatfoot gait, a toe–heel, or equinus (toe–toe) gait. If spasticity exists in the peroneal muscle, then a severe valgus foot may result while spasticity of the inverts, with weakness of the everts of the foot will result in a supinated varus attitude.

Spastic paraplegia will involve the lower extremities and will result in severe adduction at the hips. This will cause the knees to cross over one another producing a "scissor type" gait. A dropping of the opposite hip (Trendelenburg gait) may also be viewed (**Figure 258**). There will also be characteristic upper extremity abnormalities including a flexed elbow, wrist flexion, flexion of the fingers, and adduction of the thumb. A child with a spastic gait will have an inability to walk a straight line by placing one foot in front of the other. If this gait is observed, a thorough neurological evaluation is warranted to determine the cause. Cerebral palsy, syringomyelia, etc. may all produce this type of gait pattern.[12–15]

Spinal Ataxic Gait

This may be the result of tabes dorsalis, multiple sclerosis, peripheral neuritis, or brain stem lesions. There is a lack of proprioceptive orientation

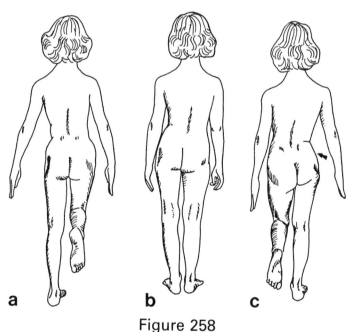

a   b   c

Figure 258

when the child is asked to close his eyes as opposed to when they are opened (Romberg test). The child will fall over or walk very awkwardly when not allowed to be able to sense his position by the visual aids. Further progression of the disorder will reveal a child walking with a broad base of gait and a slapping of the foot from heel to toe when ambulating.[13,15]

Cerebellar Ataxic Gait

This is caused by a disease process in the cerebellum affecting the coordination mechanism of the child. Different than the spinal ataxic gait, the cerebellar ataxic gait occurs with the eyes either open or closed. The gait is a similar staggering broad-based gait with an inability to walk a straight line. The slapping foot characteristic is also present.[13,15]

Equinus Gait

An equinus gait is characterized by a tip-toe walking or running pattern in a child (**Figure 259**). Spasticity may occur in the gastrocsoleus complex

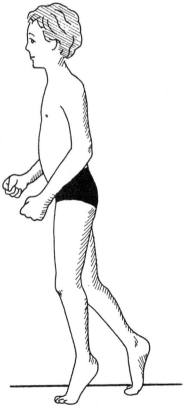

Equinus gait   Figure 259

resulting in a toe-walking gait pattern. Not always is this type of gait characteristic of a neuromuscular abnormality. Children who are just beginning to walk may present with a toe-walking gait. This will usually resolve in 4–8 months. Persistence of the condition would obviously warrant further investigation. Please read the section on *Equinus* (Chapter 7) for a more complete understanding of the causes, evaluation, and treatment. It is important to differentiate a local cause for an equinus gait from that of a neuromuscular cause. It may often take several months of evaluation to properly discern the exact etiology.[1,13,14,15]

Trendelenburg Gait

This gait is characterized by the opposite side of the pelvis dropping down in relation to the weight-bearing side (**Figure 258**). Normally a person standing on one leg will have the contralateral side of the pelvis elevate. This is the result of the strong ipsilateral hip abductor muscles that are functioning. A positive Trendelenburg gait is the result of a weakness in the hip abductor muscles. The weakness may be neurological (compression of the spinal nerves innervating this muscle group) or muscular (atrophy of the gluteus medius muscle) or a congenital hip dislocation.[2,12–15]

Drop Foot Gait

The existence of weakening paralysis of the tibialis anterior, extensor digitorum longus, and/or peroneus longus or brevis will result in a drop foot gait. These muscles cannot, in these cases, dorsiflex the foot at the ankle through the swing phase of gait. The loss of this muscle strength will result in a compensatory lifting of the limb to allow it to pass through this phase of gait. This is accomplished by flexing the hip, raising the leg by flexing the knee, and externally rotating the limb to avoid catching the tips of the toes on the ground. This type of gait can be found in cases of peroneal nerve damage, muscular dystrophy, poliomyelitis, and Charcot–Marie–Tooth disease.[13,15]

Waddling Gait

This is the same as the Trendelenburg gait. There will be weakness in the musculature or a congenital hip dislocation producing this condition. Muscular dystrophy or occasionally other myopathies willl characteristically produce this type of gait pattern. A test to see if the child is able to get up from a supine position on the floor is important in diagnosing a muscular dystrophy. The *Gowers' sign* occurs in a positive lower limb muscular dystrophy and is exhibited by the child climbing up his legs to stand (**Figure 260**). He will, from a prone position, place his hands on his knees and move up to the hips to brace himself while he is attempting to stand up. Difficulty in climbing

Gower's sign for muscular dystrophy

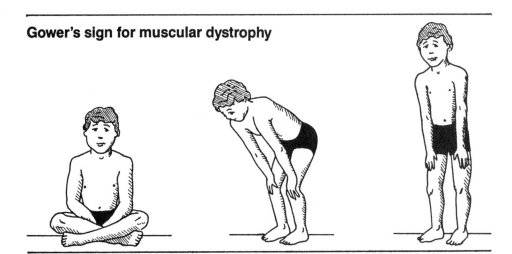

Figure 260

stairs is also very characteristic of a muscular dystrophy due to the weakness in the quadriceps and gluteus maximus.[7,13,15]

Common Gait Appearances and Their Cause(s)

When observing a child's gait, several areas must be viewed to appropriately evaluate the ambulatory function. Observing the head position downward to the foot position is necessary for a proper interpretation. Having the child walk with and without shoes is also beneficial in determining if the weight or type of shoes is affecting the gait pattern. Trying to observe the child's gait when he does not know you are looking is also extremely advantageous. This can usually be accomplished when the child is first entering the office or treatment room, or while you are talking to the parent(s) and watching his ambulation in the room.

Observe the shoulder and head position, swinging of the arms, movement of the trunk, curvature of the spine, movement of the hips either up and down or swinging forward and back, knee and patellae position, leg position and attitude, and foot function. Certain types of gait patterns have been characteristically observed with certain structural deformities. Examples of these include:

A true limb length difference will exhibit a shoulder drop and pelvic drop on the shorter side assuming there has been no compensatory scoliosis (**Figure 261**). The longer limb may show some degree of genu valgum with the foot on this limb revealing a greater degree of collapse in the architecture, i.e., a flatfoot appearance. The shorter limb will have a normal or even cavus (high arch) foot structure.

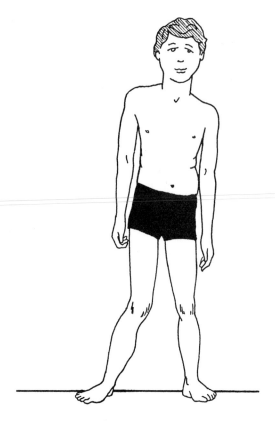

Limb shortage appearance   Figure 261

A scoliosis may produce a limb shortage which could then cause the shoulder to drop on one side and the hip to drop on the opposite side. Observing the child without a top or shirt on would better allow for an evaluation of any spinal curvatures.

Femoral torsional or versional problems will often be observed by evaluating patellar position in gait. If the patellae are marked and then viewed during walking and running, their position will reveal any abnormality in the hip joint area. Inward positioning of the patellae with in-toeing of the limb on either side could indicate a femoral antetorsion or anteversion. Further evaluation would reveal which one or both are existing. Outward positioning of the patellae and an out-toeing gait could indicate a retrotorsion or retroversion. A combination of either a retrotorsion–anteversion or an antetorsion–retroversion could place the knee and patellae on the frontal plane. It therefore is necessary to coordinate your findings with a proper and comprehensive clinical evaluation to determine these counterbalancing abnormalities (**Figure 262**).

Tibio–fibular torsion or genicular position abnormalities will produce an in-toeing or out-toeing gait without affecting the patellar position. If a child is observed in-toeing or out-toeing and the patellae are on the frontal plane,

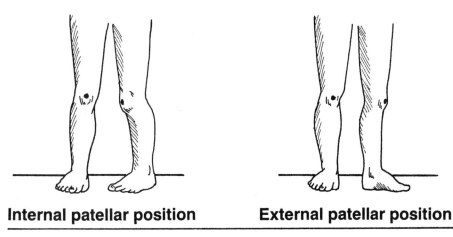

Internal patellar position   **External patellar position**

Figure 262

then one can assume the deformity lies below the femur and hip. A careful examination for a tibio–fibular torsion abnormality, a genicular position condition, an imbalance in the musculature to the foot, metatarsus adductus or pronation syndrome to determine the cause for the in-toeing or out-toeing gait is necessary (**Figure 263**). There is again the case where an abnormal retro-torsion–anteversion or antetorsion–retroversion condition may exist which would place the patellae on the frontal plane and still be considered a pathologic condition.

Children presenting with an *overpowering tibialis anterior and posterior muscle(s)* and/or a *metatarsus adductus deformity* will in-toe more in shoes than out of shoes. It therefore is paramount to observe the gait of a child with shoes on and off to help make a better diagnosis of the cause. The weight of

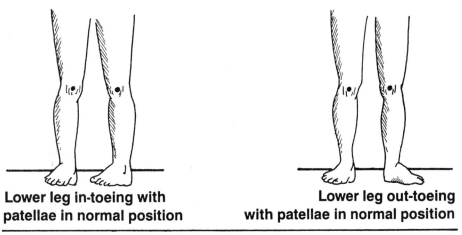

Lower leg in-toeing with   **Lower leg out-toeing**
patellae in normal position   **with patellae in normal position**

Figure 263

the shoe will allow the musculature medially to overpower the weaker lateral groups, thus causing an in-toeing gait. In metatarsus adductus a child without shoes will allow more pronation in the foot. This pronation will mask the true degree of metatarsus adductus deformity existing.

True *flatfoot conditions* will reveal an almost apropulsive gait with a valgus heel and a positive Helbing sign (lateral curvature of the Achilles tendon due to valgus position of the heel). One should observe any midtarsal collapse or breeching with propulsion. The degree of abduction is also significant in evaluating the degree of collapse. Toe purchase and extensor muscle function are also to be observed in gait. Resupination during propulsion or while the child is standing and asked to raise up on the ball of the foot is important to differentiate a rigid or flexible condition. The ability to raise up on the heel and ball of the foot and invert and evert the foot also provides an excellent understanding as to the muscle strength and joint movement.

When analyzing the gait of children, remember that up to the age of 3–5 years they are apropulsive and functioning with a knee flexed attitude. They therefore cannot be compared or evaluated using the same principles of biomechanics as in older children or adults. Additionally, gait analysis should be used as a coordinated tool in evaluation of a child and not as an independent diagnostic measure. Used in conjunction with a proper physical evaluation, it will provide a much clearer picture of the problem(s) existing and the results of the treatment programs instituted.

References

Gait Analysis:

1. Blake, R.L., Ross, A.S., Valmassy, R.L.: Biomechanics in gait evaluation. *J.A.P.A.*, 71:Number 6, June 1981.
2. Fields, L.: The limping child. *J.A.P.A.*, 71:Number 2, February 1981.
3. Jordan, R.P.: The neuromotor development of bipedal locomotion in the normal infant. *J.A.P.A.*, 71:Number 2, February 1981.
4. Jordan, R.P., Cooper, M., Schuster, R.O.: Ankle dorsiflexion at the heel-off phase of gait. *J.A.P.A.*, 69:Number 1, January 1979.
5. Mann, R.N., Hagy, J.: Biomechanics of walking, running and sprinting. *Am. J. Sports Med.*, 8:1980.
6. Perry, J.: The mechanics of walking. A clinical interpretation. *Physical Therapy*, 47:Number 9, 1962.
7. Reinherz, R., Mann, I.: Lower extremity involvement in Duchenne's muscular dystrophy. *J.A.P.A.*, 67:Number 11, November 1977.
8. Saunders, J.B.M., Inman, V.T., Eberhart, H.D.: The major determinants in normal and pathological gait. *Journal of Bone and Joint Surgery*, 35-A:1953.
9. Sgarlato, T.E.: A compendium of podiatric biomechanics. *California College of Podiatric Medicine*, San Francisco, CA, 1971.
10. Shoenhaus, H.D., Fold, M., Hylinski, J., Keating, J.: A preliminary report of computerized analysis of gait. *J.A.P.A.*, 69:Number 1, January 1978.
11. Simon, S.R., Mann, R.N., Hagy, J.L., Larsen, L.: Role of the posterior calf muscles in normal gait. *Journal of Bone and Joint Surgery*, 60-A:1978.

12. Sutherland, D.H., Cooper, L.: The pathomechanics of progressive crouch gait in spastic diplegia. *Orthopedic Survey,* 2: Number 1, July/August 1978.
13. Tachdjian, M.O.: *Pediatric Orthopedics.* W.B. Saunders Co., Philadelphia, PA, 1972.
14. Tax, H.R.: Locomotion and the child patient. *J.A.P.A.,* 67:Number 2, February 1977.
15. Tax, H.R. *Podopediatrics.* Williams and Wilkins Co., Baltimore, MD, 1980.

Chapter 15

IN-TOEING AND OUT-TOEING
GAIT PROBLEMS

In-toeing (Pigeon Toeing)

*T*his common gait abnormality may be the result of several causes or combination of causes. This section will primarily outline the possible areas that may produce this gait deformity. Reference to an appropriate section(s) in this text for a complete explanation and treatment program is also provided.

Causes for an In-toeing Gait

Antetorsion—a twist in the femur that results in an inward rotation of the limb when the head and neck of the femur are seated perpendicular to the acetabular socket. This is a structural deformity that does not require treatment and will usually resolve with development and growth. See Chapter 4 for additional information.

Anteversion—a positional change in the hip joint resulting from either an anterior positioning of the acetabular socket and/or contractures in the pubofemoral–ileofemoral ligaments and internal hip rotator muscles along with the capsule. The acetabular position will usually correct by the time a child begins weight-bearing and therefore needs no concern. The soft-tissue contractures, however, may persist and produce a limitation in the amount of external rotation. This will result in an in-toeing gait. Stretching will often resolve this soft-tissue problem if employed properly. See Chapter 4 for further information.

Internal genicular position—Surrounding the knee joint are muscular attachments that may affect the tracking of the tibia on the femur. Anatomically, there are five muscle groups that internally rotate the tibia on the femur, and only one muscle that externally rotates. As a result of positional development, the internal rotators are allowed to contract excessively, producing a limitation of external rotation at the knee. The result will be an in-toeing gait secondary to these contractures. This condition must not be confused with true tibial torsion which affects the bone directly. See Chapter 5 for additional information.

Internal tibiofibular torsion—The definition of torsion is a true twist in the bony structure. This condition should be more appropriately termed internal tibiofibular torsion than just internal tibial torsion to account for the effects of the fibula, tibiofibular syndesmosis, and ankle mortise on the relative position of the foot and therefore the gait pattern. Care must be taken to properly examine for the presence of an internal torsional abnormality without confusing it with an internal genicular positional problem. Like antetorsion in the femur, tibiofibular torsion usually corrects itself with sufficient development and requires no direct treatment. See Chapter 6 for additional information.

Overpowering tibialis anterior–posterior and abductor hallucis muscles— Similar to the condition of internal genicular position, the overpowering of the adductor muscles of the foot can also produce an in-toeing deformity. Contractures, abnormal innervation, spasticity, or an unequal development in the central nervous system may cause an imbalance in these muscle groups. This condition often will present in combination with one of the other aforementioned in-toeing abnormalities or in conjunction with a metatarsus adductus deformity. The examiner is cautioned to recognize this entity and appropriately treat it along with any other evident cause. This will certainly ensure a more rapid and desirable correction. See Chapter 11 for further information.

Metatarsus adductus (varus or adductovarus)—A medial displacement of the respective five metatarsals will produce an inward gait pattern when present. The cause for the medial displacement may be the result of intrauterine pressure and development, an overpowering or abnormally inserted abductor hallucis muscle, and/or from the contribution of an abnormal sleeping position. Early treatment is mandatory to avoid the sequel that most assuredly will result. See Chapter 11 for a complete explanation.

Treatment

Approaching an in-toeing gait abnormality is challenging and oftentimes frustrating. It, however, will be gratifying to the patient and yourself to see the results of your efforts. Care must be taken in the examination of child to determine the potential etiologies that may produce this inward gait. Once the examiner feels comfortable that all the causes are discovered, then and only then should a treatment program be developed. When reviewing each of the causes and the treatment programs, remember that a logical approach to total care can and should be formed. As an example, if a one-year-old child was to present with a metatarsus adductus, internal genicular position, and an antetorsion deformity, then your treatment program should comprise of the following: casting the metatarsus adductus first until adequate reduction; stretch casting the internal genicular position while maintaining the corrected metatarsal position; assuring the parents that the antetorsion will reduce in time. The patient should, however, be followed up in an out-toeing heel stabilizer. The stabilizer is to control the foot and avoid any secondary pronation. Additionally, it will encourage an out-toeing gait pattern. If the child was assuming an improper sleeping position, then a night splint would also be used as a follow-up to discourage the improper sleeping attitude.

Another case example could be a 4-year-old child in-toeing as a result of anteversion, internal tibiofibular torsion, and an overpowering tibialis anterior and posterior muscle. Taking into account the age of the child and the etiologies producing the in-toeing, two treatments would be simultaneously instituted. The first would be an exercise program to stretch the soft-tissue contractures surrounding the hip joint (i.e., sitting in an Indian position while pushing on the knees to stretch the respective ligaments and musculature) and second, employing an orthotic control. The orthosis could be a type D heel stabilizer to encourage out-toeing while resisting the tendency toward pronation. The stabilizer would be stressing and stretching the tibialis anterior and posterior tendons reducing their medial tension. The existence of the internal tibiofibular torsion would also be discussed with the parents. It should be explained that these bones have not developed to the same age as the child but statistically the torsion will catch up with sufficient time and development. The parents should further understand that the orthotic control will help to protect the foot while waiting for the rotation to occur but will not correct the deformity by its use.

These examples should hopefully help to understand how one may approach a problem with multiple causes and still treat them concomitantly and appropriately.

Out-toeing (Duck Walking)

Similar to an in-toeing gait abnormality, an out-toeing gait may be the result of several areas that are abnormally functioning or existing during gait. We will attempt to highlight these areas and advise the reader to read carefully the appropriate section(s) corresponding to the deformity(s) described.

Causes for an Out-toeing Gait

Retrotorsion—The result of a twist in the femur that externally rotates the leg when the head of the femur is placed into the acetabulum at a perpendicular position. The rotation is inherent in the bone structure and therefore only time and development will alter its architecture. See Chapter 4 for additional information.

Retroversion—Like anteversion, retroversion is a positional alteration in the hip joint as a result of a posterior positioning of the acetabular socket and/

or from contractures in the ischiofemoral ligament, external hip rotator muscles, and posterior capsule. Since the acetabular position usually resolves by the time weight-bearing occurs, it does not require any concern. Stretching of the soft-tissue contractures will often resolve this problem. See Chapter 4 for a complete explanation.

External genicular position—Theoretically this condition may exist; in practice, however, this author has not found its presence as an etiology for an out-toeing deformity. Therefore if it does present, it will be a rare finding.

External tibiofibular torsion—Not an uncommon finding, it will produce a marked abduction in gait. Unfortunately, this condition is an overrotation of the respective bones and therefore does not reverse itself with growth and development. If a significant functional impairment does exist, then a surgical derotation of the tibia and fibula may be required. See Chapter 6 for a detailed discussion.

Flatfoot (pronation) deformity—Whatever cause(s) may produce a collapse in the architecture of the foot, the result will be an abduction in gait. Ligamentous laxity, compensatory pronation, and muscular imbalance may all contribute to this positioning. Control and in some cases surgical realignment may be necessary to avoid the consequences of this deformity. See Chapter 8 for further information.

Treatment

As was discussed under *Treatment* for in-toeing deformities, out-toeing conditions must be properly diagnosed and a program appropriately formulated to treat the condition(s) existing. The only conditions that are amenable to direct treatment are: retroversion, external genicular position, and a flatfoot deformity. Stretching is employed for retrotorsion and external genicular position. Stretching can be utilized when a talipes calcaneovalgus deformity exists with an out-toeing gait in a young child. Orthotic control is primarily the source of treatment employed in all these situations to establish an appropriate functioning position while buying time for any of the torsional conditions to resolve and the soft-tissue structures to achieve an even balance. Certainly there are situations where an appropriate surgical realignment may be necessary, but this is left for the older child who has completed most of his development.

INDEX